Environmental Social Sciences: Methods and Research Design

The relationship between human communities and the environment is extremely complex. In order to understand this relationship, interdisciplinary research combining natural sciences, social sciences, and humanities is necessary. Here, specialists summarize methods and research strategies for various aspects of social research devoted to environmental issues. Each chapter is illustrated with ethnographic and environmental examples, ranging from Australia to Amazonia, from Madagascar to the United States, and from prehistoric and historic cases to contemporary rural and urban ones. The volume discusses climate change, deforestation, environmental knowledge, natural reserves, politics and ownership of natural resources, and the effect of differing spatial and temporal scales. Contributing to the intellectual project of interdisciplinary environmental social science, this book demonstrates the contributions it can make to environmental studies and to larger global problems, and thus will be of interest to social and natural scientists and to policy-makers.

ISMAEL VACCARO is Assistant Professor in the Department of Anthropology and the School of Environment at McGill University, Montréal. He is also Director of the Neotropical Program, managed in collaboration with the Smithsonian Tropical Institute.

ERIC ALDEN SMITH is Professor in the Department of Anthropology at the University of Washington. He has published extensively on systems of production and reproduction in various small-scale societies, and currently codirects an NSF IGERT program.

SHANKAR ASWANI is Associate Professor in the Department of Anthropology at the University of California, Santa Barbara. A recipient of the prestigious Pew Fellowship in Marine Conservation (2005), he has worked with local communities to establish a network of locally managed Marine Protected Areas and small-scale rural development projects in the Soloman Islands.

Environmental Social Sciences

Methods and Research Design

Edited by

ISMAEL VACCARO
McGill University

ERIC ALDEN SMITH
University of Washington

SHANKAR ASWANI
*University of California,
Santa Barbara*

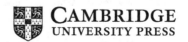

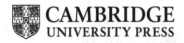

Shaftesbury Road, Cambridge CB2 8EA, United Kingdom

One Liberty Plaza, 20th Floor, New York, NY 10006, USA

477 Williamstown Road, Port Melbourne, VIC 3207, Australia

314–321, 3rd Floor, Plot 3, Splendor Forum, Jasola District Centre, New Delhi – 110025, India

103 Penang Road, #05–06/07, Visioncrest Commercial, Singapore 238467

Cambridge University Press is part of Cambridge University Press & Assessment,
a department of the University of Cambridge.

We share the University's mission to contribute to society through the pursuit of
education, learning and research at the highest international levels of excellence.

www.cambridge.org
Information on this title: www.cambridge.org/9780521125710

First published 2010

A catalogue record for this publication is available from the British Library

Library of Congress Cataloging-in-Publication data
Environmental social sciences : methods and research design / [edited by] Ismael
    Vaccaro, Eric Alden Smith, Shankar Aswani.
        p. cm.
    Includes index.
    ISBN 978-0-521-11084-6 (hardback) – ISBN 978-0-521-12571-0 (pbk.)
    1. Human ecology–Research–Methodology.   I. Vaccaro, Ismael.   II. Smith, Eric
    Alden.   III. Aswani, Shankar   IV. Title.
    GF26.E585 2010
    304.2–dc22   2010027385

ISBN   978-0-521-11084-6   Hardback
ISBN   978-0-521-12571-0   Paperback

Contents

Contributors

Shankar Aswani
Department of Anthropology
University of California
Santa Barbara, CA, USA

Oriol Beltran
Departament d'Antropologia Social
Universitat de Barcelona
Barcelona, Spain

Eduardo S. Brondízio
Department of Anthropology
Indiana University, Bloomington
Bloomington, IN, USA

Carole L. Crumley
Department of Anthropology
University of North Carolina
Chapel Hill, NC, USA
and
Stockholm Resilience Centre
Stockholm, Sweden

Lisa L. Gezon
Department of Anthropology
University of West Georgia
Carrollton, GA, USA

Denise M. Glover
Department of Comparative Sociology
University of Puget Sound
Tacoma, WA, USA

Clarence C. Gravlee
Department of Anthropology
University of Florida
Gainesville, FL, USA

David C. Griffith
Institute for Coastal Science and Policy and Department of Anthropology
East Carolina University
Greenville, NC, USA

Raymond Hames
Department of Anthropology
University of Nebraska
Lincoln, NE, USA

Jeffrey C. Johnson
Institute for Coastal Science and Policy and Department of Sociology
East Carolina University
Greenville, NC, USA

Emily Lena Jones
Department of Sociology, Social Work, and Anthropology
Utah State University
Logan, UT, USA

Eric C. Jones
Department of Anthropology
University of North Carolina at Greensboro
Greensboro, NC, USA

D. Seth Murray
Program in International Studies
North Carolina State University
Raleigh, NC, USA

Amy R. Poteete
Department of Political Science
Concordia University
Montreal, Canada

Rinku Roy Chowdhury
Department of Geography
Indiana University, Bloomington
Bloomington, IN, USA

Michael D. Scholl
Department of Sociology and Anthropology
Wagner College
Staten Island, NY, USA

Jennifer Sepez
Resource Ecology and Fisheries Management Division
NOAA Alaska Fisheries Science Center
Seattle, WA, USA

Candace Slater
Department of Spanish and Portuguese
University of California, Berkeley
Berkeley, CA, USA

Eric Alden Smith
Department of Anthropology
University of Washington
Seattle, WA, USA

Veronica Strang
Department of Anthropology
University of Auckland
Auckland, New Zealand

Ismael Vaccaro
Anthropology Department
McGill University
Montreal, Canada

Amber Wutich
School of Human Evolution and Social Change
Arizona State University
Tempe, AZ, USA

Laura Zanotti
Department of Anthropology
Purdue University
West Lafayette, IN, USA

Foreword

This book, *Environmental Social Sciences*, represents the best of what's happening in social science right now: (1) it exemplifies the movement toward interdisciplinary research; (2) it rejects the pernicious distinction between qualitative and quantitative in the conduct of social research; and (3) it makes clear the value for all social scientists of training in a wide range of methods of collecting and analyzing data. I treat these in turn.

1. Interdisciplinary social science. Environmental science has always been an interdisciplinary effort. The *Science Citation Index* lists 163 journals in the category of environmental science. Look through the top 10 journals (the ones with an impact factor of 4.0 or more) and the range of disciplines is clear: biologists, chemists, meteorologists, paleontologists, geologists ... Increasingly, it is common to see articles – like one by Clougherty (2010) on gender analysis in the distribution of the effects of air pollution, or one by Knoke *et al.* (2009) on reconciling the subsistence needs of farmers in Ecuador with the need for conserving forests, or one by Rosas-Rosas and Valdez (2010) on the impact of fees from deer hunts on the willingness of landowners in Mexico to suspend killing of pumas and jaguars – articles that can only be described as social science. (We see this as well in medical science, where the very best journals now also routinely publish articles that also can only be described as 100% social science.)

Environmental *social* science is developing quickly within the environmental sciences, with Ph.D. programs in several universities, a major textbook (Moran 2010), and, now, this book on research methods.

2. Rejecting the qual–quant distinction. Whether it's anthropology or sociology or geography, social scientists are often asked – no, required – early in their careers, to choose between humanistic and

scientific approaches to the subject matter of their discipline and between collecting and analyzing qualitative or quantitative data. Even worse, they are taught to equate science with quantitative data and quantitative analysis and humanism with qualitative data and qualitative analysis. This denies the grand tradition of qualitative approaches in all of science, from astronomy to zoology. When Galileo first trained his then-brand-new telescope on the moon, he noticed what he called lighter and darker areas. The large dark spots had, Galileo said, been seen from time immemorial and so he said, "These I shall call the 'large' or 'ancient' spots." He also wrote that the moon was "not smooth, uniform, and precisely spherical" as commonly believed, but "uneven, rough, and full of cavities and prominences," much like the Earth. No more qualitative description was ever penned (Galileo 1610: 3).

3. The need for training in a range of research methods. The chapters in this book make clear the importance for environmental social scientists of extensive training in methods. How much methods training is enough? No one can be expert in all methods of research, but increasingly, research projects demand expertise in multiple methods, including methods for collecting and analyzing qualitative data. Methods tend to be associated with disciplines, but they can never belong to disciplines. Anthropologists developed the method of participant observation, for example, but this method is now part of every social science. Sociologists are most associated with the questionnaire survey, but this method, too, is part of every social science. All social scientists, in my view, need training in research design, in several kinds of data collection (structured and unstructured interviewing, for example), and in data analysis. Anyone who works with survey data needs good skills in statistical analysis. Working with interviews or narratives or images requires training in text management.

We properly disagree with one another about epistemology – first principles in how we know anything at all – and about whether biological or material or cognitive forces predominate in explaining any given human phenomenon. Most social scientists, however, share a commitment to empiricism – to recording observations about how people think, behave, and feel. This shared commitment is made wonderfully clear in this book on methods in the environmental social sciences.

Dr. Russell Bernard

REFERENCES

Clougherty, J. E. 2010. A growing role for gender analysis in air pollution epidemiology. *Environmental Health Perspectives* **118**: 167–176.

Galileo Galilei 1610. The Starry Messenger. http://www.bard.edu/admission/forms/pdfs/galileo

Knoke, T. B., N. Calvas, R. M. Aguirre, *et al.* 2009. Can tropical farmers reconcile subsistence needs with forest conservation? *Frontiers in Ecology and the Environment* **7**: 548–554.

Moran, E. 2010. *Environmental Social Science: Human–Environment Interactions and Sustainability.* Malden, MA: Wiley-Blackwell.

Rosas-Rosas, O. C. and R. Valdez 2010. The role of landowners in jaguar conservation in Sonora, Mexico. *Conservation Biology* **24**: 366–371.

Preface

This book resulted from our desire to achieve two goals. First, we wanted to assemble a volume that could help researchers and students interested in the social aspects of environmental issues to identify the methodological possibilities offered by social sciences. Second, we wanted to present the pluralistic, interdisciplinary mix of methods, and qualitative and quantitative approaches, found in contemporary research in this area. We hope readers will find our attempts successful.

We want to acknowledge our intellectual debt to the colleagues and teachers who have helped us understand the dynamic range of possibilities in environmental social science. Ismael and Eric specifically offer tribute to the Graduate Program in Environmental Anthropology at the University of Washington. Although now moribund, the "EA Program" flourished for over a decade and provided its participants (students and faculty alike) with a dynamic intellectual and social environment for exploring diverse and non-dogmatic approaches to environmental social sciences. In comparison to a decade ago, there are now a growing number of vibrant programs for environmental social science, and an expanding scholarly and applied literature.

Finally, we want to thank William Balée, Ashwini Chhatre, Steven Goodreau, Michael Gurven, Karen Lupo, Ronald Niezen, David Nolin, Laura Ogden, Laura Rival, Raja Sengupta, and Richard Stepp for their excellent contribution as external reviewers of the chapters included in this volume.

1

Introduction

ISMAEL VACCARO AND ERIC ALDEN SMITH

ENVIRONMENTAL SOCIAL SCIENCE

Environmental social science has its roots in several disciplines and research traditions, ranging from anthropology to zoology Disciplinary identities and frameworks continue to play a significant role: environmental anthropology, political ecology (centered in geography), environmental social science, and similar named entities in several other disciplines have their own associations, scholarly journals, and sets of issues. But increasingly there is convergence, transdisciplinary interaction, and the forging of a coherent if loosely bounded research community, with scholars and practitioners from many different disciplines in the social sciences, humanities, and applied fields engaged in fruitful dialogue and collaboration. This volume aims to foster this emerging field by presenting authoritative summaries of central research methods in a manner accessible to all. In the next section, we summarize the organization of the volume and the content of each chapter; but first, in the present section, we wish to situate this emerging field in a broader intellectual and historical context.

There are many factors that helped generate environmental social science, but two are prominent. The first was the realization that landscapes and the multitude of components they contain cannot be understood without serious consideration of past and present human communities. It is now widely understood that most terrestrial and near-shore environments are profoundly shaped by human actions – they are "socionatural" systems (Balée 2006; Denevan 1992; Smith and

Environmental Social Sciences: Methods and Research Design, ed. I. Vaccaro, E. A. Smith and S. Aswani. Published by Cambridge University Press. © Cambridge University Press 2010.

Wishnie 2000). These anthropogenic impacts are not limited to large-scale societies, but extend back to the initial dispersal of *Homo sapiens* some 60 000 years ago, and include effects that both enhanced and diminished biodiversity and ecosystem functions.

The second key stimulus for environmental social science is the recognition that human societies cannot be understood without analyzing their interactions with the environments that supported them. There is a long tradition of social analysis of the complex relationships between humans and environment, ranging from the philosophical accounts of Montaigne (1595), Montesquieu (1748), Voltaire (1759) to Malthus (1798), and Boserup (1965) on the relationships between demography and resources, with other classics Morgan (1877) and White (1959) on technology, Engels (1884) and Wittfogel (1956) on environmental drivers of social complexity, and Ratzel (1882), Wissler (1926), Steward (1955), and Rappaport (1984) on ecological adaptation. Some useful reviews and collections include Borgerhoff Mulder and Coppolillo (2005), Haenn and Wilk (2006), Johnson and Earle (2000), Orlove (1980), and Vayda and Rappaport (1968).

Initially, environmental social science emphasized economic factors as key mediators of human–environment relationships (cultural ecology). Economic perspectives, however, were soon joined by analyses of the social construction of knowledge (ethnobiology and science studies), politics and ideology (political ecology), and institutions (property theory and collective action theory), among many others. Although most of the contributors of this volume are anthropologists, this edited book has been explicitly designed to be useful to practitioners interested in the environment from all types of social sciences and humanities. Indeed, none of the tools or frameworks presented here are the exclusive patrimony of a single discipline.

Environmental issues, in any case, have proven to pose extremely complex theoretical and methodological demands. For instance, what is a forest habitat? There is no unique and uncontested answer to this question. To foresters, a forest is a productive unit that should be managed to produce its maximum sustainable yield. To urban dwellers, this same forest constitutes a dramatic and picturesque landscape suitable for camping and contemplation. Local farmers may perceive a forest as wasteland, since it occupies space that is not being cultivated; or they may perceive it as a storehouse of useful wild plants and animals, or (in the case of swidden farmers) the site of once and future gardens. The very same forest, to biologists, may be the habitat that sustains species that they are trying to conserve in a protected area, or the ecosystem that generates important "services" for people and other living things. The forest is all of these things and more, but the perspective and values of any one individual or "stakeholder" group is necessarily partial. Any analysis of forests must recognize this subjectivity, and the potentially conflicting views and interests this implies. That being said, the analysis is likely to improve if, thanks to ecological analysis, we know it is a tropical rain forest with high species diversity and rapid nutrient turnover, if it has few or many introduced species, what kind of disturbance regime (from fire, wind, etc.) it is characterized by, and so on. In addition, a quantitative analysis of the extraction of timber and non-timber resources, a demographic analysis in and around the forest, and an examination of tourism in the area will offer useful complements to narratives about the forest provided by the various social actors.

In sum, the methodological complexity of socioenvironmental issues emerges in two different dimensions. First, analysis of these issues benefits from the combination of diverse methods and concepts from both natural and social sciences (Abel and Stepp 2003; Borgerhoff Mulder and Coppolillo 2005; Crumley 1994; Scoones 1999). Second, different disciplines and research traditions within the social sciences have developed diverse methodologies to approach the social components of environmental issues that often complement each other. This edited book focuses on the second point, or the need for methodological heterogeneity. The social sciences and humanities have developed a very diverse set of methodologies devoted to producing data on social issues connected, in one way or another, with the environment. This heterogeneity has resulted in qualitative and quantitative approaches that combine localized and multi-sited research, synchronic and diachronic perspectives, and discursive, statistical, or spatial analyses.

Most research projects can be thought of as including three basic elements: (1) an epistemology, or set of assumptions about how to construct, evaluate, and articulate knowledge; (2) a methodology, which is understood as a conceptual and analytical framework; and (3) a set of specific methods used to collect specific types of information, which are hopefully linked to (justified by) the first two elements. The goal of this volume is to introduce students and professionals to diverse methodologies and methods which are currently used in various environmental social sciences. Because the relationships between environment and society are extremely complex, and the methods for studying them have developed in diverse field settings and disciplines, there is no single methodological framework uniting this work (or the chapters in this volume). Any environmental issue can be studied from a multiplicity of perspectives, causality can be studied from different angles, and information can be extracted from different areas or about different aspects of the issue. Thus, the diversity of theoretical and methodological approaches has resulted in production of information distributed within many different dimensions, often with little cross-referencing (let alone integration) and often highly dependent on the theoretical or research goals of the investigator.

This book presents a representative (if not complete) sample of environmental social science methods and methodologies. The intent is to provide readers with an introduction to several important analytical options for society–environment research. The chapters also highlight case studies that illustrate the application of these methods. Overall, we hope to show how complementary these different approaches and types of information can often be. A research design that incorporates several of the proposed methods may be better equipped to generate a more nuanced approach to a particular issue. This last goal, however, is not easy, as demonstrated by the difficulties we encountered in designing this very book. The last 25 years of social sciences and humanities research have been characterized by considerable theoretical confrontation. The starkest theoretical divide has opposed scientific or positivist approaches to critical, subjectivist, or postmodern schools, with obvious epistemological and methodological consequences. The subjectivist approaches, to simplify the terminology here, have tended to emphasize qualitative approaches in general and discursive analysis in particular. Positivist approaches have gravitated towards systematic collection and statistical analysis of quantifiable information. This book, however, is designed to challenge this dichotomy by incorporating chapters from both sides of the divide, and by explicitly emphasizing multiple levels of complementarity between quantitative and qualitative methods. In fact, we suggest that this plural approach to environmental social research design is required by the complexity of environmental issues.

OVERVIEW OF THE VOLUME

As noted above, this volume is designed to offer researchers and students an array of analytical approaches and associated methods that are available to study different social dimensions of environmental issues. We believe it covers a gap in the available literature, and will prove useful for both research and teaching. Each chapter emphasizes the nuts and bolts of research design and methods in a different analytical framework. Due to length limitations, we do not expect to train researchers in each of the described methods or research strategies, but rather to make readers aware of their existence, their explanatory potential, and how research using any of them looks, as well as to provide an entry into the published literature in each area.

We have selected 14 themes that we believe cover the most important fields related to environmental social research. While not exhaustive, we believe these themes reflect the main methodological trends available in social sciences (and to some degree the humanities) in relation to environmental issues. The chapter topics, perhaps reflecting the content of the environmental social sciences, include a diverse combination of subjects. These are necessarily covered at varying levels of detail; for example, ethnobiology is a rather more compact field that political economy, which has a massive literature in both Marxist and non-Marxist varieties. A chapter devoted to the socioenvironmental uses of geographic information systems is not necessarily equivalent to one devoted to the environmental aspects of demographic studies. In other words, readers should not expect a homogeneous book, because the field is not a homogeneous one. Even the narrative strategies utilized by the different contributors differ considerably, matching their own epistemological orientations. As editors, we have attempted to provide as much similarity across chapters as possible while not forcing the contributors to adopt styles alien to them or the literature they discuss. Some chapters use a case study as an explanatory vehicle, others have used multiple examples to illustrate the methods they discuss.

In his chapter, Oriol Beltran offers a broad approach to historical demography, discussing its methodological advantages and challenges. He discusses the environmental aspects of human population dynamics, emphasizing demographic distribution, history, and correlated resource use. The chapter surveys demographic variables and their potential uses for landscape interpretation, and provides examples of various demographic patterns such as concentrated versus dispersed inhabitation patterns, as well as migration flows.

Raymond Hames presents some key methods used to describe and analyze household microeconomics – labor inputs and resource outputs. Patterns of resource use and labor allocation exhibit both cross-cultural regularities and historically and culturally specific features. Borrowing from ecology and economics, ecological anthropology has developed a powerful set of tools to measure and analyze fine-grained productive practices. This chapter explicates key methods such as time allocation, income flows within and between households, and selection of resources and environmental patches.

Utilizing a specific study case in Botswana, Amy Poteete introduces readers to institutional analysis and property theory. This chapter focuses on analysis of the institutions that regulate rights to productive resources, and the forms of natural resource management. It highlights the significance of ownership regimes (from open access to commons to state or private property) and the ways in which these articulate with various political and institutional factors.

Centering his analysis on the impacts of climatic change and hazardous events, Eric C. Jones returns us to the field of economic analysis, connecting social agency to markets and their associated political frameworks. From the perspective of political economy this chapter aims to situate individual and collective economic decisions in both environmental and political contexts, and to explicate the methodologies and conceptual frameworks that have been developed to analyze these systems.

Every human community, from small-scale subsistence-based ones to industrial mega-states, has developed knowledge that is fundamental to its members' livelihoods, and for how they both understand and utilize particular environments. The chapter by Laura Zanotti, Denise Glover, and Jennifer Sepez introduces us to ethnobiology, the study of locally produced environmental knowledge. Ethnobiology has developed a specialized set of techniques to collect and analyze this context-dependent body of knowledge in diverse sociocultural settings. This chapter explains methodologies such as free listing, pile sorting, and participatory mapping, as well as their pragmatic uses in resource management and community-based conservation.

Veronica Strang describes the challenges and the enormous potential of ethnohistory and ethnomapping to collect historical, locally relevant, information about a given environment. The sources of information of environmental anthropology are often oral texts. Dealing with ethnohistory and oral narratives presents specific challenges of fundamental importance for ethnographic research. Using examples from her own fieldwork in Australia, Professor Strang discusses the methods developed for collecting oral accounts and assessing their robustness.

Environmental conflicts are often constructed and debated via written texts. These texts result from and interact with previous textual depictions of the same or similar conflicts, and are fundamental sources of information to the researcher. Focusing on different media depictions of a recent event with strong environmental undertones, the alleged recent "discovery" of a Lost Tribe in the Amazon, Candace Slater introduces us to the subtleties and analytical potential of literary analysis of environmental discourses.

In a useful complement to the more qualitative methods discussed by Strang and Slater, Amber Wutich and Clarence Gravlee summarize a combination of qualitative and quantitative methods for analyzing textual data. Basic issues discussed include techniques for identifying themes, developing and using codebooks, and suggestions on how to produce qualitative descriptions, make systematic comparisons, and build and formally test models. An extended example is presented that concerns environmental and social aspects of water use in an urban desert context.

In recent years network analysis has emerged as a powerful tool for the analysis of the composition, directionality and intensity of social, economic and political relationships between individuals and groups. In their chapter, Jeffrey C. Johnson and David C. Griffith address the potential of network analysis for understanding complex social and environmental systems. They show how network analysis can reveal patterns that would not be evident to less systematic methods, as well as how it can be used to test explanations about the causes of such patterns.

In an increasingly interconnected world, with unprecedented flows of capital, commodities, information, and labor, numerous scholarly works have emphasized the need for ethnographic research that takes into account the delocalized or multi-sited character of many contemporary social phenomena. Focusing on the analysis of a commodity chain originating in Madagascar, Lisa Gezon describes the methods and challenges of multi-sited research. This chapter explains different ways in which this interconnectness has been addressed, and how it can connect to environmental factors such as local agricultural decision-making or deforestation.

In their chapter, Eduardo Brondízio and R. Roy Chowdhury provide an extended discussion of the usefulness of spatial analysis in environmental social science. The emergence of geographic information systems (GIS) as a powerful and widely accessible tool has revolutionized the analytical potential of social sciences to document and explain how human communities interact with the landscape. Environmental research produces multi-level scalar data that provides a spatial component to social practices. This chapter discusses how GIS is employed to display ecological and ethnobiological data, highlighting its potential for uncovering data correlation.

The chapter by Emily L. Jones discusses the methods and concepts archaeologists use to analyze long-term interactions between societies and their environments. The specific investigational context of archaeological research (no direct access to agents and processes, dependence on physical remains, and time-averaging) has forced archaeologists to devise specific methods for unveiling how past societies have both shaped and been shaped by their environments. At the same time, the archaeological record provides unique diachronic depth and detailed information on material components of human–environment interaction. This chapter discusses specific archaeological methods such as faunal analysis and paleoecological reconstruction that are useful to understanding both past and contemporary environmental dynamics and problems.

The full potential of environmental social science requires a thorough understanding of the ecology of the area under study, and the role of humans in this ecology. In the last two decades, historical ecology has emerged as an integrative framework for this endeavor. The chapter by Michael D. Scholl, D. Seth Murray, and Carole L. Crumley outlines the basic tenets of historical ecology. They discuss a wide array of issues, including the need to articulate interdisciplinary teams that can manage natural and social sciences alike.

As a way of a synthesizing the diverse themes of this volume, the last chapter, written by volume co-editor Shankar Aswani, provides an example of research located in the Solomon Islands that incorporates several of the methodological approaches described in other chapters. Research by Aswani's team has produced a wealth of data that is being used to design conservation policies which respect the intimate understanding Solomon Islanders have of their environment, as well as taking into account the local political realities and institutional frameworks for policy deployment.

CONCLUSION

In summary, the 14 chapters that follow describe the most important methodological frameworks and techniques currently available in the environmental social sciences. Indeed, this is the book we wish had been available when we were designing our own dissertation research projects. It is our sincere hope that students and researchers in this exciting and rapidly developing field will find it useful for their own projects that analyze the social aspects of environmental issues.

In conclusion, we want to highlight again the point that environmental issues are extremely complex, especially in their social dimensions, and that this complexity requires diverse and multifaceted analytical approaches. It is our strong belief that many of the methods or methodologies presented here that have been considered incompatible in the past are complementary. In fact, we would argue that these diverse approaches have great potential to become synergistic, such that when combined they produce far more than the sum of what they can offer in isolation.

In any case, environmental social scientists must increasingly become fluent in several methodological languages, either because they need to implement them themselves, or because they need to collaborate with researchers trained in other methodological traditions than their own. We hope this volume will encourage a fruitful dialogue between those using different methods, as well as stimulating individual researchers to diversify their own portfolio of methods for investigating socioenvironmental topics.

REFERENCES

Abel, T. and J. R. Stepp 2003. A new systems ecology for anthropology. *Conservation Ecology* **7**(3): 12.

Balée, W. 2006. The research program of historical ecology. *Annual Review of Anthropology* **35**: 75–98.

Borgerhoff Mulder, M. and P. Coppolillo 2005. *Conservation: Linking Ecology, Economics, and Culture*. Princeton, NJ: Princeton University Press.

Boserup, E. 1965. *The Conditions of Agricultural Growth*. Chicago, IL: Aldine.

Crumley, C., ed. 1994. *Historical Ecology: Cultural Knowledge and Changing Landscapes*. Santa Fe, NM: SAR Press.

Denevan, W. 1992. The pristine myth: the landscape of the Americas in 1492. *Annals of the Association of American Geographers* **82**: 369–385.

Engels, F. 1942 [1884]. *The Origins of the Family, Private Property, and the State*. New York: International Publishers.

Haenn, N. and R. Wilk 2006. *The Environment in Anthropology: A Reader in Ecology, Culture, and Sustainable Living*. New York: New York University Press.

Johnson, A. and T. Earle 2000. *The Evolution of Human Societies: From Foraging Group to Agrarian State*. Stanford, CA: Stanford University Press.

Malthus, T. R. 1999 [1798]. *An Essay on the Principle of Population*. Oxford, UK: Oxford University Press.

Montaigne, M. 1993 [1595]. *The Complete Essays*. New York: Penguin.

Montesquieu, C. 1977 [1748]. *The Spirit of the Laws*. Berkeley, CA: University of California Press.

Morgan, H. L. 1985 [1877]. *Ancient Society: Researches in the Lines of Human Progress from Savagery through Barbarism to Civilization*. Tucson, AZ: University Arizona Press.

Orlove, B. 1980. Ecological anthropology. *Annual Review of Anthropology* **9**: 235–273.

Rappaport, R. A. 1984. *Pigs for the Ancestors: Ritual in the Ecology of a New Guinea People*. New Haven, CT: Yale University Press.

Ratzel, F. 2000 [1882]. *Anthropogeographie*. Berlin: Adamant Media Corporation.

Scoones, I. 1999. New ecology and the social sciences: what prospects for a fruitful engagement? *Annual Review of Anthropology* **28**: 479–507.

Smith, E. A. and M. Wishnie 2000. Conservation and subsistence in small-scale societies. *Annual Review of Anthropology* **29**: 493–524.

Steward, J. 1955. *The Theory of Culture Change: The Methodology of Multilinear Evolution*. Urbana, IL: University of Illinois Press.

Vayda, A. P. and R. A. Rappaport 1968. Ecology, cultural and non-cultural. In J. A. Clifton, ed., *Introduction to Cultural Anthropology*. Boston, MA: Houghton-Mifflin, pp. 476–498.

Voltaire 2003 [1759]. *Candide or Optimism*. New York: Barnes and Noble.

White, L. 1959. *The Evolution of Culture*. New York: McGraw-Hill.

Wissler, C. 1926. *The Relation of Nature to Man in Aboriginal America*. New York: Oxford University Press.

Wittfogel, K. 1956. *The Hydraulic Civilizations*. In William L. Thomas, ed., *Man's Role in Changing the Face of the Earth*. Chicago, IL: University of Chicago Press.

2

People, numbers, and natural resources: demography in environmental research

THE DEMOGRAPHIC FACTOR IN ENVIRONMENTAL ANTHROPOLOGY

Population and demographic dynamics are characteristic traits of modern environmental anthropology. In contrast to the ambiguity of the terms used in the discipline's earliest studies of the relations between human groups and their environment, the trend towards defining these groups as populations in the 1960s introduced a higher degree of precision into the analysis. The accuracy of ethnographic observations, the attention to the dynamics of change, and the use of a terminology derived from the natural sciences soon emerged as clear advantages of the use of the categories and models of demographic studies in anthropology (Howell 1986; Kertzer and Fricke 1997).

The issues addressed from a demographic perspective in the study of human environmental relations, as well as the terminology used in the studies, have varied greatly depending on the theoretical priorities of the moment. In this sense, most classical monographs considered demographic variables as mere data, lacking any explanatory power. In common with many other cultural and environmental variables, factors such as the size or territorial distribution of human groups were simply noted as characteristics, and no consequences were drawn for the interpretation of the issues under consideration (e.g., Forde 1934).

Environmental Social Sciences: Methods and Research Design, ed. I. Vaccaro, E. A. Smith and S. Aswani. Published by Cambridge University Press. © Cambridge University Press 2010.

With the advent of cultural ecology, population traits emerged as indicators of the environmental relations of specific human groups. Alongside the technology used, the economic patterns and the social organization, demographic patterns now established themselves as part of the most important cultural factors, and the variation in these patterns was seen to be dependent on the quality, abundance and distribution of the natural resources used by human groups. The comparative studies of Julian Steward (1936) highlighted the importance of demographic patterns in environmental research. From this perspective, the seasonality in the distribution and abundance of natural resources will define a set of population patterns that is characterized by variable concentration and mobility.

Through these efforts to stress the interest in the environmental aspects of anthropology and to provide the discipline with a sounder empirical basis, work undertaken within the framework of what was known as ecological anthropology gave the study of demographic factors a decisive push forward (Lee 1979; Rappaport 1967). Instead of the traditional stress on the concept of culture, Vayda and Rappaport (1968: 494) proposed that anthropologists involved in environmental studies should take from ecology the concept of *population* (as a group of organisms from the same species or variety located inside a given area) to define the basic units of analysis. For these authors, using the same frameworks of reference as ecologists helps to clarify the contribution of specific aspects of culture to survival or the successful operation of the wider systems of which these aspects are part: it also helps to quantify and measure human environmental phenomena and allows them to be described in reasonably precise terms (Rappaport 1971).

The temptation to consider population quantitative data as exact adaptation indicators, however, is considerable. Intercultural comparison, though, reveals the relative nature of demographic statistics and the need for their interpretation in context. In this regard, the size of a specific human group (or its structure by sex and age, or the size and arrangement of its settlements) is not an index of its adaptive success. In the area of the social sciences, the value of demographic data in isolation is limited, although they are very useful for generating hypotheses and for discussing ethnographic information as a whole.

The problem we find when applying the concept of *carrying capacity* to human ecology, as compared to its usefulness in the study of the environmental behavior of other species, can be used to illustrate the validity of this statement. In human ecosystems the maximum population that a specific territory can sustain is not a simple function of the abundance and characteristics of its natural resources. The determination of the resources needed, including food, is not fixated but defined culturally and subject to change (Bartels, Norton, and Perrier 1993). Likewise, the engagement of human populations with their environment is not passive but active. Indeed, a characteristic trait of our species' adaptation is the capacity to increase the resources available. Access to resources and their distribution also constitute a social function. Finally, human environmental relations are not restricted to the area around temporary or permanent settlements: exchange relations between groups make us consider their environment as an open area, with varying levels of use and dependence, but without immutable limits. This is the context of the debate on the effects of demographic pressure on the change of production techniques and economic relations (Cohen 1977). In short, in anthropology the concept of carrying capacity basically has a heuristic value (Brush 1975).

The interest in the relation between demographic factors and production systems, encouraged by Ester Boserup's work (1965) on the development of agriculture, drew attention to the emphasis on stability and integration that characterized environmental research until the mid 1970s. The study of population was to make a decisive contribution to remedying these shortcomings, by introducing an interest in dynamics and change into this area of research (Orlove 1980).

SOURCES AND CONCEPTS

Problems of delimitation and scale

The indicative nature of population data is not the only problem facing the use of demography as an analytical tool in environmental research. Population data require contextual examination and their value in intercultural comparisons is relative. The units of analysis themselves, which have been defined as populations, are subject to difficulties of delimitation which will have an important influence on the interpretations. We must acknowledge this point at the beginning to avoid overestimating the contributions of demographic information, and to emphasize that the difficulty in establishing discrete limits in the units of observation is a common and fundamental problem found in all human and social sciences. However, the limits of a given population can always be discussed more reasonably and efficiently than those of a society or culture.

Generally speaking, delimiting a human group as a population always implies an unavoidable initial ambiguity that must be borne in mind throughout the analysis (Johnson-Hanks 2007). In part, the operationality of demographic analysis rests on the fiction of considering human populations as discrete entities, although no historical group has existed over time closed upon itself, and exceptionally few have existed within a secluded and exclusive territory. To determine the units of analysis in demography one must use criteria that are consistent with the issues addressed and the situation under consideration, and apply them provisionally and always critically. As units of observation in ethnography, populations are often delimited in geographical terms (i.e., individuals and groups that share the same living space, considered at a restricted local scale or at a larger regional level), although broader economic or cultural criteria may also be involved. In environmental research, factors such as natural resource use or the complementary nature of different spaces in a single territory are of particular relevance. The forms of settlement (sedentary residential clusters or temporal aggregates associated with nomadism) are also first-class indicators.

Associated with the problem of their delimitation, the determination of units of analysis in demography also confronts the issue of scale. In addition to questions of consistency and rigor (which are key criteria in the establishment of representative samples), demography demonstrates a greater efficiency in both diagnosing and predicting social reality in larger populations than in smaller groups. The same happens with the statistical processing of data: as opposed to the relative consistency of the indices and rates obtained for larger populations, the values for smaller local groups present greater stochastic variation, and should be examined using specific methods of analysis with the support of ethnographic data such as medical information or kinship (see Early and Headland 1998; Howell 1979). The information on demographic behavior should allow, through the analysis of primary data from different levels of aggregation, the combination of scalar approaches in the same way as in ethnography (at an individual, household, local or regional scale, and at a monographic or comparative analytical level): a close-up analysis, favoring contextualization and a deeper understanding of the nature of a specific population, and a more distant approach, which reveals the existence of more general trends and behaviors.

Administrative boundaries inside which official census data are usually collected cannot be accepted uncritically as units of analysis.

Although the ways in which the available data have been collected and organized can contribute to establish the units to be considered, the effect they are likely to have on each specific research context should also be evaluated.

The production of primary data

As in any other scientific area, the analytical value of demographic factors in environmental research will ultimately depend on the empirical consistency of the primary data. Generally speaking, researchers face two possible contexts, each presenting its own problems. In some study locations, if census data are lacking or unavailable, researchers themselves will have to collect demographic information on which to base their analysis. In this case, preparing an ethnographic census is often one of the first tasks of fieldwork (Townsend 2000). Depending on the population size, it may be possible to collect information on all the individuals of a specific population or alternatively it may be advisable to choose a random sample or a sample based on a representative criterion in order to study the whole. In both cases, however, information should be collected individually, and as close to the source as possible, by questioning each specific social actor or through qualified informants (for example, an adult from each household). Residential units provide a useful basis for carrying out systematic censuses. In environmental analysis, in addition to biographical data (name, age, place of residence, place of birth, data on parents, siblings, spouses and descendants, and other socially relevant data in specific cultural contexts), information on residential patterns and economic organization (e.g., household composition, access to productive resources, and practices), and possibly also information on the health and biophysical characteristics of individuals (such as illness, body weight, and height), is in general significant in order to study the nutritional status of populations (Moran 1993).

If population records are available, preliminary data collection may not be necessary, but this does not preclude the need for meticulous and critical study of the sources used. Though limited and unreliable in certain environmental research scenarios, most contemporary states keep close control of population through a variety of records used to regulate citizens' rights, tax economic activities, regional planning or conscription, and so on. Alongside administrative census data, the records kept by other institutions and organizations can also provide useful information on particular aspects. Church sources such as records of baptisms, marriages, and deaths, for example, have made a huge contribution to historical demography studies in Europe of periods before official government records existed (Netting 1981; Wrigley 1969). In all these cases, though, researchers must assess the reliability of the sources with great care. The data collection methods may not have been optimal, the recording may have been carried out with a particular purpose in mind, or the records may be far from complete (Reher and Schofield 1993; Willigan and Lynch 1982): tax records, for instance, rarely include full information on the activities, wealth, or even the number of members in each census unit.

Fieldwork can provide invaluable qualitative indicators that make it possible to analyze population behaviors beyond census statistics ("demography without numbers," to quote Scheper-Hughes 1997), as well as a contextual interpretation of the decisions and choices that determine demographic change (Fricke 1997). Brandes (1984), for example, has shown how the official census of Spain in the mid twentieth century systematically concealed certain practices that were considered socially shameful, such as suicide or cohabitation. Census information may also distort our understanding of living arrangements, if it considers couples that in fact share a dwelling as separate entities. Data on employment may overlook "moonlighting" (by concentrating on a subject's main occupation or by applying standard criteria). Equally, the patterns of residential mobility (either seasonal or permanent) are very difficult to classify under the headings drawn up by census agents. Ethnographic knowledge thus allows us to evaluate more specifically the data contained in the records by comparing the information obtained through a variety of strategies with a combined quantitative and qualitative approach which should be applied throughout the research process (Basu and Aaby 1998).

A critical approach to the procedures and documentary sources used, the wide variety of the factors considered, and great care in the processing of data are not exclusive requirements of demographic methods, but they are defining traits of scientific ethnography. However, due to the apparent exactitude of the statistical information (Van der Geest 1998), the study of population possibly requires an even greater rigor than other areas of environmental analysis.

Basic forms of analysis

The data on the characteristics of a population can be subjected to two different types of analysis. These should be complementary in order to obtain a complete and exhaustive demographic examination. But this will depend on the information obtained through fieldwork and documentary work, and also, obviously, on the environmental issues which are the object of study and the hypotheses raised in the discussion. A population, as an entity subject to constant evolution, can be approached either by examining it at a specific moment of its historical development or by examining its development over a specific period of time (Pressat 1961; Preston, Heuveline, and Guillot 2001; Tapinos 1985; Shryock and Siegel 1973). As the following section will show, both emphases have great potential for environmental research both in anthropology and in the social sciences as a whole.

Population status

The static analysis of a population not only highlights its structural traits at a specific moment of its existence, but also provides useful hints regarding its history and its future. Its *size* or abundance (total volume) is possibly the most immediate trait in the characterization of a population, in spite of its limited explanatory ability. Thus, although it is important to know the number of individuals in a group, this information in itself is not indicative of the environmental issues or of the behaviors that have evolved in order to face them.

From a comparative perspective or inside a broader contextual framework, population size can become more significant, although it will always depend on the delimitation criteria established. Cross-cultural analyses, for example, show a significant correlation between certain types of subsistence practices and the size of the human groups involved (Bates and Lees 1996; Ellen 1997). Historically, food production encouraged the appearance of larger population groups than in hunter–gatherer societies (Johnson and Earle 2000). The abundance factor is often related to the territory, on the basis of *population density* (the number of inhabitants per surface unit). As mentioned above, establishing the limits of a given population can be problematic, and establishing the criteria for delimiting a territory when calculating its level of geographic concentration is even more difficult. From an environmental perspective administrative divisions or those deriving from land ownership are always arbitrary in groups that are not self-sufficient. Hardesty (1977: 126) also suggests the need to establish a more exact calculation than gross density, which considers specifically the proportion of individuals in a useable territory (leaving out unproductive areas). Although ethnographic research allows us to identify the more important resources for a specific population, identifying, at the same time, its territoriality, one cannot establish a single universal criterion to determine what is and what is not a productive resource (Narotzky 1997: 10).

Data about population structure are less problematic, and are more given to analysis and comparison. Demographers have usually considered two main factors in their characterizations of demographic structures – age and sex – and used them to refer to the *age* and *sex structure*. This structure varies according to the rates at which new individuals join a population and others leave it (as a consequence of births, deaths, and migratory movements). It is usually represented in the form of a *population pyramid*. The vertical axis represents the different age groups (usually in 5-year intervals, with the 0–4 year interval at the base) with bars representing the number of individuals in each group. Each bar is divided into two segments according to sex: the male population is shown on the left of the horizontal axis and the female population on the right. The use of percentages (instead of absolute volumes) and a single representation (a 2/3 relation between the vertical and the horizontal axis) standardizes the graph and improves its interpretation and comparison.

The age pyramid summarizes the chronological and sexual structure of a population and its shape provides information on the population's history and mode of growth. Broadly speaking, demographic studies usually differentiate between pyramids with a broad base (indicating a young population with a rapid growth rate), those that are wider at the top (showing a lack of generational renewal and population reduction), those with similar values for the different age groups (indicating stagnation), and those with a clear pyramidal structure, evidence of a population with a balanced replacement between deaths and births. The existence of strongly different values for certain age groups reflected in the pyramid shape indicates the effects of past episodes that may have a specific environmental significance (such as migratory movements, epidemics or war, and so on) (Figure 2.1).

The chronological structure can also be analyzed through indicators calculated on the basis of the demographic information available. The *ageing index* (the number of individuals over 65 years old per 10 divided by the number under 14) defines populations as ageing or young, and the *dependency ratio* (the rate of individuals under 14 years old and over 60 divided by the individuals between 15 and 59 years old) indicates their capacity for work. However, these measurements should be specified for each particular cultural context; in the second

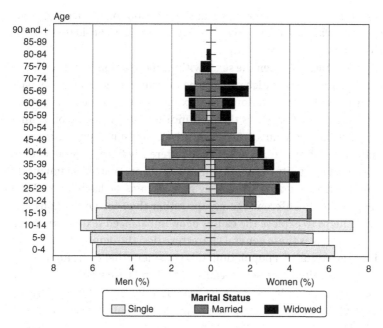

Pyramid 1924

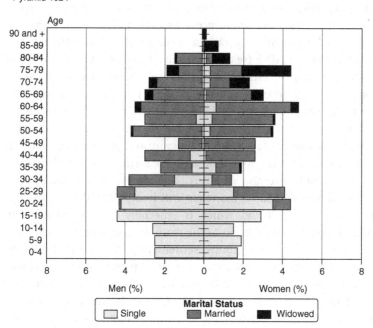

Pyramid 1986

Figure 2.1   Population pyramids in El Poal, 1924 and 1986.
Source: Estrada 1998: 82 and 92.

case, for example, it is obvious that the contribution of each age group to a population's productive capacity cannot be considered on the basis of a universal concept.

The ratio between the sexes within a population is another structural characteristic which can also be measured exactly and may have environmental connotations. The *sex ratio* (the ratio of men relative to women per 100) allows the identification of the degree of balance between the sexes. Imbalances may arise as a result of practices where individuals of both sexes are treated differently from childhood, or as a result of mortality or migration, and so on, and may have important consequences for aspects such as growth rates or labor roles. Their calculation for different age groups rather than for populations as a whole helps to explore the causes of an imbalanced sexual structure.

As well as these general characteristics, the demographic analysis of the status of a population may consider other indicators which are more limited precisely because of their relative significance. Both the existing records and records created in the context of a particular research study can provide much more information about the individuals within a population than just their age and sex. Depending on the specific object of study, this information can be very significant. Official censuses often record aspects such as main economic activity, educational level, race, and marriage status. Although this information should be treated critically, it allows the formulation of hypotheses and the establishment of research initiatives that can be compared with other evidence. Behaviors relating to marriage, for example, which have received special attention in European historical demography (e.g., Henry 1980), have been interpreted as regulatory mechanisms of demographic pressure and growth in a context in which marriage is the socially acceptable setting for reproduction.

Alongside size and structure, the analysis of a population at a specific moment in its existence will finally include the study of its *geographic distribution*, which is especially relevant in environmental research. In addition to the main distinction drawn between nomadic and sedentary groups, settlement location, the itineraries followed and the degree of concentration of population in each place of residence are fundamental elements in the relations of human populations with their environment. Cross-cultural analysis reveals that the modes of exploitation of natural resources are the main determining variable of settlement patterns, to the extent that they can be considered a basic factor among the strategies of use of these resources (Chang 1962; Martínez Veiga 1978). Resource location,

Table 2.1 *Household structure in Alagna, 1935 and 1980.*

	1935		1980	
	N	%	N	%
1. Solitaires	34	20.5	46	28.9
2. No family	15	9.0	7	4.4
3. Simple-family households	93	56.0	100	62.9
4. Extended-family households	18	10.8	4	2.5
5. Multiple-family households	6	3.6	2	1.3
Total	166	99.9	159	100.0
Complex households (4+5)	24	14.4	6	3.8
Mean household size		2.99		2.62

Source: Status animarum of 1935 and Viazzo's census of 1980 (Viazzo 1989: 97).

abundance and seasonality, however, are not the only environmental determining factors of the types of settlement. Alongside other physical factors (for instance, altitude or particular geographical features) human groups will be very sensitive to the elements related to the social environment (which includes political borders, administrative demarcations, communication networks, and the location of exchange centers).

Given its scale, the analysis of the types of territorial distribution of population goes beyond mere statistical treatment, and requires more complex types of graphic representation (see Brondízio and Roy Chowdhury, Chapter 12 in this volume). Similarly, data must allow for a high degree of disaggregation (from the types of residential units to the different organizational levels of the groups that can be identified) so as to avoid generalizations and to encourage a deeper understanding of territorial behaviors. In this regard, the analysis of types of residence carried out by the historical anthropology of the family (Laslett 1972) can provide highly relevant indicators in certain research contexts (Table 2.1).

Demographic dynamics

The study of demographic growth reveals a population's dynamics over time. In terms of the variations in the number of its individual members (which is usually reflected in its structure as well as in its forms of distribution), a population will experience positive or negative growth according to the changes in its birth and death indices and the migratory movements that affect it. Environmental factors may be an important element to explain the causes of these demographic changes, and the variations will in turn imply modifications in the relations established by the groups with their environment (Swedlund 1978). This consideration of demographic evolution encourages the understanding of human environmental relations in terms of their complexity.

Demographic research has developed many methodological tools for the study of population growth. The models that derive from its study, and especially what is known as the *demographic transition model*, continue to be the object of special attention (Johnson-Hanks 2008). However, as opposed to the interest aroused by phenomena associated with *natural growth* (birth and death), migratory movements (immigration and emigration), which are particularly difficult to record rigorously, have usually been less studied in spite of their significance in certain contexts. As we stated above, no historical population has developed over time entirely closed upon itself.

The measurement of the rhythms of demographic change uses a variety of indices (Preston, Heuveline, and Guillot 2001: 92–116). Generally speaking, the *natural growth rate* derives from the difference between the *fertility rate* (number of births during a year per 1000 inhabitants) and the *mortality rate* (number of deaths during a year per 1000 inhabitants). The lack of correspondence between the real variation in a population size at two different moments and the natural growth rate will provide an approximation of the effects of the migratory movement. Therefore, in the analysis of this phenomenon it is easier to calculate the *migratory rate* than to evaluate exactly the number of arrivals and departures occurring during a specific period of time. When studying the processes involving growth, as in the case of demographic analysis as a whole, the accuracy of the data and the possibility to disaggregate into different groups of individuals will make research more consistent making it easier to assess the relation between population and the environment. For example, as opposed to the merely approximate nature of the *gross fertility rate* (that is, calculated for the whole of a given population), the *age-specific fertility rate* allows a better observation of behaviors associated with reproduction. The total fertility rate (TFR, number of births during a year per 1000 women between 15 and 49 years old) is one of the most commonly calculated birth indices. The *infant mortality rate* is a good indicator of the health of a population, as children less than 1 year old are very sensitive to factors such as food quality and abundance and infectious diseases.

Table 2.2 *Age at first marriage in Törbel, 1700–1974.*

	Average age	
	Females	Males
1700–49	28.33	30.85
1750–99	27.11	31.33
1800–49	28.48	30.05
1850–99	29.10	33.44
1900–49	28.85	32.55
1950–74	27.13	30.60
Mean	28.24	31.49

Source: Netting 1981: 135.

Data provided by transversal observation of population can be refined by its longitudinal analysis (the analysis of its cohorts). A *cohort* is the group of individuals that have simultaneously lived the same event during the same period of time (i.e., people born during the same year or all the women married in a given year). The analysis of generations allows for a better interpretation of demographic phenomena such as marriages or fertility, as it avoids the distortions added by the differential dimensions of each age group over the totality of the considered population.

The possibility of relating several indicators will provide a better understanding of the demographic phenomena taken as a whole. Several aspects related to fertility (such as the *mean age of women at birth of first child* or the *abortion rate*) and marriage rates (such as the *definitive celibacy rate*, the *mean age at first marriage*, the *total divorce rate*), for example, can be decisive in interpreting the mechanisms involved in the social regulation of demographic growth (Table 2.2). The conditioning of the participation of women in reproduction by accelerating or delaying marriage, for instance, is a formula widely used to modify demographic pressure thanks to its flexibility and reversibility (Harris and Ross 1990).

THE SOCIAL AND ENVIRONMENTAL CONTEXT
OF DEMOGRAPHIC BEHAVIORS

In the dialectic process of any empirical research in environmental anthropology, demographic data can suggest many questions and many solid hypotheses, and also provide the opportunity to explore in a simple, direct way the causes of the behaviors observed regarding the problems under study. A brief presentation of some of the applications of this approach will show the methodological and analytical potential of demographic studies in environmental research.

The two cases we will discuss here are part of a research project conducted in the central area of the southern Pyrenees, a mountainous region in southern Europe. In a series of studies of human ecology in this area (Beltran 1995; Beltran and Vaccaro in press), our work has combined an interest in the local ways of life in the past (especially, from the end of the eighteenth century onwards) and attention to the social and political aspects that define contemporary landscape uses (particularly tourism and the protection of natural areas) in the context of a process defined as the production of natural heritage (Vaccaro and Beltran 2007). Including ethnographic fieldwork carried out at different local sites, the study focuses particularly on documentary evidence of the area's political, legal, and economic organization, as well as its demography, thanks to the large quantity of historical records preserved in the local archives.

Our research has focused on the Catalan districts of the Val d'Aran (with a surface area of 63 360 ha, at the head of the Garonne, which flows into the Atlantic Ocean) and the Pallars Sobirà (with a surface area of 137 792 ha, formed by the headwaters of the river Noguera Pallaresa, a tributary of the Ebro which flows into the Mediterranean). In spite of their geographical and historical differences, the two districts share many common traits. Until the mid twentieth century, the local economy was mostly characterized by agriculture and livestock farming organized on the basis of family farms and the joint ownership of pastures and forests. While the mountainous environment limited agricultural production (which was basically for private consumption and required regular supplies of goods produced elsewhere), the abundance of seasonal pastures encouraged surplus stock farming to produce meat, wool, and draft animals, which were marketed further afield. From the end of the 1940s onwards, the construction of many hydroelectric power stations that fed the industrial growth of the Mediterranean towns sped up the integration of the two districts into the regional market and marked the end of an economy based on subsistence production. Two decades later, the opening of ski resorts in the area brought in tourism, which has now become the main economic activity of the local population. The locals now provide the services needed for white and green tourism; they become guides and guards, they staff hotels and ski resorts, and build second homes (Beltran and Vaccaro 2007).

The spatial distribution of the population

The Pallars Sobirà is a good example of the potential of population studies in environmental analysis. Our analysis was based on the use of the *nomenclátor*, a record issued periodically by the Spanish government from 1860 onwards; unlike the official census, it records all the existing population groups and entities, and not only the categories recognized in the official territorial divisions (the smallest administrative unit, the municipality, may be formed by a population centered in a single nucleus or according to much more complex arrangements). Data collection was centered on the number of individuals and households located in each population center. This information was complemented by other data (toponyms, cartographical studies, and local ethnographic knowledge) and allowed a detailed analysis of the inhabited areas in the district and their changes over time, thus providing a much fuller picture than the official population census.

Broadly speaking, the changes in the district's population show a strong contrast which goes beyond the steady fall in the total volume of inhabitants reflected in the demographic evolution taken as a whole (from 18 762 inhabitants in 1857 to 6883 in 2005). Until the beginning of the twentieth century, the population was distributed regularly throughout the territory over a large number of small settlements located in the valleys or high plains, with only a few larger settlements located at the bottom of the main valley. Records indicate the existence of 116 populated clusters most of which (as many as 68) had 20 houses at the most. On the other hand, in 1991, when the lowest population figures in modern times were recorded, the effects of economic change had substantially modified the district's human landscape. The population had abandoned the higher valleys en masse, where the climate is more extreme, productivity is limited, and communications are more difficult, and had concentrated in the few settlements located in the lower part of the valleys (Figure 2.2). The strong growth of the administrative capital (Sort), which by the late twentieth century was home to a fifth of the total population of the district, is a good indicator of this process.

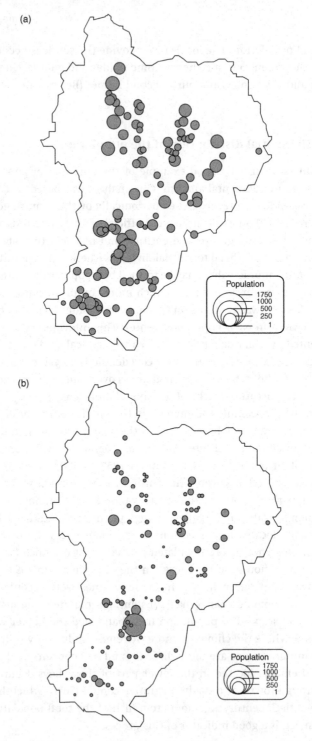

Figure 2.2   Population distribution in the Pallars Sobirà, (a) 1857 and
(b) 1991.
Source: Nomenclátor 1857 and 1991.

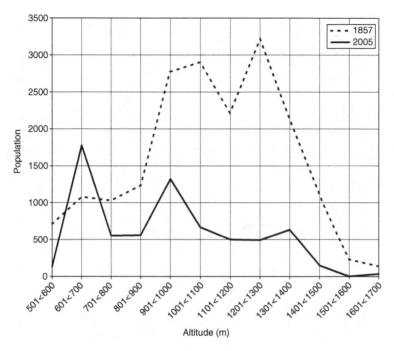

Figure 2.3   Pallars Sobirà's population depending on altitude,
1857–2005.
Source: Nomenclátor 1857–2005.

Throughout the twentieth century, in a process which acceler-
ated from the 1960s, the population living at an altitude above 1000 m
decreased from 63 to 38.9 percent (Figure 2.3) and the population living far from the main communication routes from 77 to 50.6 percent
(Figure 2.4). In fact, the number of inhabitants of the villages accessible by road today is practically the same as 150 years ago, while the
mountain slopes accumulate most of the demographic decay regis-
tered during this period with loses amounting to 80 percent of their
population.

The two extreme types of human landscape found in the Pallars
Sobirà are indicative of the changes experienced in the relations of
the local population with the environment of the district. Whereas
in the past the use of the existing natural resources for agriculture
and livestock farming required spatial dispersal (seasonal migrations
of livestock and temporary residence at higher altitudes), nowadays
the existence of large uninhabited areas encourages the extensive
establishment of natural protected areas and tourist infrastructures
devoted to urban population's consumption.

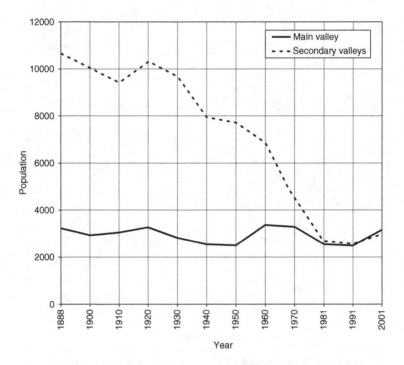

Figure 2.4   Population in the main and secondary valleys in Pallars Sobirà, 1888–2001.
Source: Nomenclátor 1888–2001.

The regulation of demographic growth

The study of the social organization of agricultural and livestock exploitation in the Val d'Aran, which focused on the analysis of the family and communal institutions regulating access to the natural resources, highlighted the important role played by migratory movements in the environmental history of the district, especially until the first decades of the twentieth century. As mentioned above, in most cases the demographic study of migrations has to be based on indirect sources of information, and exact data are impossible to obtain. However, the oral information gathered from informants and from the many references found dispersed in the historical and administrative archives suggested that the issue deserved specific attention.

The population census provided a certain amount of evidence. The censuses carried out by the state from the mid nineteenth century onwards record the presence or absence of individuals, and also include temporary residents. The reliability of these data is only

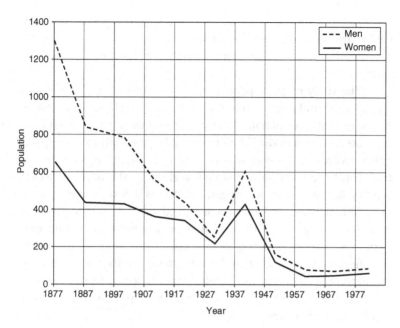

Figure 2.5 Evolution of absent population in censuses of the Val d'Aran, 1877–1981.
Source: Beltran 1995: 93.

relative, as they depend on the criteria applied by the census agent, but a detailed examination combined with an appraisal of information from other sources gives an idea of the demographic behavior that they reflect. The record from 1877, for example, indicates that one of every five persons who was resident in the valley was absent when the census was made. This phenomenon continued significantly until at least 1920, when 8 percent of the population was absent at the time of the census elaboration (Figure 2.5). The variations between villages in the district, as well as the examination of the individual character-istics of the absentees (basically sex, age, marital status and position within the household) provided equally interesting information.

Although in some cases these absences would have been due to chance, or might have anticipated more permanent changes, for the most part they reflected a common practice: seasonal migration. Because of the intense seasonality of the local climate, workforce requirements varied at different times in the year; by sending away some of its members temporarily, households could gain some flexi-bility and were able to adopt diversified economic patterns. During the long winter months, when the livestock were housed in the stables and the fields were covered in snow, the strongest young men traveled across the border to France, thus reducing the load on household consumption and providing an opportunity to earn some additional income.

The study of other population-related data identified a second type of structural migration in the Val d'Aran population and allowed its quantitative evaluation. Alongside the study of the demographic censuses, research in the Val d'Aran included the analysis of the population records of a representative sample of the villages in the district. Until the creation of the civil registry in the mid nineteenth century, data on births, marriages, and deaths in Spain were recorded in church archives. The analysis of basic data (such as dates of birth, marital status, or age of the deceased, for example) made it possible to study significant aspects of demographic behavior in depth, such as the calculation of the birth and death rates. The differential between the natural growth and the absolute data reflected in the censuses revealed the importance of permanent migrations in the demographic regulation of the district.

Thus, in addition to circumstantial migratory movements (such as the one caused by the Spanish Civil War in the late 1930s), the scarcity of natural resources locally available in an agro-ranching economy provided incentives to generate a series of mechanisms to regulate the demographic pressure. These mechanisms often encouraged the expulsion of a number of individuals of the community from each generation. From a juridical perspective, for instance, the fact that at each generation only one of the descendants of each family would inherit the complete household patrimony and the family's communal rights would promote this outbound mobility. Like the inheritance patterns, marriage patterns were fundamental in the social control of demographic growth. The differences in behavior regarding elements such as marrying age, second marriages in case of premature death of the spouse, or permanent celibacy had, like migratory movements, an effect on the different systems of pressure on the resources (Figure 2.6). These behaviors were explored through a rigorous analysis of the data available from birth, marriage and death records in the church and administrative archives.

DEMOGRAPHY AS AN ENVIRONMENTAL INDICATOR

The importance of demographic analysis in environmental research ultimately relies on two main factors. First, population types and

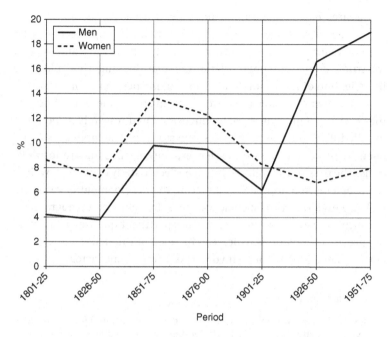

Figure 2.6   Definitive celibacy in the Val d'Aran, 1801–1975.
Source: Beltran 1995: 87.

dynamics are not independent variables in the environmental relations of human groups: on the contrary, aspects such as the rhythm
of growth, the type of settlement, or even the demographic structure
should be analyzed as active mechanisms through which a given population reacts to the problems and opportunities posed by its environment. The debate on the impact of demographic pressure on the
intensification of food production has often obviated the impact of
sociocultural behaviors on population growth.

Second, demography has some immediate methodological advantages over other factors and variables also relevant in environmental
studies such as the study of natural resource use and management.
Although it must be based on especially meticulous data collection
and critical data analysis, and must avoid an absolute identification
between the complex phenomena of environmental anthropology
and some of their isolated manifestations, it is clear that the quantitative evaluation of the aspects that relate to the study of populations
achieves higher levels of precision than other indicators. Demographic
analysis provides a kind of "road map" of a population on the basis of
which we can correlate the ethnographic data obtained through other

procedures. Basic demographic indicators (such as chronological structure or density) become the touchstones that can improve the information on economic and political behaviors within the framework of the study of environmental relations, and at the same time allow the investigation of the factors that shape landscapes and their change.

The two examples presented here suggest some of the possibilities of demographic analysis for environmental research. Although it usually follows formal procedures, the study of populations, as is frequently the case in the social sciences, does not fit standard formulations. The possibilities offered by each specific study context, as well as the problems and approaches directing the development of research, will suggest a variety of specific solutions. In summary, demography is a fruitful research field for formulating pertinent questions and making precise observations which can broaden our understanding of the environmental phenomena involving anthropogenic factors.

REFERENCES

Bartels, G. B., B. E. Norton, and G. K. Perrier 1993. An examination of the carrying capacity concept. In R. H. Behnke, I. Scoones and C. Kerven, eds., *Range Ecology at Desequilibrium. New Models of Natural Variability and Pastoral Adaptation in African Savannas*. London: Overseas Development Institute, pp. 89–103.

Basu, A. M. and P. Aaby 1998. Introduction: approaches to anthropological demography. In A. M. Basu and P. Aaby, eds., *The Methods and Uses of Anthropological Demography*. Oxford, UK: Clarendon Press, pp. 1–21.

Bates, D. G. and S. N. Lees, eds. 1996. *Case Studies in Human Ecology*. New York: Plenum Press.

Beltran, O. 1995. *Es aranesi. Adaptació a l'entorn i organització social al Pirineu Central*. Barcelona: Universitat de Barcelona.

Beltran, O. and I. Vaccaro 2007. El paisaje del Pallars Sobirà: pastores, centrales hidroeléctricas y estaciones de esquí. In I. Vaccaro and O. Beltran, eds., *Ecología política de los Pirineos. Estado, historia y paisaje*. Tremp, Spain: Garsineu, pp. 139–56.

Beltran, O. and I. Vaccaro in press. *Parcs als comunals. La patrimonialització de la muntanya al Pallars Sobirà*. Barcelona: Generalitat de Catalunya.

Boserup, E. 1965. *The Conditions of Agricultural Growth: The Economics of Agrarian Change under Population Pressure*. Chicago, IL: Aldine.

Brandes, S. H. 1984. Nombres que enganyen: cinc problemes en la interpretació de dades censals en l'Espanya rural. *Quaderns de l'Institut Català d'Antropologia* **5**: 28–43.

Brush, S. B. 1975. The concept of carrying capacity for systems of shifting cultivation. *American Anthropologist* **77**(4): 799–811.

Chang, K. C. 1962. A typology of settlement and community patterns in some circumpolar societies. *Arctic Anthropology* **1**: 28–39.

Cohen, M. N. 1977. *The Food Crisis in Prehistory: Over Population and Origins of Agriculture*. Yale, CN: Yale University Press.

Early, J. D. and T. N. Headland 1998. *Population Dynamics of a Philippine Rain Forest People: The San Ildefonso Agta*. Gainesville, FL: University of Florida Press.

Ellen, R. 1997. Modes of subsistence: hunting and gathering to agriculture and pastoralism. In T. Inglod, ed., *Companion Encyclopedia of Anthropology. Humanity, Culture and Social Life*. London: Routledge, pp. 197–225.

Estrada, F. 1998. *Les cases pageses al Pla d'Urgell. Família, residència, terra i treball durant els segles XIX i XX*. Lleida, Spain: Pagès.

Forde, C. D. 1934. *Habitat, Economy and Society*. London: Methuen.

Fricke, T. 1997. Culture theory and demographic process: toward a thicker demography. In D. I. Kertzer and T. Fricke, eds., *Anthropological Demography. Toward a New Synthesis*. Chicago, IL: University of Chicago Press, pp. 248–277.

Hardesty, D. L. 1977. *Ecological Anthropology*. New York: John Wiley & Sons Inc.

Harris, M. and E. B. Ross 1990. *Death, Sex, and Fertility: Population Regulation in Preindustrial and Developing Societies*. New York: Columbia University Press.

Henry, L. 1980. *Techniques d'analyse en démographie historique*. Paris: Institut National d'Études Démographiques.

Howell, N. 1979. *Demography of the Dobe !Kung*. New York: Academic Press.

Howell, N. 1986. Demographic anthropology. *Annual Review of Anthropology*, **15**: 219–246.

Johnson, A. W. and T. Earle 2000. *The Evolution of Human Societies. From Foraging Group to Agrarian State*. Stanford, CA: Stanford University Press.

Johnson-Hanks, J. 2007. What kind of theory for anthropological demography? *Demographic Research* **16** (1): 1–26.

Johnson-Hanks, J. 2008. Demographic transitions and modernity. *Annual Review of Anthropology* **37**: 301–315.

Kertzer, D. I. and T. Fricke 1997. Toward an anthropological demography. In D. I. Kertzer and T. Fricke, eds., *Anthropological Demography. Toward a New Synthesis*. Chicago, IL: University of Chicago Press, pp. 1–35.

Laslett, P. 1972. The history of the family. In P. Laslett and R. Wall, eds., *Household and Family in Past Time*. Cambridge, UK: Cambridge University Press, pp. 1–90.

Lee, R. B. 1979. *The !Kung San. Men, Women, and Work in a Foraging Society*. Cambridge, UK: Cambridge University Press.

Martínez Veiga, U. 1978. *Antropología ecológica*. La Coruña, Spain: Adara.

Moran, E. F. 1993. *La ecología humana de los pueblos de la Amazonia*. Mexico: Fondo de Cultura Económica.

Narotzky, S. 1997. *New Directions in Economic Anthropology*. London: Pluto Press.

Netting, R. M. 1981. *Balancing on an Alp. Ecological Change and Continuity in a Swiss Mountain Community*. Cambridge, UK: Cambridge University Press.

Orlove, B. S. 1980. Ecological anthropology. *Annual Review of Anthropology* **9**: 235–273.

Pressat, R. 1961. *L'analyse démographique. Concepts, méthodes, résultats*. Paris: Presses Universitaires de France.

Preston, S. H., P. Heuveline, and M. Guillot 2001. *Demography: Measuring and Modeling Population Processes*. Malden, MA: Blackwell Publishing.

Rappaport, R. A. 1967. *Pigs for the Ancestors. Ritual in the Ecology of a New Guinea People*. New Haven, CN: Yale University Press.

Rappaport, R. A. 1971. Nature, culture, and ecological anthropology. In H. Shapiro, ed., *Man Culture, and Society*. New York: Oxford University Press, pp. 237–267.

Reher, D. S. and R. Schofield, eds. 1993. *Old and New Methods in Historical Demography*. Oxford, UK: Clarendon Press.

Scheper-Hughes, N. 1997. Demography without numbers. In D. I. Kertzer and T. Fricke, eds., *Anthropological Demography. Toward a New Synthesis*. Chicago, IL: University of Chicago Press, pp. 201–222.

Shryock, H. and J. Siegel 1973. *The Methods and Materials of Demography*. Washington, DC: US Government Printing Office.

Steward, J. 1936. The economic and social basis of primitive bands. In R. Lowie, ed., *Essays in Anthropology Presented to A. L. Kroeber*. Berkeley, CA: University of California Press, pp. 331–345.

Swedlund, A. C. 1978. Historical demography as population ecology. *Annual Review of Anthropology* **7**: 137–173.

Tapinos, G. 1985. *Éléments de démographie*. Paris: Armand Colin.

Townsend, P. K. 2000. *Environmental Anthropology. From Pigs to Policies*. Long Grove, IL: Waveland Press.

Vaccaro, I. and O. Beltran 2007. Consuming space, nature and culture: patrimonial discussions in the hyper-modern era. *Tourism Geographies* **9**: 254–274.

Van der Geest, S. 1998. Participant observation in demographic research: fieldwork experiences in a Ghanaian community. In A. M. Basu and P. Aaby, eds., *The Methods and Uses of Anthropological Demography*. Oxford, UK: Clarendon Press, pp. 39–56.

Vayda, A. P. and R. A. Rappaport 1968. Ecology, cultural and non-cultural. In J. A. Clifton, ed., *Introduction to Cultural Anthropology*. Boston, MA: Houghton-Mifflin, pp. 476–498.

Viazzo, P. P. 1989. *Upland Communities. Environment, Population and Social Structure in the Alps Since the Sixteenth Century*. Cambridge, UK: Cambridge University Press.

Willigan, J. D. and K. A. Lynch 1982. *Sources and Methods of Historical Demography*. New York: Academic Press.

Wrigley, E. A. 1969. *Population and History*. New York: McGraw-Hill.

3

Production decisions and time allocation: a guide to data collection

RAYMOND HAMES

INTRODUCTION

In this chapter I deal with methods for collecting behavioral and economic data on productive inputs and outputs. Any attempt at the collection of quantitative data requires that the researcher should ideally
have prior knowledge of the full range of economic activities and perform preliminary evaluations of the accuracy of data collection procedures and coding schemes. This will prevent false starts, increase
cross-cultural comparability, and lead to a more systematic account of
activities. Whenever possible, I encourage researchers to rely on observational data as a kind of gold standard: it produces data amenable
to sophisticated quantitative analysis, is crucial for theory testing, is
more easily used for cross-cultural comparison than qualitative observations, and reduces the known errors in recall data (see Stange *et al.*
1998 for an illuminating account of recall errors compared to direct
observation). Nevertheless, because of intrusiveness, labor intensive-
ness, and cultural sensitivities in direct observation, recall data are
oftentimes required, but may be integrated into behavioral records.
Techniques for reducing recall error (e.g., short time frames) and cross-
checking are recommended in such cases.

Conventionally, economic activities may be defined as behaviors
whose end result is the production of a material good (e.g., food or
artifact), maintenance of an object (e.g., tool repair), or provisioning of
a service (e.g., assisting a neighbor building a house). Production activities can be easily characterized along a set of input measures (time,

Environmental Social Sciences: Methods and Research Design, ed. I. Vaccaro, E. A. Smith and
S. Aswani. ublished by Cambridge University Press. © Cambridge University Press 2010.

energy, or even risk) but output measures are more complex. In food production outputs are conventionally weight, kilocalories, or macro-nutrients (carbohydrates, fats, and proteins) and represent common denominators for comparative and analytic purposes. Which of these currencies is appropriate will depend on the research question posed.

However, in non-market economies without exchange value currencies there are many common productive activities that are difficult to reduce to a common output denominator even though they have clear economic values (water and fuel collection). If one works to collect and mash *nara* (a Yanomamö term for a red plant pigment used as a cosmetic) or builds a musical instrument then the output is red coloring or a flute. The only common denominator they have with other economic activities is the time and energy it takes to produce them. But time and energy are limited, and the ability to produce such goods may demonstrate that one has sufficient margin in food and other necessary kinds of production to spend time in other kinds of production. Employing costly signaling theory, Bliege Bird and Smith (2005) propose that the production of some goods (e.g., elaborate houses or flutes) serves to signal personal attributes ranging from "physical vigor to cognitive skills to coalition size and cohesion. While the precise benefits to signalers and receivers have not been measured in most cases, the leading contenders include obtaining better mates, forming valuable alliances, and avoiding the costs of violent competition" (p. 237). The hypothesis, then, is that "luxury" goods production demonstrates that the individual is easily able to produce life essentials (akin to Veblen's [1899] "conspicuous consumption").

Costly signaling analyses show that what constitutes economic or productive data has broadened over the years, especially with the introduction of evolutionary approaches to human ecology. In behavioral ecological analyses the focus is on activities that lead to the growth, reproduction, and maintenance of offspring and relatives. Therefore, what constitutes productive activities is much broader, since it can include such things as the care of offspring or the cultivation of inedible trophy yams (Bliege Bird and Smith 2005: 228). In addition, as will be shown below, behavioral ecology is also concerned with the development of economic competencies among children and therefore does not restrict itself to the activities of adults. The advantage of behavioral observation in its focus on the behavior of individuals, regardless of what they may be doing (except in the case of focal follows described below) or how old they are, is that it leads the researcher to describe behavior more comprehensively. Such an inclusive approach allows an analyst, whatever his or her theoretical persuasion, to select which behavior he or she wishes to classify as economic so long as codes are reasonably detailed for all behavior (an issue discussed below). This broadens the appeal and cross-cultural power of behavioral observations.

In the pages below I describe current techniques used to collect input and output production data, the strengths and weaknesses of different approaches, and ways to insure the collection of an unbiased sample. In addition, I show how techniques of behavioral observation have been artfully extended to include ways to measure labor and resource exchanges as well as environmental impacts of subsistence activities.

OBSERVATION AND RECALL

A researcher can acquire quantitative data on time allocation through direct observation or through informant recall. The method one chooses will depend on a complex set of factors, and each approach has particular strengths and weaknesses. Informant recall, sometimes called the time diary method or 24-hour recall, requires informant literacy and familiarity with a 24-hour day. At the end of the day, an informant is asked to record all activities typically divided into half-hour time increments. Reseachers collect these subject-generated forms on a regular basis. This approach is standard among sociologists and others who work in literate societies (Paolisso and Hames in press). In many ethnographic contexts this method is difficult to implement since local notions of time of the day are not easily divisible into half-hour intervals, and even if the population is literate, use of forms based on general Western cultural concepts may prove difficult to implement. Alternatively, recall could be generated by interviewing informants at the end of the day (e.g., Aspelin 1979). This is not to say that recall methods should not be used; rather their uses are limited to specific activities. Those interested in an extensive discussion of the strengths and weakness of each method should consult Paolisso and Hames (*in press*). Here I focus exclusively on observational techniques and reveal that they occasionally rely on informant recall.

DIRECT BEHAVIOR OBSERVATION

There is a robust literature on various techniques of direct behavior observation. General reviews are found in a classic paper by Altmann

Basic Observational Techniques

		Sampling Rules	
		Group	Individual
Recording Rules	Instantaneous (event)	Instantaneous scan	Instantaneous focal
	Continuous (state)	Continuous scan	Continuous focal

Figure 3.1   Sampling and recording rules in behavior observations.

(1974) and in Martin and Bateson's (1993) textbook with a focus on psychology and ethology, and in anthropological applications by Gross (1984), Johnson and Sackett (1998), Borgerhoff Mulder and Caro (1985) and Hames (1992). By direct observation, I mean observations that are generated by a researcher. As with recall research, the goal of direct observation is to collect a wide variety of quantitative data on behavior that can be used to statistically test hypotheses or to more precisely describe patterns of behavior. It may lead to the discovery of patterns of behavior that may not have been apparent to the observer or subject, and it may completely reverse an ethnographer's subjective perceptions of what occurs on a daily basis (Erasmus 1955).

Following Martin and Bateson (1993: 84–86), I distinguish between sampling rules (who or what is observed) and recording rules (whether behavior is recorded continuously or instantaneously). Any behavior measurement is a combination of a sampling rule and a recording rule. A simplified picture of how sampling and recording rules are combined is presented in Figure 3.1 (see Martin and Bateson 1993: 88, Figure 6.1 for a more elaborate scheme).[1] I will briefly characterize the logic behind using different sampling rules and then turn to a much more detailed consideration of recording rules reflecting dominant ethnographic interest and research.

---

[1] I do not discuss ad libitum sampling, a kind of behavior sampling, which involves the unsystematic recording of "interesting" behaviors and is only useful for initial investigation or, perhaps, rare but important events.

A researcher can elect to sample either a behavior itself or individuals or groups. If a behavior is selected (termed behavior sampling or "one-zero") then one records whether or not a particular behavior occurred during a recording period. Who is sampled is solely determined by whether the individual expresses the behavior. This procedure can be done on individuals or groups. Once the group or individual (or even place) is selected and the sampling period is determined (e.g., a 10 minute block of time) the observer selects a time interval (e.g., every minute) and records whether the behavior occurs or does not occur (hence one-zero, or yes-no) independent of how many times it occurred. Like instantaneous sampling (see below) the unit of observation is dimensionless. So long as the sampling intervals are short (e.g., sampling every minute versus every 5 minutes) this method produces reasonably accurate measures (Martin and Bateson 1993: 55).

Behavior sampling is useful for recording behaviors that are rare but significant and would be otherwise missed using alternative sampling and recording schemes, although it is sometimes used in conjunction with other sampling and recording rules. Behavior sampling is frequently used in primatology (e.g., Mitani and Watts 2005) to study crucial behaviors such as agonistic interactions, grooming, and sex that researchers believe are central for understanding social relations, status position, dominance and subordination, and reciprocal relations. However, it is rarely used by ethnographers (see Marlowe 2005 on parental care of Hadza children for an exception).

If one makes individuals the unit of observation then one must decide whether to focus on a group or an individual. *Focal sampling* is employed when the focus is on a single individual for an extended period of time (focal observation or a focal follow). The individual's behavior may be recorded instantaneously or continuously (see below) within a particular time frame. This does not mean that others with whom the focal individual interacts are not necessarily recorded. In contrast, in *scan sampling* one observes a group with several individuals who are in close enough spatial proximity for them to be recorded simultaneously (group observation, with dyads being the most common). Scan observations pose obvious difficulties in terms of a researcher's ability to accurately monitor the behavior of more than one individual. This limitation is made more severe if one attempts to make continuous observations instead of instantaneous observations. Scan observations are limited to closely interacting dyads such as a parent and offspring (Ivey 2000; Ivey Henry *et al.* 2005; Fouts and Lamb 2005) or spatially delimited groups, such as a group involved in a ritual, a shouting match (Flinn 1988) or cooperative agricultural labor (Hames 1987). A solution to the problem of attempting to record more than several individuals on a continuous basis would be to use video equipment to record group members, followed by review of the video to carefully extract data for analysis, as in Takada's (2005) work on mother infant interactions among !Xun foragers. An alternative strategy of observing a group would be to code the behavior very generally. For example, if a group of people were gathered for a ritual performance one could record some of them as watching and others performing instead of more precisely coding behavior as watching while talking, waiting to perform while watching, or performing a specific ritual act.

Clearly use of focal or group sampling depends on the research question posed and the recording rule (see below) employed. If one is interested in detailed and sequential characterization of a behavior or a behavior complex (e.g., details of hunting when it is necessary to code for travel, search, rest, pursuit, and return) regardless of social context (e.g., Bliege Bird and Bird 2002) or how much time is allocated to foraging is particular locations (Aswani 1998 on Pacific fishing), then focal sampling is best, while group sampling is the method of choice when the emphasis is on social interaction or the collection of population level measures on age and sex differences.

RECORDING RULES

Recording rules are of two broad kinds. *Continuous* recording is the moment-by-moment description of certain behaviors within a fixed time interval. It is fine-grained and permits measurement of duration, latency, and other measures discussed below. *Instantaneous* sampling, as the name suggests, simply records the behavior of the individual the instant he or she is observed. It is a "dimensionless" measure since it has no duration. As such, the only statistics that can be compiled are counts of the various behaviors recorded, but such counts can be legitimately transformed into real time measures under certain conditions and with certain assumptions. For example, if one samples behavior during waking hours, say a 14-hour day, and one knows that 15 percent of observations were in food preparation activities, then one could reasonably conclude that 2.1 hours per day were spent in this activity. (Of course, this assumes that this behavior only occurs during the daylight sampling period, see Scaglion 1986 on nighttime sampling.) Although simple counts may seem like a severe limitation, instantaneous (commonly called instantaneous scan sampling) is the most commonly used recording method in anthropology, for a number of reasons I will describe below.

A way to conceptually differentiate between continuous and instantaneous recording is to think of continuous sampling as akin to recording behavior with a video camera while instantaneous records behavior uses a still camera. I will first begin with a characterization of strengths, weakness, and appropriateness of continuous recording and follow it with a consideration of instantaneous recording. Since instantaneous recording is by far the most commonly used technique in anthropology I will present a more detailed examination of the methodological literature behind it and novel extensions of the technique.

Continuous recording

Continuous recording is employed whenever the research question requires detailed information on multiple dimensions of behavior. Under continuous recording the following dimensions of behavior may be collected:

- Frequency: how frequently a behavior occurs within a particular time period
- Intensity: how energetically or forcefully the behavior is acted. There are numerous field and laboratory experimental studies (e.g., Hipsley and Kirk 1966; Durnin and Passmore 1967; Montgomery and Johnson 1976) that can be adapted to one's field data to create good estimates of caloric expenditures of effort
- Latency: the period of time prior to the onset of a behavior
- Duration: how long a behavior lasts
- Sequence: the ordering of behaviors through time or in relation to external contexts.

Instantaneous recording

As mentioned, instantaneous recording only permits the collection of behavior frequency and intensity while continuous recording allows one to collect all of the above dimensions of behavior. At first glance it would seem obvious that continuous recording would be the best choice; but continuous recording has a number of limitations. As I have already mentioned, it is normally linked to focal sampling, making it extremely difficult to record the continuous behavior of more than one individual at a time unless the individuals are immediately adjacent to one another (as is the case, for example, in studies of parent–infant interactions). The second problem is that it is very intrusive, such that a subject may alter his or her behavior when observed on a continuous basis at close quarters. The third is that it is very expensive of a researcher's time. Quantitative analysis depends on a reasonably large sample of individuals in different contexts and at different times of the day and who have an adequate range of demographic qualities (old, young, female, male). Gaining a representative sample using continuous sampling is thus difficult for a single researcher. But for certain kinds of questions such a method is indispensable. For example, if one is concerned with how responsive parents are to infant vocalizations, duration of nursing bouts, and responses to fretting and crying (Konner and Worthman 1980; Fouts and Lamb 2005) then continuous observations are required. By way of contrast, if one's research question is who cares for infants and toddlers then instantaneous sampling will provide richer data (the full range of caretakers under a variety of conditions) at a much lower cost of researcher time (Hames 1988; Marlowe 2005; Henry Ivey *et al.* 2005). For a good sample of research on childcare using both methods, singly and in combination, see the volume edited by Hewlett and Lamb (2005).

In many instances a researcher may benefit from using both instantaneous and continuous sampling procedures. For example, Marlowe (2005) and Bird and Bliege Bird (2005) used a combination of instantaneous and continuous methods to study care-taking and the foraging activities of infants and children respectively. The goal of these studies was to generate general time allocation data on a large number of individuals coupled with more precise measures of specific activities and patterns of parent–infant interaction.

Commonly called "spot checks" (after Johnson 1975), "scan sampling" or "instantaneous scan sampling" (Borgerhoff Mulder and Caro 1985; Hames 1988), instantaneous recording is by far the most commonly used method of behavior sampling in ethnography. The procedure consists of recording a subject's behavior the moment the subject is observed at randomly determined intervals. Additionally, as in other approaches, one often notes contextual information such as location, the presence of other individuals, date, and time of day. In village-based ethnographic studies it usually consists of serially visiting households in a village or section of a village and recording the behavior of everyone present at the moment (instant) that the individual is viewed by the ethnographer. After the recording is done the ethnographer proceeds to the next house and repeats the procedure until the entire village is sampled (but see below on "block sampling").

Instantaneous recording has considerable popularity among ethnographers from a variety of theoretical perspectives. Under the leadership of Allen Johnson, numerous researchers who had collected data employing instantaneous recording contributed to the establishment of a time allocation digital database and universal coding scheme along with cultural descriptions (Johnson 1990).[2] Instantaneous recording has a number of advantages. It is very economical in terms of an ethnographer's research time. An outcome of the economy of the approach is that it permits a large number of different individuals to be sampled. Frequently, all members of a village of more than 100 individuals, which more easily permits an analyst to ask questions about differences in behavior as they vary by age, social status, and sex. In some cases, over the course of a year some ethnographers have made more than an average of 300 observations per person in a village of more than 100. Finally, it is less obtrusive to subjects, such that they are less likely to modify their behavior compared to the constant scrutiny of continuous observation. In continuous observation, researchers may literally dog the footsteps of their informants to collect behavioral information.

METHODOLOGICAL ISSUES AND PROBLEMS

In recent years methodological reports have emerged where researchers describe problems they have encountered in using behavior observations, and their solutions. These studies candidly assess the practical, methodological, and observer effects that may not be apparent to a neophyte. In these methodological reflections, the goal is to ensure the accurate and unbiased collection of data through self-criticism. More specifically, Hawkes *et al.* (1987) deal with the problem of overestimating the frequency of easily visible group behavior, Betzig and Turke (1985) on intentional versus observed behavior, and Borgerhoff Mulder and Caro (1985) on a variety of problems such as coding, seasonal and diurnal patterns, verbal reports, and inter-observer reliability. Johnson and Sackett (1998) along with Borgerhoff Mulder and Caro

---

[2] A full list of the publications from this project are available at http://www.yale. edu/hraf/publications_body_completepublist.htm#Time%20Allocation%20Series

(1985) are two sources anyone planning to use behavior observations should read; they provide an excellent summary of problems, options, and solutions in a wide variety of situations.

Observational problems

A researcher should always strive to observe behaviors candidly, develop techniques that ensure that all relevant behaviors have an equal opportunity to be observed, and that the presence of the observer and the methods used do not affect the behavior of the observed. Of course, a culture's preferences for privacy, openness, and observability may require the researcher to modify these requirements tactically in order to achieve an unbiased sample of observations. In many cultures it is inappropriate for a researcher to unexpectedly enter a house to observe behavior even though unpredictability (to the observed) ensures that what is observed is not modified in anticipation of the ethnographer's presence. In other instances, restrictions owing to the observer's or subject's sex or social status may create problems.

In many instances the goal of instantaneous sampling is the creation of a random sample of a large number of subjects representative of all social divisions. Although a large sample size is always desirable, improperly building it may lead to bias. Peregrine *et al.* (1993) illuminate this point. They used a video tape recorder to create a 32-hour continuous record of activities of preschoolers in a nursery setting. Using that continuous record as the base, they drew samples analogous to those employed by ethnographers using behavioral observation techniques. They found that attempting to make longer observations (recording all behavior for a 1-hour period instead of numerous visits of shorter duration totaling 1 hour) led to results that deviated significantly from the 32-hour record. This and other studies clearly indicate that in order to generate a random sample a researcher must be able to make observations at any time of the day, under all conditions, and independent of social situations. More to the point, researchers may be unaware of how choices made about when, where, and who to sample may lead to sampling biases. If a researcher chooses subjects, times, or locations because of cooperativeness or convenience then bias may be introduced (Borgerhoff Mulder and Caro 1985: 325). It is clear that no ethnographer has free and instantaneous access to all individuals in their sample. Consequently, purely random observations are difficult. Nevertheless, there are a variety of procedures that one can use to ensure as close to a random sample as possible.

In some small communities it is feasible to include all house-. holds in a single sampling round making instantaneous observations very economical. However, if households are widely dispersed across the landscape, travel time becomes so great that it is inefficient to attempt to observe all households in a single sampling round. Block sampling is designed to overcome this problem, and was first devised by Behrens (1981). He divided the households in his Shipibo community into several contiguous household clusters separated from one another by several kilometers. He stayed in each cluster for 4 hours and sampled all households in the cluster every 30 minutes (for a similar procedure see Gurven and Kaplan 2006). Block sampling is obviously useful in an urban context where subjects may be widely dispersed.

All researchers have faced the problem of showing up to make observations only to discover that the subject or subjects are not present. One solution to the problem is to simply ask someone who should know (e.g., a present household member) to report where the subject is. The report is then used as an "observation" when in reality it is a report. If so, the researcher should record this fact (Borgerhoff Mulder and Caro 1985). Whether or not such second-hand information can be used depends on the accuracy of reports and the degree to which such reports have sufficient resolution to satisfy research goals. The correspondence between reports and actual behavior should be ascertained prior to research and monitored during research. In one study, for example, at the end of the day I tracked down individuals on whom reports had been given and asked them what they were doing at the time when the report was generated (Hames 1979). I found a greater than 95 percent correspondence between reports by others and the subject's own recall. Consequently, I felt that reports were reliable but continued to periodically check the accuracy of reports by interviewing those reported on at the end of the day.

Observations, whether continuous or instantaneous, are typically made during daytime hours and sometimes extend into early evening or morning. In many places sampling during nighttime hours is either dangerous or unwelcome. In a pioneering piece of research, Scaglion (1986) sampled behavior during nighttime hours (7:00 p.m. to 6:00 a.m.) and discovered that in 26 percent of observations his New Guinea subjects were awake, and in approximately 75 percent of these instances they were engaged in ritual activities. When nighttime observations are pooled with daytime observations and then compared to daytime observations, some underestimates and overestimates of behaviors are evident (see Scaglion, 1986, Table 4: 542). Researchers must determine the importance of nighttime activities, and modify their observational hours accordingly.

Coding Problems

Recording a behavior classified as an instance of "X" entails a coding decision. Issues in coding seem to resolve around three major issues: (1) the problem of simultaneity; (2) what and how finely to code; and (3) functional versus structural descriptions. To the uninitiated, nothing could seem easier than describing the behavior of another. Having to do so in rapid-fire sequence can be a humbling experience, however. For example, in observing the Ye'kwana it was not uncommon for me to come upon a woman sitting on the lever of a manioc press (to express the juice from the pulp) while nursing a child and conversing with an adjacent woman. How should I code what was she doing? Johnson and Sackett (1998: 327) call this the simultaneity problem, and describe the strengths and weaknesses of six possible solutions. All the solutions are reasonable, but the one I favor is to code the behaviors as primary, secondary, and tertiary, thus preserving the richness of the observation. This creates another problem: which behavior is primary, etc. Context can help one decide. In this case the woman had gone to the press to express the juice. So a particular kind of food preparation would be the primary activity. She had brought her child with her which makes childcare a secondary activity. Another woman happened to be there, so conversation becomes the tertiary activity. Preservation of such complexity may be cumbersome, but I believe it is worth the effort. For example, in the case above, if one were interested in knowing who cares for children, valuable data would be lost if the mother's secondary behavior was not recorded.

Researchers should carefully consider the problem of behavior coding even if economic behavior is their sole interest. The first thing to realize is that any code is an abstract and limited characterization of a complex act. Furthermore, researchers should not neglect careful classification of so-called non-economic behavior because different research questions may have a more expansive definition of economically productive behavior. A good example of this is seen in Lee's initial measures of work among the San when he documented that they worked but 2.2 to 2.4 hours per day, a figure widely cited in the literature (Lee 1968, 1969). However, Lee restricted his definition of labor to direct food production (hunting and gathering) and left out much of what is arguably a more reasonable array of economic activities such as food processing, artifact production, and fuel and water collection. When all these activities were added, labor time jumped to 6.4 hours per adult day in Lee's fuller account (1979). A solution to this problem is to make random observations of behavior such that the behavior of a subject is recorded independently of what the subject is doing. If one follows the standard protocols outlined above for continuous or instantaneous recording, then all behaviors will be recorded and an analyst, given his or her research interest, can decide what to include or exclude as relevant economic behavior.

How behavior is described is critical for cross-cultural comparisons. Whether one employs functional versus structural descriptors in codes (following Hames 1992) or descriptions by consequence or physical descriptions (following Borgerhoff Mulder and Caro 1985) is an important issue. Structural/physical codes describe the bodily actions, stances, orientations, etc. of the observed, and can be quite detailed since one may be describing a very complex pattern of behavior. Functional/consequence codes focus on the purpose or design of the behavior, are simple, and conform to our intuitive understanding of behavior. For example one might structurally describe a behavior as squatting on the ground while striking plants with a machete at ground level, and occasionally tossing plants into a pile. Functionally, one would write "weeding." Coding structural descriptions is akin to writing a telegraphic sentence (e.g., squat, machete, swing, toss plant) which can make analysis difficult. Functional codes like "weeding" are more tractable. But sometimes our intuitions regarding function may be highly inaccurate, particularly in novel cultural environments. Accurate functional descriptions presuppose that the researcher has an excellent grasp of local behavioral intentions and variability and it is therefore imperative that a researcher takes time to ask informants about what he or she is observing. An excellent discussion of this problem can be found in Borgerhoff Mulder and Caro (1985: 327–328) and should be read by anyone planning behavior observations. One solution to the problem is to double code the behavior following structural and functional rules.

Finally, another dimension of coding is how finely codes are constructed. I believe the best procedure is to code behavior as finely as practicable, using a hierarchical scheme. For example, one could call a variety of related behaviors "food preparation" without coding for the kind of food or the preparation step involved. But lack of detail causes the loss of valuable information and the corresponding inability, for example, to answer the simple question of what food resource demands the most processing and which step is the most time consuming. Bock (2002) and Gurven and Kaplan (2006) made analytic use of such detail to assess the roles of strength and skill in the allocation of labor activities through the life course. Johnson and Sackett (1998) propose a flexible and widely used cross-cultural coding scheme used by many.

BEYOND SIMPLE BEHAVIOR: TIME, LOCATION, INTERACTION, AND RESOURCE FLOWS

Many assume that behavior observations are primarily designed to provide static or dynamic information on basic activities broken down by social attributes (e.g., sexual division of labor). However, the strength, flexibility, and utility of behavior observations goes far beyond the recording of an individual's behavior in its simple behavioral and time coordinates. Many interesting questions can be quantitatively answered depending on how one constructs the data record as well as what time and space mean in a specific cultural context. For example, Sugawara (1988) used the location variable to document gender differences in inter-camp visiting among San foragers, and Ohtsuka et al. (2004) were able to use the location variable to understand gender-based differences in exposure to environmental toxins. Winking et al. (2009) used the location variable to determine the conditions under which husbands assist wives in childcare. Below I show how detailed recording of locational and other variables open new areas of research through behavioral observations.

A location variable is useful for a variety of questions that focus on whether the behavior is done inside or outside the home, or individually or collaboratively. Use of a location variable depends on what location may mean for a particular group. For example, Hames (1987) used the location to determine whose garden an individual was working in order to create measures of garden labor exchange among the Ye'kwana. In another study (Hames and McCabe 2005) on the Ye'kwana, the location variable was used to measure meal sharing patterns. In both cases, when someone was observed to work in a garden not his or her own or eat a meal in another household, the owner of the field or household was known, and these cases were scored as measures of labor and food exchange, respectively. Yasuoka's work (2006) is a particularly excellent example of how behavior observations tied to locational information can be employed to answer important ecological questions such as the ability of Pygmy populations to forage independently of horticulturalists. There are many other uses of the locational variable that have to do with basic patterns of association that may be used to characterize fundamental aspects of social organization and networks. Below are further examples of uses of quantified behavioral observations beyond standard time allocation accounts.

Instantaneous recordings have been employed to study the flow of food resources between individuals and families, a fundamental dimension of economic organization. The method was pioneered by Kaplan *et al.* (1984) in a study of resource sharing among Ache hunter-gatherers and replicated in many other studies (see Gurven 2004 for a review). The traditional method for studying food exchange is for the researcher to interview household members and ask them to recall food received or given from or to other households during specific time intervals (e.g., Aspelin 1979), or to make direct observations of distributions (Hames 1990). Although these techniques have important advantages (e.g., accurate information on weights or volumes given and received), they also have limitations. They rely on recall which may be inexact, provide no measure of how much each family member is impacted, and miss many of the casual and spontaneous exchanges that are common in many societies, such as meal sharing (Hames and McCabe 2007). While recording instantaneous observations in an Ache camp, any time an individual was observed to eat, researchers (Kaplan *et al.* 1984) asked the food consumer who gave the food and who produced it (through hunting or gathering). This allowed them to effectively measure the flow of food resources, many of which would not have been captured by traditional methods. Since eating is a common activity and the Ache share a great deal, sample size was large enough for extensively detailed analysis as it related to a whole host of variables relevant to testing different theories of exchange.

ESTIMATING PRODUCTION

Using a life historical perspective, time allocation techniques have recently been applied to investigating the (sex-specific) age at which humans achieve self sufficiency (producing as much as they consume), what qualities must be achieved (strength, skill, and knowledge) to make this transition to a productive adult, and the degree to which families can satisfy their consumptive needs over the demographic cycle. In investigating these questions researchers have developed more intensive techniques to measure variation in productivity and have extended their analyses to all age groups.

Problems associated with measuring production differ between immediate return activities (foraging) versus delayed return activities (agriculture and pastoralism). Furthermore, accurately measuring production is difficult because it can vary dramatically depending on age and sex. Consequently, simple time allocation measures are usually not adequate proxies for production (Bird and Bliege Bird 2005; Bock 2002; Gurven and Kaplan 2006). Early research on hunting, for example, used a combination of interviews and direct measurement of production (e.g., Lee's well known studies of San foraging productivity (1968, 1969) to calculate measures of economic performance). Hunters were interviewed at the end of the day or every week to ask how long they hunted and what they captured or even how many large animals they had taken in the last year. Alternatively, some researchers collected instantaneous data on all activities and coupled them with daily interviews to measure hunting yields (Hames 1979). While these approaches are satisfactory for certain kinds of activities and their efficiency in data collection can generate large samples, they may be problematic. Hunters may over- or underestimate what they acquired, fail to include the assistance of others, make divisions after a kill, or may not note that hunting was combined with other activities.

Today, focal follows coupled with weighing of acquired resources are increasingly employed to gain very precise output/input measures, especially as it relates to changes in efficiency over the life course. Using focal follows and continuous sampling, Bird and Bliege Bird (2005) were able to collect data on the foraging productivity of all Meriam aboriginals. Collecting this fine-grained data is time-consuming. Bird and Bliege Bird (1997; 2005: 244) made 358 focal follows on 75 individuals between the ages of 4 and 75 for a total of 518 hours of foraging observation. During each of the continuously observed focal follows they collected a large array of data such as tools used, weight of resources taken, successful versus unsuccessful resources acquisitions, and time devoted to searching, travel, and pursuit. This wonderfully fine-grained research permitted them to answer critical questions revolving around the productivity of children and adults as it relates to strength and endurance or the development of skills that pay-off in enhanced adult productivity as well as how foraging choices made by children differed from adults yielding a nuanced test of diet breadth.

In delayed-return activities such as horticulture and pastoralism, estimating production for individuals is far more difficult. This is because total production inputs represent a series of interconnected activities over a long time period, often characterized by a division of labor such that numerous individuals are responsible for each stage of production, while the ultimate outputs may occur months after the original inputs. In horticulture it is common for men to clear fields, women to plant; both may harvest, and women process the food for immediate consumption and storage, but women and men do these tasks at different efficiencies. In addition, the costs of tool production and maintenance must be factored, which may be difficult since many tools are multi-purpose (a machete can be used to butcher meat, cut thatch, slash undergrowth, weed a garden, etc.). A simplified solution to this problem promoted by Kramer (2002: 311) is the use of discount coefficients for various tasks required in agriculture (see also Kaplan 1994 and Gurven and Kaplan 2006). Using continuous observations, she examined the rate of work accomplished in a variety of fundamental productive tasks by children at several age intervals and adults (Kramer 2005). For all but the simplest activities the efficiency of children was considerably less than adults. The next step was to estimate the entire caloric needs of the household using standard caloric expenditure references (e.g., Durnin and Passmore 1967) for particular tasks, and then compare this to the net efficiency (resources produced per unit time by different age/sex categories) and daily time allocated to these tasks by household members. Since there is almost no food or labor sharing among the Maya (Kramer 2005) it was assumed that all food consumed by household members was produced by household members.

At this point, this sort of estimation procedure seems to be the best that has been devised for delayed production systems. Kramer (2002: 310) notes that the difficulty in gaining reasonably accurate production estimates is a serious problem. In her own study Kramer notes that 80 percent of labor is for food production, but necessary activities such as drawing water and hauling firewood are not included. Although the Maya engage in little inter-household resource exchange her estimation procedure would be problematic if such exchanges are common, which may be the rule in more traditional horticultural systems (Gurven 2004).

Much hinges on accurate estimates of productivity; variation in age at economic independence (the age at which an individual produces more than he or she consumes) is a critical question in life history theory, and of interest to economic and development anthropologist. For example, Kaplan shows (1994: 781–783) that among the Piro and Machiguenga individuals did not achieve economic independence until about the age of 20. Similar approaches have been employed by Kaplan's students and colleagues to generate age-related production and consumption curves for the Hiwi, Ache, and Maya (Gurven and Kaplan 2006). Productivity measures were also critical for establishing the fact that some households (i.e., those with many dependent children) cannot meet their own consumption needs through their own efforts (Gurven and Walker 2006; Hill and Hurtado in preparation). Such families appear to be subsidized by co-resident households, and this finding represents an important new area of research. Just as importantly, behavior measurements on production and consumption have helped toward a better understanding of intergenerational "wealth flows." In development economics and demography, the reigning paradigm has been that poor farmers desire many children so they will have support in their old age. In contrast, the evolutionary theory of parental investment, and research using behavioral observations, showed that even where children were economically productive, the flow of resources was largely from parents to children and grandchildren (Turke 1989; Kaplan 1994). Finally, the question of when and how humans become competent economic producers has spawned a number of high quality studies on time allocation and production oftentimes combining continuous and instantaneous techniques. An entire issue of *Human Nature* (2002, **13**(2)) was devoted to examining the development of economic competence.

Behavior observations have been essential in the examination of how humans impact the environment and the related question of conservation among tribal populations. As noted by behaviorally oriented researchers (Hames 1991; Alvard 1998) early claims of conservation were supported by analyses of ideological systems and practices. The assumption was that beliefs guide behavior. However, a variety of studies demonstrated that beliefs had little impact on conserving game resources (Aunger 1994). More to the point, the actuality of conservation depends on patterns of game harvesting. Researchers using behavior observations to examine hypotheses deduced from conservation in diet breadth, prey selectivity, areal patterns of exploitation, and long-term game yields have rather conclusively demonstrated that conservation is exceptionally rare where ever investigated (Alvard 1998; Hames 2007).

CONCLUSION

I have attempted to show that direct and indirect behavior observations are important for answering crucial questions surrounding economic production and human environmental impacts. The behavior observation techniques reviewed were initially employed to simply measure time allocation patterns. Through time, the technique has grown in sophistication and it is now employed to measure the exchange of goods and services, the development of productivity through the life course, production data, areal patterns of exploitation, and resource selectivity. The development of behavior observation techniques has been mandated by hypothesis testing from foraging, life history, and other evolutionary theories that require the collection of high quality empirical data. In other scientific arenas researchers have made sophisticated modifications of observational techniques to address issues of sea tenure (Aswani 2002), food consumption surveys (Umezaki *et al.* 2002), and energy balance in high altitude regions (Panter-Brick 1996). I believe that considerable improvement can be made in behavioral techniques if researchers would more carefully describe the procedures they use so they could be more fully evaluated and more easily replicated by others. To some extent journal page limits prevent this from happening. Be that as it may, I expect that direct observation techniques will be increasingly used as we begin to ever more carefully and fully describe issues in ecological anthropology.

REFERENCES

Altmann, J. 1974. The observational study of behavior. *Behaviour* **48**: 1–41.
Alvard, M. 1998. Evolutionary ecology and resource conservation. *Evolutionary Anthropology* **7**: 62–74.
Aspelin, L. 1979. Food distribution and social bonding among the Mamainde of Mato Gross, Brazil. *Journal of Anthropological Research* **35**: 309–327.
Aswani, S. 1998. Patterns of marine harvest effort in southwestern New Georgia, Solomon Islands: resource management or optimal foraging. *Ocean and Coastal Management* **40**: 207–235.
Aswani, S. 2002. Assessing the effects of changing demographic and consumption patterns on sea tenure regimes in the Roviana Lagoon, Solomon Islands. *Ambio* **31**: 272–284.
Augner, R. 1994. Are food avoidances maladaptive in the Ituri Forest of Zaire? *Journal of Anthropological Research* **15**: 54–72
Behrens, C. A. 1981. Time allocation and meat procurement among the Shipibo Indians of eastern Peru. *Human Ecology* **9**: 189–220.
Betzig, L. and P. Turke 1985. Measuring time allocation: observation and intention. *Current Anthropology* **26**: 647–650.

Bird, D. W. and R. Bliege Bird 1997. Contemporary shellfish gathering strategies among the Meriam of the Torres Strait Islands, Australia: testing predictions of a central place foraging model. *Journal of Archaeological Science* **24**: 39–63.

Bird, D. W. and R. Bliege Bird 2005. Martu children's hunting strategies in the Western Desert, Australia. In B. Hewlett and M. Lamb, eds., *Hunter–Gatherer Childhoods: Evolutionary, Developmental and Cultural Perspectives*. New Brunswick, NJ: Transaction Publishers, pp. 129–146.

Bliege Bird, R. and D. Bird 2002. Constraints of knowing or constraints of growing? *Human Nature* **13**: 239–267.

Bliege Bird, R. and E. A. Smith 2005. Signaling theory, strategic interaction, and symbolic capital. *Current Anthropology* **46**: 221–48

Bock, J. 2002. Learning, life history, and productivity. *Human Nature* **13**: 161–197.

Borgerhoff Mulder, M. and T. Caro 1985. The use of quantitative observation techniques in anthropology. *Current Anthropology* **26**: 232–262.

Durnin, J. and G. Passmore 1967. *Energy, Work, and Leisure*. London: Heinemann.

Erasmus, C. J. 1955. Work patterns in a Mayo village. *American Anthropologist* **57**: 322–333.

Flinn, M. 1988. Parent-offspring interactions in a Caribbean village: daughter guarding. In L. Betzig, M. Borgerhoff Mulder, and P. Turke, eds., *Human Reproductive Behaviour*. Cambridge, UK: Cambridge University Press, pp. 189–200.

Fouts, H. N. and M. E. Lamb 2005. Weanling emotional patterns among the Bofi foragers of Central Africa: the role of maternal availability and sensitivity. In B. Hewlett and M. Lamb, eds., *Hunter–Gatherer Childhoods: Evolutionary, Developmental and Cultural Perspectives*. New Brunswick, NJ: Transaction Publishers, pp. 309–321.

Gross, D. R. 1984. Time allocation: a tool for the study of cultural behavior. *Annual Review of Anthropology* **13**: 519–558.

Gurven, M. 2004. To give and to give not: the behavioral ecology of human food transfers. *Behavioral and Brain Sciences* **27**: 120–155.

Gurven, M. and H. Kaplan 2006. Determinants of time allocation across the lifespan: a theoretical model and an application to the Machiguenga and Piro of Peru. *Human Nature* **17**: 1–49.

Gurven, M., H. Kaplan, and M. Gutierrez 2006. How long does it take to become a proficient hunter? Implications for the evolution of extended development and long life span. *Journal of Human Evolution* **51**: 454–470.

Gurven, M. and R. Walker 2006. Energetic demand of multiple dependents and the evolution of slow human growth. *Proceedings of the Royal Society, B* **273**: 835–841.

Hames, R. 1979. A comparison of the efficiencies of the shotgun and bow in neotropical forest hunting. *Human Ecology* **7**: 219–252.

Hames, R. 1987. Relatedness and garden labor exchange among the Ye'kwana. *Evolution and Human Behavior* **8**: 354–392.

Hames, R. 1988. the allocation of parental care among the Ye'kwana. In L. Betzig, M. Borgerhoff Mulder, and P. Turke, eds., *Human Reproductive Behaviour*. Cambridge, UK: Cambridge University Press, pp. 237–254.

Hames, R. 1990. Sharing among the Yanomamö. Part I: the effects of risk. In E. Cashdan, ed., *Risk and Reciprocity in Tribal and Peasant Economics*. Boulder, CO: Westview Press, pp. 89–106.

Hames, R. 1991. Wildlife conservation in tribal societies. In M. Oldfield and J. Alcorn, eds., *Biodiversity: Culture, Conservation, and Ecodevelopment*. Denver, CO: Westview Press, pp. 172–199.

Hames, R. 1992. Time allocation. In E. A. Smith and B. Winterhalder, eds., *Evolutionary Ecology and Human Behavior.* Chicago, IL: Aldine de Gruyter, pp. 203–236.

Hames, R. 2007. The ecologically noble savage debate. *Annual Review of Anthropology* **36**: 177–190.

Hames, R. and C. McCabe 2007. Meal sharing among the Ye'kwana. *Human Nature* **18**: 1–21.

Hawkes, K., K. Hill, H. Kaplan, and M. Hurtado 1987. Some problems with instantaneous scan sampling. *Journal of Anthropological Research* **43**: 239–247.

Hewlett, B. S. and M. E. Lamb, eds. 2005. *Hunter–Gatherer Childhoods: Evolutionary, Developmental, and Cultural Perspectives.* New Brunswick, NJ: Aldine de Gruyter.

Hill, K. and A. Hurtado In preparation. Cooperative breeding in South American hunter–gatherers. School of Human Evolution and Social Change, Arizona State University, Tempe, AZ.

Hipsley, E. H. and N. E. Kirk 1966. *Studies of dietary intake and the expenditure of energy by New Guineans.* Vol. 147. Noumea, New Caledonia: South Pacific Commission Technical paper no. 147.

Ivey, P. 2000. Cooperative reproduction in Ituri forest hunter-gatherers: Who cares for Efe infants. *Current Anthropology* **41**: 857–866.

Ivey Henry, P. K., G. A. Morelli, and E. Z. Tronick, eds. 2005. Child caretakers among Efe foragers of the Ituri Forest. In B. S. Hewlett and M. E. Lamb, eds., *Hunter–Gatherer Childhoods: Evolutionary, Developmental and Cultural Perspectives.* New Brunswick, NJ: Transaction Publishers.

Johnson, A. 1975. Time allocation in a Machiguenga community. *Ethnology* **14**: 301–310.

Johnson, A. 1990. Time-allocation research: the costs and benefits of alternative methods. In B. L. Rogers and N. Schlossman, eds., *Intra-Household Resource Allocation: Issues and Methods for Development Policy and Planning.* Tokyo: United Nations University Press, pp. Chapter 10.

Johnson, A. and R. Sackett 1998. Direct systematic observation of behavior. In H. R. Bernard. Ed., *Handbook of Methods in Cultural Anthropology.* Walnut Creek, CA: Altamira Press, pp. 301–330.

Kaplan, H. 1994. Evolutionary and wealth flows theories of fertility: empirical tests and new models. *Population and Development Review* **20**: 753–791.

Kaplan, H., K. Hill, K. Hawkes, and A. Hurtado 1984. Food sharing among Ache foragers of Eastern Paraguay. *Current Anthropology* **25**: 113–115.

Konner, M. J. and C. M. Worthman 1980. Nursing frequency, gonadal function, and birth spacing among !Kung hunter-gatherers. *Science* **207**: 788–791.

Kramer, K. 2002. Variability in the duration of juvenile dependence: the benefits of Maya children's work to parents. *Human Nature* **13**: 299–325.

Kramer, K. 2005. Children's help and the pace of reproduction: cooperative breeding in humans. *Evolutionary Anthropology* **14**: 224–237.

Lee, R. 1968. What hunters do for a living: or how to make out on scarce resources. In R. Lee and I. DeVore, eds., *Man the Hunter.* Chicago, IL: Aldine, pp. 30–45.

Lee, R. 1969. !Kung Bushman subsistence: an input-output analysis. In D. Damas, ed., *Ecological Essays*, vol. 230. Ottawa: Nat. Museum of Canada.

Lee, R. 1979. *The !Kung San: Men, Women, and Work in a Foraging Society.* Cambridge, UK: Cambridge University Press.

Marlowe, F. W. 2005. Who tends Hadza children?, In B. Hewlett and M. Lamb, eds., *Hunter–Gatherer Childhoods : Evolutionary, Developmental and Cultural Perspectives.* New Brunswick, NJ: Transaction Publishers, pp. 177–190.

Martin, P., and P. Bateson 1993. *Measuring Behavior*. Cambridge, UK: Cambridge University Press.

Mitani, J. C. and D. P. Watts. 2005. Correlates of territorial boundary patrol behaviour in wild chimpanzees. *Animal Behaviour* **70**: 1079–1086.

Montgomery, E. and A. Johnson 1976. Machiguenga energy expenditure. *Ecology of Food and Nutrition* **6**: 97–105.

Ohtsuka, R., N. Sudo, M. Sekiyama, *et al.* 2004. Gender difference in daily time and space use among Bangladeshi villagers under arsenic hazard: application of the compact spot-check method. *Journal of Biosocial Science* **36**: 317–332.

Panter-Brick, C. 1996. Seasonal and sex variation in physical activity levels of agro-pastoralists in Nepal. *American Journal of Physical Anthropology* **100**: 7–21.

Paolisso, M. and R. Hames (in press). Methods for the systematic study of human behavior. *Field Methods*.

Peregrine, P., D. R. Drews, M. North, and A. Slupe 1993. Sampling techniques and sampling error in naturalistic observation: an empirical evaluation with implications for cross-cultural research. *Cross-Cultural Research* **27**: 232–246.

Scaglion, R. 1986. Importance of nighttime observations in time allocation studies. *American Ethnologist* **13**: 537–545.

Stange, K., S. Zyzanski, T. Fedirko Smith, R. Kelly, *et al.* 1998. How valid are medical records and patient questionnaires for physician profiling and health services research? A comparison with direct observation of patient visits. *Medical Care* **36**: 851–867.

Sugawara, K. 1988. Visiting relations and social interactions between residential groups of the Central Kalahari San: hunter–gatherer camp as a micro-territory. *African Study Monographs* **8**: 173–211.

Takada, A. 2005. Mother-infant interactions among the !Xun: analysis of gymnastic and breastfeeding behaviors, In B. Hewlett and M. Lamb, eds., *Hunter-Gatherer Childhoods: Evolutionary, Developmental and Cultural Perspectives*. New Brunswick, NJ: Transaction Publishers, pp. 123–144.

Turke, P. 1989. Evolution and the demand for children. *Population and Development Review* **15**: 61–90.

Umezaki, M., T. Yamauchi, and R. Ohtsuka 2002. Time allocation to subsistence activities among the Huli in rural and urban Papua New Guinea. *Journal of Biosocial Science* **34**: 133–137.

Yasuoka, H. 2006. Long-term foraging expeditions (*Molongo*) among the Baka hunter-gatherers in the northwestern Congo Basin, with special reference to the Wild Yam Question. *Human Ecology* **34**: 275–295.

Veblen, T. 1899. *The Theory Of The Leisure Class. An Economic Study in the Evolution of Institutions*. New York: Macmillan.

Winking, J., M. Gurven, H. Kaplan, and J. Stieglitz 2009. The goals of direct paternal care among a South Amerindian population. *American Journal of Physical Anthropology* **139**: 295–304.

4

Analyzing the politics of natural resources: from theories of property rights to institutional analysis and beyond

AMY R. POTEETE

TOOLS FOR INSTITUTIONAL AND POLITICAL ANALYSIS

How do patterns of socioeconomic and political organization affect access to, control over, and the sustainability of natural resources? How does access to and control over natural resources influence livelihoods, inequality, and political relationships? Who controls natural resources? What accounts for the extent and form of cooperation and conflict over natural resources? Can patterns of natural resource access and control be altered to promote better social, economic, political, and ecological outcomes? Scholars concerned with these and related questions about natural resources have developed tools for institutional and political analysis. The scope of this chapter does not allow a comprehensive review of these approaches. The focus is on economic theories of property rights, the new institutionalism, and forms of political analysis concerned with cooperation, contestation, and power.

Property rights

Property rights define a variety of rights and assign them to particular actors or categories of actors. Examples include rights of access,

Environmental Social Sciences: Methods and Research Design, ed. I. Vaccaro, E. A. Smith and S. Aswani. Published by Cambridge University Press. © Cambridge University Press 2010.

withdrawal, management, exclusion, and alienation. Over the years, scholars have developed and revised typologies of property rights and distinguished between the nature of the property rights, the identity of the holder of property rights, and the characteristics of the resource subject to property rights. Research on property rights seeks to understand the emergence and development of property rights and how various allocations of property rights influence the efficiency and sustainability of natural resource use.

The early economic scholarship categorized property rights as private, state, or communal (Alchian and Demsetz 1973; Demsetz 1967). According to this typology, private property exists when rights are held by individuals or private firms, state property involves state control of rights on behalf of the public, and communal rights describe situations in which all potential users enjoy rights of access and withdrawal, but rights of exclusion have not been allocated. By definition, resource users could not capture the full returns from their investments in resources under communal property, nor did they bear the full costs of their use of the resource. Thus, inefficient use leading to degradation or depletion appeared inevitable for resources under communal property unless demand for a resource was quite low. Hardin (1968) famously described this situation as the "tragedy of the commons."

The association of common property with over-exploitation reflects a conflation of common property with the absence of property rights. Ciriacy-Wantrup and Bishop (1975) argued that "common property" should be used *only* to describe collectively held rights to exclude others, and that situations characterized by the absence of rights to exclude should be referred to as "open access" (see also Ostrom 1990; Bromley 1992). In essence, common property is a form of private property, in which private or exclusive rights are held by a group instead of an individual or household. Unsustainable resource use *is* expected under conditions of open access, because effective property rights are lacking, but can be avoided under common property because collective rights-holders can control resource use.

When demand for a resource grows, its increased value stimulates efforts to define property rights more clearly and in a more exclusionary manner. Privatization often involves individualization of rights but – as suggested by the distinction between common property and open access – can also entail the (more precise) definition of criteria for claiming rights associated with common property. The transformation of property rights is an inherently conflict-ridden process, as more secure rights for some implies the dispossession of others. Sometimes institutional change is blocked. Even if formal institutions change, it can be difficult to enforce more exclusive rights. Under these conditions, levels of resource use may become unsustainable and levels of investment in maintenance or more efficient production techniques may be depressed.

Institutional analysis

Earlier economic theories of property rights equated common property with an absence of property rights because they focused on formal rights backed by law. Many common-property systems, however, developed independently of government and have never been formalized. Informal systems of property rights exist for diverse natural resources, including fisheries, forests, land, wildlife, and water.[1] Growing recognition of the prevalence and importance of informal institutions for all sorts of social interactions contributed to the emergence of the new institutionalism in the 1980s.

The new institutionalism refers to a family of approaches that share an understanding of human behavior as conditioned by institutions, formal and informal, whether associated with government or not (Hall and Taylor 1996; March and Olsen 1984).[2] Institutions refer to commonly understood rules of what one must, may, or must not do in particular situations (Ostrom 1990) or, as North puts it, "the rules of the game in a society" (1990: 1). Institutions influence social outcomes because they shape the expected costs and rewards associated with various actions. Because these incentive structures are commonly understood, institutions also influence expectations about the behavior of others (North 1990). In applications to natural resources, institutional analysis expands upon and challenges theories of property rights. It accepts the importance of formal property rights, but does not assume their priority. The approach lends itself to evaluations of efficiency and sustainability, the most common dependent variables for the property rights school. But institutional analysis can also address a variety other concerns, including equity, risk management, and conflict management.

---

[1] For reviews, see Baland and Platteau (2000, Part II) and Poteete, Janssen, and Ostrom (2010). See De Soto (2000) on other types of informal property systems.

[2] The "old institutionalism" of the early twentieth century focused on formal legal arrangements.

For institutional analysts, property rights represent *sets* of institutions. Schlager and Ostrom (1992), for example, distinguish among rights of access, withdrawal, management, exclusion, and alienation and offer a typology of property rights based on the range of rights held. A variety of actors – and types of actors – may hold different, often overlapping sets of rights related to a shared resource or resource system (e.g., Edwards and Steins 1998; Schoonmaker Freudenberger 1993). Even if the state claims all rights except alienation, for example, members of a community may exercise rights of access and withdrawal. Greater recognition that rights may be held by many actors gave rise to new questions about the consequences of different combinations of rights for investment, efficiency, sustainability, and other outcomes. Although policy analysts often depict rights of alienation as critical (De Soto 2000; Deininger and Binswanger 1999), empirical studies suggest that sustainability hinges on the ability to exclude (Agrawal and Ostrom 2001; Netting 1981).

Institutional analysts see property rights as *a subset of the wide range of institutions* that influence the use of natural resources (Oakerson 1992). Other relevant institutions include those that define group boundaries, criteria for the distribution of benefits and burdens associated with management, rules for making collective decisions and settling conflicts, and relations with the other actors, organizations, and the government (Ostrom 1990). Ensminger's (1996) study of institutional change in a Kenyan community of pastoralists shows how economic and political institutions interact to influence patterns of natural resource use, market exchanges, settlement patterns, and socioeconomic equality. The development of long-distance trade, the growth of sedentary villages, and the decline of migratory herding were not simply responses to changes in relative prices. They also reflected the changing role of the government in enforcing contracts, regulating weights and measures, limiting the authority of traditional Orma leaders, and mediating interactions between rival groups of pastoralists. Institutional arrangements related to the bureaucracy also affect natural resource use (Gibson 1999; Poteete 2003a, b).

Institutional analysis provides tools for analyzing the effects of specific institutional arrangements and the dynamics that affect institutional stability and change. Gibson and Marks (1995), for example, criticize the *design* of programs for community-based natural resource management because, by providing benefits to the community as a group, these programs *fail to create incentives* for individual community members to support conservation. The challenges of multi-level

governance and other types of interactions across institutions represent another area of concern (Hooghe and Marks 2003). Large-scale
institutions are required to address ecosystem dynamics and interactions across localities, but often are not sufficiently responsive to
local conditions and concerns (Young 2002). Disappointments with
programs for decentralized natural resource management have been
attributed to institutional interactions that undermine local discretionary authority and encourage upward accountability (Ribot 2003).
Interactions among institutions at the same scale of organization also
influence outcomes. Rivalries, whether involving general-purpose and
special-purpose local organizations (Manor 2004) or different policy
areas and associated ministries (Poteete 2009b), are common. Poor
coordination or active efforts at sabotage can generate disappointing
outcomes. Changing problematic institutions depends on the resolution of collective action problems, with the prospects for collective action conditioned by the characteristics of groups of would-be
rights-holders and of the natural resources (Baland and Platteau 2000;
Ostrom 1990).

Politics: cooperation, contestation, and power

While institutional analysis draws attention to questions with significant distributional consequences, the focus on incentives and collective action problems can obscure sources of discord. Yet institutional
choice, reproduction, and change are conflict-ridden processes (Knight
1992). In addition to struggles for collective action among those with
shared goals, actors with divergent interests compete with each other.[3]
Political analysis highlights conflicting material interests, the symbolic connections between natural resources and identity politics, and
competition for authority.

As noted above, natural resource systems encompass multiple
elements and are used for many purposes. The same land may be used
for timber production, the collection of non-timber forest products,
grazing, wildlife, recreation, and many other purposes. Likewise, rivers
support fisheries, enrich soils through seasonal floods, act as conduits
for transportation, and can contribute to irrigation, electricity production, and the supply of drinking water. Some activities do not overlap
or may even be complementary. When herds graze on fields after the
harvest, for example, there are opportunities for mutually beneficial

---

[3] See examples below.

exchange of crop residues for manure (e.g., Agrawal 1999: Chapter 5). Other forms of resource use are inherently incompatible. To cite just two examples, land cleared for crops ceases to serve as a source of forest products, and dams for irrigation and energy production interfere with fishing and flood-plain agriculture. Conflicts often concern the priority to be given to different management goals and associated forms of use: conservation versus production, subsistence versus commercial use, single- versus multi-purpose use, and so forth. Distributional conflicts arise even among actors with shared management goals, such as between farmers at different locations along an irrigation canal or pastoralists who use the same pastures.

Access to natural resources and specific forms of natural resource use are often tied to community membership (Berry 1993; Peters 1984; Schwartz 2006). Issues of identity and institutions that affect natural resources are thus entangled. Property rights and other institutions determine who participates in decision-making, who benefits from natural resources and on what basis. These institutional choices signal political choices among political communities or alternative definitions of community (Boone 2007; Poteete 2009b; Ribot, Chhatre, and Lankina 2008). Conflicts over institutional choices and natural resources often pit local against national interests; they also frequently involve clashes between territorial, residential, or ethno-linguistic definitions of local community membership.

Conflict is all the more likely because multiple institutional arrangements coexist and compete with each other. Institutional and legal pluralism is widespread (Berry 1993; Moore 2001). Especially in post-colonial and post-socialist settings, actors within the state attempt to consolidate power and secure a position of predominance relative to other organizations, such as traditional authority structures, religious organizations, and other social networks (Migdal 1988; Sikor and Lund 2009). Other actors and organizations seek to maintain and expand their own areas of autonomy and control, and thus resist the state's efforts to achieve hegemony (Lund 2006). Rival actors and organizations seek to control natural resources as a way to build, defend, or expand their authority. Competition for authority pertains not only to physical control of natural resources, but also to control over access to natural resources and opportunities to convert natural resources into other types of benefits (e.g., through processing, trade, or social exchanges) (Ribot and Peluso 2003).

Political analysts examine interactions between material interests, political organization and competition, and natural resource use and management. How does competition between different economic interests, political organizations, and political communities influence the choice of institutional arrangements, or contribute to institutional continuity or change? How do institutions affect the form of contestation and the consolidation of authority at the local and national levels? How do political competition and institutional changes affect identity politics? What are the implications of economic, political, and identity-based competition for natural resource use and management? Institutions, including property rights, feature prominently in these questions. But property rights and other institutions represent only one of many mechanisms through which relationships of cooperation and contestation operate.

In sum, the analysis of property rights, institutions, and politics directs attention to several related questions. Property rights theory emphasizes the importance of shifts in relative prices in driving efforts to change formal rights of exclusion and alienation. Institutional analysis draws attention to informal institutions and emphasizes the difficulty of enforcing rights, whether defined formally or informally. The difficulty of exclusion presents perhaps the most significant challenge for sustainability, albeit one that varies across natural resources. The definition and enforcement of exclusive rights is not simply a technical matter. Collective action is required to achieve institutional change, maintain shared infrastructure, and defend collective resources. And collective action is itself problematic. Individuals are often wary of investing in collective endeavors without assurance that others will also contribute. Furthermore, people and organizations do not necessarily have common goals or want to work together; they often compete to control natural resources. Beyond their material value as sources of livelihood and marketable products, natural resources have symbolic value as markers of identity. Because of their material and symbolic value, political actors can use control over natural resources to build or reinforce authority. Thus, political and symbolic as well as material interests influence contestation over natural resources.

METHODOLOGICAL ISSUES

A scholar embarking on institutional and political analysis related to natural resources faces a number of methodological challenges. I emphasize issues related to the definition of a project, the observation and measurement of informal and intangible phenomena, interactions across fields of action and scales of organization, and the difficulty of controlling for confounding factors. For illustrations, I draw on my own field-based and largely qualitative research on policies and politics related to three natural resources – rangelands, wildlife, and minerals – in Botswana. This chapter does not discuss issues related to cross-national research involving statistical analysis of a large number of observations.

In Botswana, policy debates have centered on the choice between individual or communal rights to resources, and whether communal rights should refer to local, district-level, or national communities. There has also been considerable contestation related to the institutional arrangements for natural resource management by communities. These conflicts are not simply over institutional arrangements; at least as important is the site of control over these resources: traditional or state authorities, national or sub-national actors, and, within the government, which of several ministries. These battles play out in village politics, bureaucratic politics, the courts, and electoral campaigns. I am thus able to address the different sorts of challenges associated with research related to diverse natural resources, institutional arrangements, and sites and forms of political contestation. My research centers unabashedly on the *politics* of natural resource management; questions of efficiency and sustainability are less prominent in this chapter than in the broader literature.

Defining the study

Research begins with definition of the unit of analysis or the unit about which observations will be made. It might be an individual, a collection of individuals of a particular type, a system (e.g., ecological, cultural, political), or a territory. If the goal is to analyze the effects of institutional arrangements, for example, the unit of analysis should be the people, territory, or resources under particular institutional arrangements. For research on the prospects for collective action, observations should focus on groups that might act collectively, such as political jurisdictions, sets of individuals with common patterns of resource use, or the set of all individuals with an interest in a resource system. The individual resource user is an appropriate unit of analysis for research related to the social and economic consequences of particular institutional arrangements. A focus on social or political units of analysis makes more sense in research on the influence of social organization or political contestation. My research on the politics of natural resource policies in Botswana has addressed three units of analysis: (1) specific policies, (2) the sub-national political jurisdictions, and (3) individuals. Over-time comparisons of policies – or other types of institutional change – support assessments of the influence of other forms of countrywide change.

If the universe of possible cases consists of two or three policies or institutional arrangements within a country, it may be possible to collect data for the entire population. Because Botswana has adopted only two policies related to the creation of private ranches, for example, studying both presented no special challenges (Poteete 2003a). For many types of research, however, the population is too large to study. I analyzed the local politics surrounding the introduction of private ranching for a sub-set of districts and priority areas for implementation within each district (Poteete 1999, 2003b). In principle, decisions about sample size reflect trade-offs between internal and external validity. More intensive data collection increases internal validity by raising confidence that indicators capture the intended theoretical concepts, observations are accurate, and that inferred relationships exist. Data collection for a larger number of observations increases external validity – if observations are representative of the larger population – by decreasing the likelihood that the idiosyncratic will be mistaken for the typical. Because there are trade-offs between intensive and extensive data collection, researchers also face trade-offs in the relative prioritization of internal and external validity.

But research priorities are not the only consideration. Decisions about sample size and selection also depend on the time and effort required for data-collection. For political and institutional analysis related to natural resources, data are often difficult to access and time-consuming to collect. The units of analysis, for example, may be difficult to identify or locate. Recognition of formal political jurisdictions or organizations such as government bureaus is straightforward. Unless there is a reliably complete and up-to-date registry, formal organizations outside the public sector are often less visible; small-scale organizations are easy to overlook.[4] Recognition of informal organizations requires considerable local knowledge. It is even more challenging to identify units of *potential* collective action, especially groups that are cooperating but have not (yet) organized formally or that have not (yet) achieved collective action (Poteete and Ostrom 2004).

---

[4] For examples of sampling based on official registries, see Landry and Shen (2005) on urban households in China, Agrawal and Goyal (2001) and Agrawal and Yadama (1997) on Van Panchayats in India, and Dayton-Johnson (1999, 2000) on irrigation groups in Mexico.

Difficulties related to the identification of units of analysis also affect sampling strategies. Random sampling, for example, requires a complete list of the entire population. If such lists do not exist or are not reliable, randomization may not be an option, particularly if the units of analysis are numerous or not easily recognized. Consider, for example, a household survey that I conducted in rural Botswana.[5] The combination of relatively undocumented settlements, settlement patterns that are difficult to map, and mobility made the development of the population lists required for random sampling prohibitive. Instead, I used a quota sample. I divided the target sample for each study area between settlements and agricultural lands based on the relative population sizes of the relevant census blocks. For each settlement and agricultural area, I set quotas for the breakdown of respondents based on the age and gender structure reported in the census. I divided these quotas evenly across wards, the territorial sub-units within villages, to guard against spatial clustering of respondents and associated biases.[6] I scheduled survey work for times of the day when different types of respondents, including those with formal employment were most likely to be available. This structured approach raised confidence in representativeness of the sample.

Measurement

Institutional and political analysis requires observations related to formal and informal institutions and organization, patterns of political competition and cooperation, and political discourse. The informal and intangible loom large. Relevant practices are not always openly acknowledged and discourses often have multiple meanings. Interpretation of the historically and culturally informed significance of political discourse as well as informal practices depends on deep local knowledge. Personal relationships of trust are critical. Trust increases access to potential respondents and opportunities for participant observation and the likelihood that people will reveal elements of the informal realm to outsiders.

Formal institutions are generally documented in official laws and regulations. These sources are relatively accessible. Evaluating the

---

[5] For other strategies, see Landry and Shen (2005), Lindberg and Morrison (2008), and Meinzen-Dick, Raju, and Gulati (2002).

[6] Prior to independence, the wards were associated with distinct families and cultural groups. The post-colonial system of land administration has eroded but not eliminated the sociopolitical significance of the wards.

extent to which formal institutions are acted upon and enforced, and identifying informal rules present bigger challenges. Even if, by definition, informal institutions are commonly understood within a given community, members of that community may not openly acknowledge them. They may be reticent to discuss institutions that lack formal recognition and may even violate official laws. Or respondents may imagine that unwritten but commonly understood rules are not worth discussing and would not be of interest to outsiders. People sometimes internalize the informal institutions in their own society to such an extent that they do not even think of them as institutions at all. People are even less likely to discuss non-institutionalized practices, especially if they violate formal norms. Such conditions and challenges affect investigations of interests in natural resources. A combination of qualitative observations and local knowledge is required to recognize and understand the linkages between natural resource use and identity or other symbolic issues.

Qualitative research hinges on access and the ability to interpret observations. For institutional and political research related to natural resources, it is important to have access to people with an interest in the natural resources, but also to the politicians, bureaucrats, and representatives of non-governmental organizations (NGOs) and donors who are involved in decision-making, management, implementation, and enforcement. Interviews or focus groups provide valuable narratives about interests, practices, and patterns of cooperation and contestation. Archival research helps pin down the timing and key features of events. Minutes of meetings or hearings reveal sets of issues around which conflict and cooperation center and provide some sense of patterns of interaction. Correspondence, official statements, and newspapers are particularly valuable sources of discourse. Of course, documents are always partial, and documents written to make an argument – including correspondence, statements, editorials, and letters to the editor – intentionally present a biased view. The difficulty of figuring out what is *not* being said is one of the greatest challenges. Direct observation of harvesting and processing, marketing, official meetings and political rallies, and informal exchanges offers opportunities to witness ordinary interactions among different types of actors. Although the presence of the researcher inevitably influences these interactions, people cannot step outside of patterned interactions entirely.

Sharp observational skills, the need for local knowledge, and the importance of trust are inherent to ethnographic research, whatever the topic or analytical approach. It is widely accepted that triangulation of different types of observations from many sources – participant observation, interviews, archival work – enhances the possibilities for reading between the lines and increases confidence in the analysis. Nonetheless, balancing multiple methods requires dexterity. The researcher must develop skill in a variety of data collection techniques and seek opportunities for access. In addition, decisions must be made about the allocation of limited time in field settings to each form of observation. The difficulty of this balancing act depends in part on whether the types of settings targeted for observation are clustered in some sense (e.g., spatially or in terms of the number or type of actors and organizations involved) or diffuse. An abiding concern with interactions across fields of action and scales of organization exacerbates the difficulty of balancing different forms of observation. The next section looks more closely at the methodological implications of this concern with interactions across fields and scales.

INTERACTIONS ACROSS FIELDS AND SCALES

Institutional and political analysis of natural resources differs from other forms of ethnographic research in that the concern with interactions between ecological conditions, economic activities, social and political organization, and culturally and historically informed discourse demands a broad frame for observations. Ultimately, the quality of interpretations of observations depends on the researcher's grasp of the structure of relationships in the field setting, broadly understood. Frameworks for institutional and political analysis emphasize the importance of interactions across fields of action and scales of organization.

Fields of action refer to realms of interaction associated with a particular set of issues, concerns, or organizations. Fields of action might refer to particular sectors, such as agricultural land, fisheries, forestry, livestock and grazing, wildlife, tourism, and so forth. Institutional fields of action might be defined with reference to particular organizations, such as the parliament, the courts, traditional authorities, local governments, a specific ministry or agency, local non-government organizations, or donors. And political fields of action include competition in elections, bureaucratic politics, and situations of legal pluralism involving competition between state agencies and non-state organizations such as traditional authority structures, cooperatives, and religious organizations.

It is almost instinctive to define a research project with reference to particular field of action. And yet, as artificial constructs, focusing on a single field of action can be misleading. Land and other natural resources are often sites of competition between the state and non-state authorities. In the years after Botswana gained independence, for example, several policies reduced chiefly control over natural resources (Poteete 2009a, 2009b). The new government almost immediately deprived chiefs of control over sub-soil resources, claiming that mineral wealth should be used for the benefit of the nation as a whole. Although Land Boards were established to replace chiefly authority over land administration shortly after independence, the transfer occurred gradually. The chiefs held ex officio positions as Land Board members for many years and, even after they lost their formal representation, they retained influence as a source of information about past land allocations. Chiefly authority over land eroded gradually as the Land Boards accumulated their own records.

Rural land accommodates many overlapping actual or possible activities: crop production, grazing, gathering of wild products (e.g., firewood, thatching grass, fruits), hunting, tourism, wildlife habitat and migration routes, and so forth. Researchers, policy-makers, and individuals with an interest in the natural resource system may view the same area through the lenses of agricultural practices and policies, wildlife habitat and biodiversity protection, or opportunities for infrastructure development (e.g., drilling wells, prospecting for mines). Indeed, policy-makers and interested parties regularly put forward alternative, competing framings. In Botswana, other departments and agencies viewed policies for the promotion of fenced ranching as an effort to extend the territorial jurisdiction of the Ministry of Agriculture and a threat to other forms of land use. The creation of wildlife management areas and the Community-Based Natural Resource Management program by the wildlife department addressed perceived problems associated with wildlife conservation, but also represented an effort to block the expansion of the Ministry of Agriculture (Poteete 2009b). Uncritical acceptance of a particular framing increases the risk of overlooking this sort of competition.

Interactions can also occur between fields that have no obvious practical relationship to each other if reframing an issue offers advantages for some set of actors. In Botswana, politicians linked debates about community-based wildlife management to policies that define rights to revenues from mineral resources (Poteete 2009b).

Bureaucratic jockeying for jurisdiction over land encouraged the introduction of rival policies for fenced ranching and wildlife management that targeted the same areas. But the major centers for mining and wildlife are located in different parts of the country. This linking involves interactions between fields of action related to distinct sectors, but also interactions between fields of electoral competition and natural resource management. These intersections transformed institutional choices related to management strategy into choices about the basis for allocating benefits associated with natural resources, and thus mobilized competition between local, district-level, and national definitions of political community.

The discourse surrounding wildlife management in Botswana hints at the interactions across local, district, and national scales of political action and organization. Cross-scale interactions frequently extend to the international arena, as well. The priorities of international donors are reflected to some extent, albeit imperfectly, in Botswana's policy choices. In the late 1960s and early 1970s, an international consensus promoted privatization of land and capital-intensive strategies for agricultural development. This consensus was reflected in both the institutional arrangements introduced by Botswana's 1975 Tribal Grazing Lands Policy (TGLP) and the discourse used to justify the policy (Poteete 2003a). The World Bank provided substantial financial support for TGLP, but its confidence in privatization as a mechanism for rural development had faded by the 1990s. Botswana's 1991 Agricultural Development Policy ran counter to a new international consensus that emphasized the importance of mobility and flexibility in rights to arid and semi-arid lands. Within Botswana's bureaucracy, opposition to the expansion of fenced ranching referred explicitly to this new consensus (Poteete 2003a).

Concerns originating in the international arena may resonate in national policy, but events and developments within a country are in no sense determined internationally. Policy-makers draw opportunistically from the international arena. This can be seen in Botswana's decision to extend fenced ranching in 1991, despite a shift in the international consensus, and in the ways that actors within Botswana domesticate policies that appear to reflect international priorities. Certainly, the government of Botswana presented its promotion of fenced ranching as a policy of privatization to halt degradation of the commons, and it emphasized the role of fencing in supporting more intensive production strategies. Yet "privatization" involved long-term, heavily subsidized leases to farmers by district-level Land Boards. In the 1970s and 1980s, many ranchers also received heavily subsidized loans from the National Development Bank. These conditions did not encourage more sustainable management of the range or more intensive forms of livestock production. They did represent highly valuable opportunities for patronage.

Similarly, Botswana adopted its program for community-based wildlife management at the urging of USAID. Although international supporters for community-based natural resource management emphasized expectations of improved wildlife protection, this approach also reflected the widespread enthusiasm for market-based strategies and a limited role for the state in the 1980s (Igoe and Brockington 2007). Yet domestic actors had their own reasons to adopt community-based management. As discussed above, it presented opportunities for the wildlife department to defend its territorial jurisdiction against incursions by the Ministry of Agriculture. In addition, the financial benefits associated with the program presented opportunities to extend patronage networks (Blaikie 2006) and shore up electoral support in locally competitive constituencies (Poteete 2009b). As electoral competition intensified nationally, these calculations changed. Politicians from areas of the country with little wildlife, who previously took little interest in wildlife management, began to depict decentralized wildlife management as a threat to the national distribution of mining revenues, and to national unity more generally. This rhetoric contributed to a partial recentralization of wildlife management in 2007 (Poteete 2009b).

The examples from Botswana reveal that interactions across fields and scales of organization and action are pervasive and, perhaps more to the point, central sites of political competition. To some extent, interactions across fields and scales are inevitable. Natural resources can be framed in diverse ways in part because ecological systems are multi-faceted. Likewise, the coexistence of organizations at various scales makes cross-scale interactions inevitable. Yet, the examples also provide evidence of intentional efforts to reframe issues and link fields of action for their own advantage. Whether created intentionally or approached opportunistically, interactions across fields and scales of action are inherently political because they represent alternative systems of value (priority) and alternative systems of meaning. They thus create opportunities for actors to justify actions with reference to one field or scale of activity without drawly attention to advantages gained in other fields or at other scales. By implication, research that focuses narrowly on one or a few fields or scales of action risks missing most of the political action. Unfortunately, a broad framing of research presents considerable practical and analytical challenges. The practical challenges, as mentioned in the previous section, concern the allocation of limited resources across diverse research activities. The analytical challenge, as discussed below, arises from the large number of variables at play across various fields and scales.

CONFOUNDING EFFECTS

Outcomes related to natural resources are influenced by many factors: ecological, social, political, and economic. The role of institutions and politics can be obscured by spatial variation in ecological conditions or across groups with different socioeconomic practices, or by temporal variation associated with ecological, social, and economic dynamics. In studies with large numbers of observations, statistical controls address this problem to some extent, although the analysis must check for the possibility of multiple causal patterns (Achen 2002; Rudel 2008). Most institutional and political research related to natural resources focuses on one or few cases, however, and relies more heavily on intentional case selection and process-tracing. The goal is to select cases that feature variation along a limited number of factors of particular analytical interest while limiting or eliminating other sources of variation. Within-case comparisons offer particularly attractive opportunities to limit variation in institutional arrangements, cultural characteristics, and macro-political conditions. No single form of comparison can fully control for all possible confounding effects, but analytical leverage can be increased through triangulation across several forms of comparison.

My research in Botswana has relied on comparisons of subdistricts, districts, time periods, and types of natural resources, as discussed above. The same government institutions – agencies, procedures, and policies – apply to all districts, but there is considerable variation in ecological conditions, socioeconomic organization and economic activities, and political organization and competition. Important forms of spatial variation also exist within districts. For example, ecological conditions vary considerably between the Okavango Delta in the northwest, the dry grasslands in the center and south of the country, somewhat more humid conditions in the east, and the very dry west and southwest. But district boundaries do not correspond to ecological zones and many districts encompass several ecological zones. The prevalence of pilot projects, donor-sponsored projects, and phased policy implementation contributes another dimension of spatial diversity.

My research on policies that promoted fenced ranching compared implementation at the district level. Although decisions about the administration of land occur at the district level, the implementation of policies that affect land usually unfolds in a phased manner. Thus, the household survey and other forms of socioeconomic and political analysis focused on smaller-scale areas designated for priority implementation by district-level officials. Each area tends to be relatively homogeneous ecologically and in terms of land use. Comparison of sub-district areas targeted for the introduction of ranching in several districts raised doubts about the generality of assessments based on research in one or few locations. The creation of fenced ranches and their allocation to individuals or small partnerships proved to be widely accepted in areas where water points had been developed relatively recently and were well spaced,[7] but roundly rejected as inappropriate where pastoralists relied on a network of surface water and wells, existing water points were closely clustered, or multi-member water point syndicates were common (Poteete 1999, 2003b). Policies or management strategies may work well in some places and yet be entirely inappropriate in many other locations.

In my research, the combination of two forms of within-case comparisons – across time periods and across spatial units – has proven particularly valuable. Comparisons of districts or at the sub-district level cannot fully control for multi-faceted spatial variation. Differences in reactions to proposals for fenced ranching in the 1990s corresponded with a complex of differences in ecological conditions, the degree of economic specialization, sociocultural organization of economic activities, political mobilization of ethno-linguistic identities, and political competition. It is impossible to assess the relative importance of these conditions based on a spatial comparison at a single time point. Many forms of spatial variation are stable over time. Spatial differences in ecological conditions remain important and, despite countrywide declines in the importance of livestock and agriculture in Botswana, spatial differences in the organization of livestock production and economic activities have also persisted. Analysis of policy sectors over time reveals the importance of developments

---

[7] Many officials opposed ranching even in areas where public opinion was favorable.

related to the state bureaucracy (Poteete, 2003a) and fluctuations in the intensity of political competition (Poteete, 1999, 2003b). Changes in national-level electoral politics have contributed to shifts in the use of mineral revenues to invest in public goods (e.g., infrastructure, education) versus benefits for particular interests (Poteete, 2009a), alternation between centralized and decentralized approaches to wildlife management (Poteete 2009b), and to a stop-go dynamic in the demarcation and allocation of fenced ranches.

Analytical strategies that seek to control variation are valuable, yet inherently limited. They are perhaps most valuable for analysis focused on a single field or scale of action. As discussed in the previous section, however, interactions across fields and scales are both pervasive and critical as sites of political action. Furthermore, case selection that controls variation focuses on correlation as an indicator of relationships. Correlation is not a reliable indicator of causation. Analysis based on correlation will miss multiple paths to the same outcome. Even if multiple causation is not an issue, explanation requires the identification of processes and mechanisms linking cause to effect. Process-tracing seeks evidence of mechanisms and processes by observing sequences of events and actions and analyzing *how* events and actions relate to each other. Process-tracing requires over-time analysis, in order to track sequences. Process-tracing raises awareness of interactions across fields and scales. At the same time, the focus on specific processes helps bound the scope of analysis so that it becomes manageable.

CONCLUSION

Institutional and political analysis guards against naïve expectations about possibilities for policy interventions, but provides little guidance on how to achieve political transformation. Ironically, although these approaches emphasize agency in the creation of institutions and in pushing strategically for political advantages, institutional and political analysis sees agency as operating within highly structured contexts. Scholars working in these research traditions recognize social and political dynamism, as well as the coexistence of dynamism with stability, as important theoretical challenges. Awareness of the limitations of current approaches and the difficulty of developing more satisfactory alternatives can be seen in the debates regarding path dependency, for example. The development of analytical tools that allow more scope for the role of agency and creativity would both greatly enhance the practical value of political analysis and provide a better understanding of the coexistence of sources of dynamism with extended periods of superficial stability.

Institutional and political analysis overlaps with narrative analysis and network analysis in ways that may help solve these theoretical puzzles. Institutional analysis within the rational choice tradition assumes a highly individualistic world, in which individuals make decisions based on self-interest and discourse and narrative are irrelevant because talk is not binding. For these scholars, narratives and networks are irrelevant. There is ample evidence, however, that these assumptions are not accurate, with the possible exception of interactions in markets and other highly competitive settings. But institutional analysis in no way requires assumptions of narrow individual rationality. Many scholars combine institutional analysis with more sociologically grounded models of behavior. These perspectives acknowledge the importance of narratives and networks in guiding responses to institutional arrangements, as well as the likelihood of coordinated action to create or change institutions.

We have seen that narratives and networks are central to political analysis. In some respects, political action is all about building networks of allies – and challenging the networks of rivals. Political actors use narrative appeals, as well as the distribution of access to material benefits, to expand their networks. The drive to build networks provides a source of dynamism. In focusing on the competitive aspects of network building, political analysis expects mobilization to prompt counter-mobilization. From this perspective, dynamism is assumed to be constant. Mobilization and counter-mobilization often result in surface stability, if no group gains the momentum required to change the balance of powers. But the ongoing processes of contestation represent an unceasing source of pressure for change.

Institutional and political analysis is also enriched by other forms of analysis, such as ecology and ethnobiology, ethnohistory and history, household production, and political economy. Institutions are embedded in a social, economic, and political context. Their symbolic value is informed by history and culture. This chapter has alluded to the importance of ecology, or at least ethnobiology (in the context of social mapping onto natural resource uses), and alternative understandings of ecological processes. Indeed, the importance of interactions across fields of action for institutional and political analysis makes attentiveness to the other forms of analysis indispensable.

The primary methodological challenge of institutional and political analysis arises precisely from its reliance upon analysis at multiple scales, using multiple methods, and being attentive to the concerns of multiple disciplines and areas of specialization. It is not reasonable to expect each individual researcher to command multiple disciplines or a wide range of methods (Poteete, Janssen, and Ostrom 2010), or even to collect observations for all relevant fields and scales of action. There is a real risk that, in trying to broaden the scope of analysis, depth and accuracy will be lost. Collaborative research offers opportunities to bring together scholars to overcome these challenges by dividing the labor, but does not fully solve the problem. Perhaps scholars should accept a fragmented approach as unavoidable, in the sense that any single study will be inevitably partial, but that a multi-faceted analysis can emerge through a body of literature.

ACKNOWLEDGMENTS

Thanks to the Republic of Botswana for permission to conduct research in Botswana; the Fulbright Foundation, the Social Science Research Council, and the University of New Orleans for financial support; the University of Botswana for institutional support; and respondents and friends in Botswana. Comments from Thomas Sikor, Ismael Vaccaro, and an anonymous reviewer helped improve the chapter; I am responsible for its limitations.

REFERENCES

Achen, C. H. 2002. Toward a new political methodology: microfoundations and ART. *Annual Review of Political Science* **5**: 423–450.
Agrawal, A. 1999. *Greener Pastures: Politics, Markets and Community Among A Pastoral Migrant People*. Durham, NC: Duke University Press.
Agrawal, A. and S. Goyal 2001. Group size and collective action: third party monitoring in common-pool resources. *Comparative Political Studies* **34**: 63–93.
Agrawal, A. and E. Ostrom 2001. Collective action, property rights and decentralization in resource use in India and Nepal. *Politics and Society* **29**: 485–514.
Agrawal, A. and G. N. Yadama 1997. How do local institutions mediate market and population pressures on resources? Forest panchayats in Kumaon, India. *Development and Change* **28**: 435–65.
Alchian, A. and H. Demsetz 1973. The property rights paradigm. *Journal of Economic History* **33**: 16–27.
Baland, J.-M. and J.-P. Platteau 2000. *Halting Degradation of Natural Resources: Is There a Role for Rural Communities?* New York: Oxford University Press.
Berry, S. 1993. *No Condition is Permanent: The Social Dynamics of Agrarian Change In Sub-Saharan Africa*. Madison, WI: University of Wisconsin Press.

Blaikie, P. 2006. Is small really beautiful? Community-based natural resource management in Malawi and Botswana. *World Development* **34**: 1942–1957.

Boone, C. 2007. Property and constitutional order: Land tenure reform and the future of the African state. *African Affairs* **106**: 557–586.

Bromley, D. W. 1992. The commons, property, and common-property regimes. In D. W. Bromley, ed., *Making the Commons Work: Theory, Practice, and Policy*. San Francisco, CA: ICS Press, pp. 3–15.

Ciriacy-Wantrup, S. V. and R. C. Bishop 1975. "Common property" as a concept in natural resources policy. *Natural Resources Journal* **15**: 713–27.

Dayton-Johnson, J. 1999. Irrigation organization in Mexican *unidades de riego*: Results of a field study. *Irrigation and Drainage Systems* **13**: 55–74.

Dayton-Johnson, J. 2000. Choosing rules to govern the commons: a model with evidence from Mexico. *Journal of Economic Behavior and Organization* **42**: 19–41.

Deininger, K. and H. Binswanger 1999. The evolution of the World Bank's land policy: Principles, experience, and future challenges. *The World Bank Research Observer* **14**: 247–276.

Demsetz, H. 1967. Toward a theory of property rights. *American Economic Review* **57**: 347–359.

De Soto, H. 2000. *The Mystery of Capital: Why Capitalism Triumphs in the West and Fails Everywhere Else*. New York: Basic Books.

Edwards, V. M. and N. A. Steins 1998. Developing an analytical framework for multiple-use commons. *Journal of Theoretical Politics* **10**: 347–383.

Ensminger, J. 1996. *Making a Market: The Institutional Transformation of an African Society*. New York: Cambridge University Press.

Gibson, C. C. 1999. *Politicians and Poachers: The Political Economy of Wildlife Policy in Africa*. New York: Cambridge University Press.

Gibson, C. C. and S. A. Marks 1995. Transforming rural hunters into conservationists: An assessment of community-based wildlife management programs in Africa. *World Development* **23**: 941–957.

Hall, P. A. and R. C. R. Taylor, 1996. Political science and the three new institutionalisms. *Political Studies* **44**: 936–957.

Hardin, G. 1968. The tragedy of the commons. *Science* **162**: 1243–1248.

Hooghe, L. and G. Marks 2003. Unraveling the central state, but how? Types of multi-level governance. *American Political Science Review* **97**: 233–243.

Igoe, J. and D. Brockington 2007. Neoliberal conservation: a brief introduction. *Conservation and Society* **5**: 432–449.

Knight, J. 1992. *Institutions and Social Conflict*. New York: Cambridge University Press.

Landry, P. F. and M. Shen 2005. Reaching migrants in survey research: The use of global positioning system to reduce coverage bias in China. *Political Analysis* **13**: 1–22.

Lindberg, S. I. and M. K. C. Morrison 2008. Are African voters really ethnic or clientelistic? Survey evidence from Ghana. *Political Science Quarterly* **123**: 95–122.

Lund, C. 2006. Twilight institutions: public authority and local politics in Africa. *Development and Change* **37**: 685–705.

Manor, J. 2004. User committees: a potentially damaging second wave of decentralisation? *European Journal of Development Research* **16**: 192–213.

March, J. G. and J. P. Olsen 1984. The new institutionalism: organizational factors in political life. *American Political Science Review* **78**: 734–749.

Meinzen-Dick, R., K. V. Raju, and A. Gulati 2002. What affects organization and collective action for managing resources? Evidence from canal irrigation systems in India. *World Development* **30**: 649–666.

Migdal, J. S. 1988. *Strong Societies and Weak States: State Society Relations and State Capabilities in the Third World.* Princeton, NJ: Princeton University Press.

Moore, S. F. 2001. Certainties undone: fifty turbulent years of legal anthropology, 1949–1999. *The Journal of the Royal Anthropological Institute* **7**: 95–116.

Netting, R. McC. 1981. *Balancing on an Alp: Ecological Change and Continuity in a Swiss Mountain Community.* New York: Cambridge University Press.

North, D. 1990. *Institutions, Institutional Change and Economic Performance.* New York: Cambridge University Press.

Oakerson, R. J. 1992. Analyzing the commons: a framework. In D. W. Bromley, ed., *Making the Commons Work: Theory, Practice, and Policy.* San Francisco, CA: ICS Press, pp. 41–59.

Ostrom, E. 1990. *Governing the Commons: The Evolution of Institutions for Collective Action.* New York: Cambridge University Press.

Peters, P. E. 1984. Struggles over water, struggles over meaning: cattle, water and the state in Botswana. *Africa: Journal of the International African Institute* **54**: 29–49, 127.

Poteete, A. R. 1999. Disaggregating state and society: Accounting for patterns of tenure change in Botswana, 1975–1996. Doctoral dissertation, Duke University.

Poteete, A. R. 2003a. Ideas, interests, and institutions: challenging the property rights paradigm in Botswana. *Governance* **16**: 527–557.

Poteete, A. R. 2003b. When professionalism clashes with local particularities: Ecology, elections, and procedural arrangements in Botswana. *Journal of Southern African Studies* **29**: 461–485.

Poteete, A. R. 2009a. Is development path dependent or political? A reinterpretation of mineral-dependent development in Botswana. *Journal of Development Studies* **45**: 544–571.

Poteete, A. R. 2009b. Defining political community and rights to natural resources in Botswana. *Development and Change* **40**: 281–305.

Poteete, A. R., M. Janssen, and E. Ostrom 2010. *Working Together: Collective Action, the Commons, and Multiple Methods in Practice.* Princeton, NJ: Princeton University Press.

Poteete, A. R. and E. Ostrom 2004. In pursuit of comparable concepts and data about collective action. *Agricultural Systems* **82**: 215–232.

Ribot, J. C. 2003. Democratic decentralisation of natural resources: Institutional choice and discretionary power transfers in Sub-Saharan Africa. *Public Administration and Development* **23**: 53–65.

Ribot, J. C. and N. L. Peluso 2003. A theory of access. *Rural Sociology* **68**: 153–181.

Ribot, J. C., A. Chhatre, and T. Lankina 2010. Introduction: institutional choice and recognition in the formation and consolidation of local democracy. *Conservation and Society* **6**: 1–11.

Rudel, T. K. 2008. Meta-analyses of case studies: a method for studying regional and global environmental change. *Global Environmental Change* **18**: 18–25.

Schlager, E. and E. Ostrom 1992. Property-rights regimes and natural resources: a conceptual analysis. *Land Economics* **68**: 249–269.

Schoonmaker Freudenberger, M. 1993. Regenerating the gum arabic economy: Local-level resource management in northern Senegal. In J. Friedmann and H. Rangan, eds., *In Defense of Livelihood: Comparative Studies on Environmental Action.* West Hartford, CT: Kumarian Press, pp. 52–78.

Schwartz, K. Z. S. 2006. *Nature and National Identity after Communism*. Pittsburgh, PA: University of Pittsburgh Press.

Sikor, T. and Lund, C. 2009. Access and property: a question of power and authority. *Development and Change* **40**: 1–22.

Young, O. 2002. Institutional interplay: the environmental consequences of cross-scale interactions. In E. Ostrom, T. Dietz, N. Dolsak, *et al.*, eds., *The Drama of the Commons*. Washington, DC: National Academy Press, pp. 263–291.

5

Extreme events, tipping points, and vulnerability: methods in the political economy of environment

ERIC C. JONES

INTRODUCTION

Integrating economic and political perspectives for the purposes of understanding daily life in human ecosystems produces particular methodological challenges for researchers. Many levels of analysis (e.g., individual, group, and other levels of social organization) and many units of analysis (e.g., behaviors, strategies, linguistic status/rank markers) may be present in any given study, and *standard* procedures for examining the political economy of environment are not common. Ecological economics provides a number of standardized analytical approaches, but does not typically address the daily life of individuals, households, and communities, nor does it try to understand "why societies are the way they are" in ecological contexts. "Why societies are the way they are" (whether at micro or macro levels) requires adding the analysis of power; thus, I wanted to conceive of this anthropological approach to economy and ecology as *the political economy of environment*.

For our purposes, the term political economy is intended to conceptualize how human populations create social order through economic production, political prestige, and ideology (Blanton *et al.* 1996). More specifically, it is largely a top-down approach that assumes that elites generally attempt to maintain power at any level of political

Environmental Social Sciences: Methods and Research Design, ed. I. Vaccaro, E. A. Smith and S. Aswani. Published by Cambridge University Press. © Cambridge University Press 2010.

organization. To do so, they focus on some aspect of economic production for which they can control scarcity and value through taxation, storage, access, or production. Often this scarcity involves environmental inputs, such as the mining of precious stones or the storage of grain. Accompanying this economic focus should be a coherent mode of garnering prestige such as via foreign dignitaries or via access to the divine by a god-king. This prestige assures processes of political continuity (e.g., continued recognition by foreign powers of a state's leaders even if they change). Finally, there will also exist a common or dominant ideology that indicates where allegiance and devotion should be directed, such as the tribal focus on kin or a state's focus on gods. These practices are integrated into the daily life of commoners and are also reversely shaped by them. This allegiance helps structure access to productive resources, such as land and other natural resources.

Various techniques allow for an accounting of these foci on production, prestige, and allegiance in contexts where this method is applied to human–environment interactions. Effort to capture the nature of these three components is present in each of the methodologies presented in this chapter. A minimum set of approaches addressed in this chapter includes:

- Human geography models of vulnerability to environmental hazards
- Societal political economic response to major environmental change
- Natural resource dependence and the role of local vs. extra-local resources
- Household livelihood strategies
- Event qualities
- Technological utopianism
- Regional analysis
- Dynamics of commons.

These methodologies are not the only ones available for a political economy of environment, but they are sufficient for a book chapter of this size and they are among ones that have been successfully employed. Systematic and identifiable traditions of data collection and analysis in this field are scarce, resulting in a need here to adapt or systematize the methodologies rather than present them exactly as conducted by researchers. Neither does my presentation of these methodologies necessarily credit long intellectual traditions that have spawned the general approaches and/or, in some cases, initial versions of the actual data collection and analytical techniques. However, the chapter does provide citations from the pieces by which I became familiar with these general approaches, several of which are based on more complete research projects found in *The Political Economy of Hazards and Disasters* (Jones and Murphy 2009).

Often, it is useful to employ these methodologies *in contexts of extreme change* in order to lay out more clearly the political economic aspects of human–environment relations. In describing these tools, I have focused more heavily on political economy than on environment, assuming that the audience is more familiar with conceptualization and measurement of ecological and environmental variables than with political and economic ones.

HUMAN GEOGRAPHY MODELS OF VULNERABILITY TO ENVIRONMENTAL HAZARDS

This section presents two very comprehensive attempts in human geography to integrate and build upon known factors and causal mechanisms for determining a population's risk. Both rely primarily on aggregated population data, such as from government censuses, but both can be improved considerably through survey, observational, or interview data that highlight how elites and commoners understand hazards and how they behave regarding them.

First, a very comprehensive model by Wisner *et al.* (2004; Blaikie *et al.* 1994) has been used conceptually by many hazards scholars. However, their model appears to have been applied systematically to any specific ethnographic case only recently by Anthony Oliver-Smith (2009). Table 5.1 presents the variables that Wisner and colleagues identified for understanding the political economy of vulnerability to environmental hazards and disasters. I have translated their conceptual Pressure and Release Model into a tabular model with greater emphasis on postulating specific relationships between variables. I have not subtracted from nor added to the variables. My goal is to stay true to their insight as to the variables that are important, but also to make these variables more useful for employing methodologically. The Pressure and Release Model basically states that the material in Table 5.1 creates vulnerability, but that actual risk (for disaster) also depends on the environmental hazards that are present and/or possible.

Briefly, Table 5.1 shows that vulnerability to environmental hazards depends mostly on location, preparedness, inappropriate or

Table 5.1 *Factors in a political economy of vulnerability to environmental hazards (adapted from Wisner et al. 2004:51).*

Root causes	Dynamic pressures	Unsafe conditions
Limited access to power (lack of freedom of press/speech, lack of ethical standards in public life)	–	–
Limited access to structures (lack of local markets, lack of local institutions)	Rapid population change, rapid urbanization	Lack of local institutions, unprotected buildings and infrastructure
Limited access to resources (lack of appropriate skills and local investment)	Deforestation, decline in soil productivity	Prevalence of endemic disease, low income levels, livelihoods at risk
Ideology of political and economic systems	Arms expenditure, debt repayment schedules	Lack of disaster preparedness, special groups at risk, dangerous locations

unprotected infrastructure, and on a number of environmental conditions and pressures that negatively affect resource availability.

Insights from Oliver-Smith's (2009) application of the model are enlightening. He compared Hurricane Katrina's impact on New Orleans with Hurricane Mitch's impact on Honduras. Here, in Table 5.2, I populate the prior table with secondary data from Oliver-Smith's narrative analysis of Hurricane Mitch based on research by Stonich (1992) and Winograd (2009). I do not include his analysis of New Orleans due to space limitations, but I encourage the comparative approach, too.

Root causes in the left column are the same in both Table 5.1 and Table 5.2. Dynamic pressures develop out of these root causes, and the dynamic pressures can result in unsafe conditions. Oliver-Smith's post-facto analysis of vulnerability for Honduras pre-Hurricane Mitch displays the utility of Wisner and colleagues' framework, resulting in very close matches between the theoretical (Table 5.1) and the empirical (Table 5.2) cases. A political economy analysis of non-traditional agricultural export (rather than arms export of debt payments as in the general model) depicts a specific arrangement of ideology, prestige,

Table 5.2 *Application of Wisner* et al. *(2004) hazard vulnerability methodology to pre-Hurricane Mitch Honduras using data from Oliver-Smith (2009).*

Root causes	Dynamic pressures	Unsafe conditions
Limited access to power (lack of freedom of press/ speech, lack of ethical standards in public life)	–	Lack of transparency in government
Limited access to structures (lack of local markets, lack of local institutions)	Population displacement, rapid urbanization	Lack of power in local institutions
Limited access to resources (lack of appropriate skills and local investment)	Intensification of land use resulting in degradation (over half of land in use at risk of landslide, drought; half of land in use also at risk of flooding)	Increased malaria, diarrhea and parasitic diseases; 70 percent of preschool children malnourished; 4th lowest GDP in Latin America; 80 percent of population below poverty level
Ideology of political and economic systems	Non-traditional agricultural exports	Dangerous locations on newly occupied hillsides and low-lying areas

and production engaged by elites. In general, pressures of land degradation and population displacement can produce disaster when coupled with limited local power, limited transparency in national governmental activities, poverty, living in dangerous areas, plus the presence of a hurricane or other hazard. Oliver-Smith suggests using this approach to understand vulnerability in growing coastal cities *before exposure* to a hazard agent. He also suggests finding ways to incorporate the potential of human agency into this methodology.

Another relatively holistic approach regarding vulnerability to hazards is the Hazards-of-Place Model of Vulnerability (Cutter 1996). The model basically dichotomizes geographic context (elevation and proximity) and social fabric (experience, perception, and built

Table 5.3 *Dimensions of social vulnerability for studying environmental hazards.*

Variable	Measure proposed by Cutter *et al.* (2003)	% variation accounted for (Cutter *et al.* 2003)
Personal wealth	per capita income	12.4
Age	median age	11.9
Density of the built environment	commercial establishments per square mile	11.2
Single-sector economic dependence	% employed in extractive industries	8.6
Housing stock and tenancy	% of units that are mobile homes	7.0
Race/ethnicity	% African American, Hispanic, Native American, Asian	19.1
Occupation	% in service occupations	3.2
Infrastructure dependence	% employed in transportation, communication and public utilities	2.9

environment) as two aspects of vulnerability. A more recent attempt to quantify the social fabric aspects of the model was conducted by Cutter, Boruff, and Shirley (2003) via a factor analysis of 42 relevant variables. In their new Social Vulnerability Index (SoVI), eight variables accounted for 76 percent of the variation in social vulnerability among all 3141 counties in the USA, as seen in Table 5.3. Data to be collected for this methodology could involve any metric that addresses the broad variables, such as those in the measure column used by Cutter and colleagues.

The conceptual approach of this model is similar to that of Wisner and colleagues, which is an attempt to integrate sociocultural and biophysical variables relevant to vulnerability.[1] Attempts to apply this model in actual hazard settings have proven more messy and

---

[1] Another holistic political economic approach to hazards from the field of human geography/anthropology is the Cascade of Impacts Model utilized by Whiteford and Tobin (2009).

preliminary than ideal (e.g., Azar and Rain 2007; Cutter *et al.* 2006; Piegorsch *et al.* 2007), and ethnographic work is often a necessary compliment to the model for local settings. However, it is clear that political decisions about housing density, other zoning issues, and support of certain economic sectors like extraction or utilities are coupled with the economic experiences of individuals of certain races, occupations, wealth levels, and ages to produce vulnerability. While the approach is not overtly political economic due to a lack of focus on political factors and on roles of governing elites, these political and economic factors are indeed part of a larger process of societal adaptation to local, regional, and global conditions – and this adaptation is guided by governing elites, as discussed in the next methodology.

SOCIETAL POLITICAL ECONOMIC RESPONSE TO MAJOR
ENVIRONMENTAL CHANGE

In terms of cross-cultural research, a typology used by Blanton *et al.* (1996) is extended here to understand how a society might react to a natural disaster based on its political economic orientation. Specifically, this methodology investigates how societal elites alter political efforts, ideological foci, and access to production in response to stability and instability caused by disasters and hazards, including weather and climate changes. However, for polity longevity, some kind of balance must be achieved between the decision-makers (the governing elite) and the larger populace (the commoners), as goods are produced, decisions are made, and life is made to be meaningful.

Based on their research and a review of literature, Blanton *et al.* (1996) make a distinction between two general but coherent and common political economic strategies that structure formal and informal institutions in the rise and fall of governing elites throughout Classic Period Mesoamerica. These two strategies are: (1) exclusionary, and (2) corporate, with the distinctions perhaps holding up better in pre-modern contexts than modern ones – although elite adherents of one system commonly employ strategies associated with the other societal type. Table 5.4 provides a general comparison of the two political economic types.

This technique is for coding general political economic strategy of elites in a society for which ethnographic information exists. These strategies need not be applied to ecological questions, but in this case it is used to examine long-term interplay between human systems and biophysical environments – specifically how political economic

Table 5.4 *A general comparison of corporate and exclusionary polities (adapted from Blanton et al. 1996).*

Society	Economic focus of elite control	Focus of ideology regarding allegiance	Political style	Example
Corporate	public goods	cosmological order	insular	Inka
Exclusionary	prestige goods	filial responsibility	international	Early Aztec

orientation is related to the level of exposure of societies to disaster cross-culturally. Any ethnographic source, whether article or book, can be used as the basis for coding. Much of this kind of research is done using the Human Relations Area Files repository of ethnographic manuscripts along with the related Outline of Cultural Materials (OCM) that provides a numeric code helpful in finding information relevant to the questions. For example, the presence of OCM 731 indicates that disasters are discussed on a given page(s) in the manuscript. Word searches and creative use of the OCM are necessary to comprehensively scan a manuscript for relevant materials for coding.

Coding societal political economic types (Blanton *et al.* 1996)

Exclusionary strategy

1. Control of labor, material and marriage exchange through polygyny, gender hierarchy, multi-generational extended households, clanship (ranked descent groups or conical clans), tribal formation, or other forms of patrimonial rhetoric
2. Elite control of production, exchange, and consumption of valuable/prestige goods
   - difficult to obtain exotic goods, substitute food, or other items in intergroup exchange systems, easier to monopolize rare goods
     - goods produced through complex technologies

- technological innovation for prestige goods rather than basic goods
- elite control of raw materials and production of prestige goods link the elite to common households as households incorporate exotic goods into exchange systems
- fluidity, competitiveness, emphasis on individual skills

3. International style
    • multinational culture between groups where competing networks also participate in cross cultural exchanges and reaffirm their positions vis-à-vis their own networks (because other networks also have rare goods)
    • missions and emissaries sent back and forth, legitimating roles as rulers
    • graphic representations of rulers
    • warfare, personal wealth, princely burials (rank distinction in burials).

Corporate strategy

1. Elite control of household agricultural production or production of staples
    • highly developed political structures without prestige goods systems
    • taxed staple goods (staple finance)
2. Cognitive orientation of solidarity and interdependence
    • specific, often hierarchical roles and statuses reduce competition and individual achievement
    • relative egalitarianism, despite hierarchy or defined statuses
    • fertility, renewal of society and cosmos in ritual and collective representations
    • graphic representations of renewal of society and cosmos
    • ethnically disparate subgroups included in society
    • patrimonial rhetoric transcended/obviated
    • communal cemeteries
    • impressive public works.

Coding criteria

99 – Missing (data available but did not code)
 0 – data not available
 1 – exclusionary society

2 – corporate society

3 – mixed exclusionary and corporate.

Quality of codes

1.   There are clear analytical statements by the author directly relat-
      ing to aspects of exclusionary orientation (patrimonial rhetoric,
      prestige goods, international style) or corporate orientation
      (public goods, communal ideology)
2.   There are clear descriptions of examples of what you the coder
      would consider exclusionary or corporate behaviors
3.   Descriptions of examples are partial.

Data Format

I set up a data file/spreadsheet/database in an appropriate database/
spreadsheet application with the parameters shown in Table 5.5. All
societies in the sample, with or without relevant data were included. I
analyzed only societies with relevant data using simple cross-tabs and
Chi-square measure of association.

In my pilot study, political economic orientation is the dependent variable and exposure to disasters/hazards is the independent
variable. I am lucky in that I got disaster codes from both Ember and
Ember (1992) and Justinger (1978).[2] However, relying on the codes of
others means I cannot control the exact criteria for coding, since it
has already been done. Having two sources is very helpful, as the two
sources agreed almost all of the time for the societies that overlap in
their samples. I dichotomized societies into high and low exposure to
disasters. Ember and Ember's codes were for recentness of incidence
of food-destroying natural disasters, and Justinger's codes were for
fear of disaster or having had a recent disaster. When codes did not
agree, I went to the electronic Human Relations Area Files to ascertain
the level of disaster exposure for the limited geographic area in which
our political economic code came from. I used at least five excerpts/
citations from each relevant ethnography in the Human Relations
Area Files before coding a society. A minimum of three ethnographies
in agreement were used per society. Of course, these societies are not

---

[2] These sources should be referred to for coding procedures for exposure to natural
disasters.

Table 5.5 *Sample data collection spreadsheet for societal political economic orientation.*

Society and time period	Author/ date/ page(s)	Political economic code	Quality of code	OCM or key word used	Notes/quotes
Klamath	Stern T. 1965 p. 96	1	2	61*	"Thus members of the Pelican Bay band sometimes shared foodstuffs"

* indicates all possible digits (0–9) to follow preceding number; in this case 610–619.

unchanging, and thus ethnographies are snapshots. I did not include the disaster code in this table so that my students and I would not have prior knowledge of which society had what level of disasters – thus avoiding a bias in coding that could come from attempting to assure predicted correlation.

How do corporate societies structure disaster vulnerability and recovery? Corporate societies structure vulnerability and resilience through: (1) strict hierarchy of role and responsibility yet often relative egalitarianism, (2) an ideological commitment to all in society, and (3) using food production to maintain that hierarchy and that commitment. The Amhara of East Africa (Ethiopia) fit the proposed pattern; they face very few disasters and thus are not forced to make a class of people vulnerable to disasters through geography, access to resources, etc. It is perhaps this stability that allows corporate societies to flourish.

How do exclusionary societies structure vulnerability and resilience? They (1) nurture connections to people with power, including through diplomacy to legitimate internal authority, (2) encourage an ideological commitment to everyone in a family/clan, and (3) use prestige goods to create social status. The Trobrianders of Papua New Guinea in Oceania/western Melanesia are an exclusionary society that experiences frequent disasters and food instability. Their ways of dealing with disaster and insecurity in terms of an exclusionary political economic orientation include indebting their neighbors to them through gifting, and including the trade of food along with the ritual trade of preciosities. The focus of exclusionary societies generally is not on investing in the skills and education of youth, but expecting young people to learn the finesse of trade and diplomacy through trial and error. Corporate and exclusionary societies face similar challenges in many cases, but also distinct challenges as a result of the ways they organize production and construe meaning in community life.

NATURAL RESOURCE DEPENDENCE AND THE ROLE OF LOCAL VERSUS EXTRA-LOCAL RESOURCES

A mix of local and extra-local resources is typically necessary to deal with ecological insecurity and environmental change. Drought, collapse of natural resource markets, etc., all require local fortitude and ingenious adaptation but also external resources in order to sustain population and lifeways in the face of such ecological disturbance or fluctuation. This approach seeks to identify how local and extra-local resources are engaged to maintain households and communities that are dependent on natural resources.

Dyer (2009) discusses a continuum of response to environmental hazards and disasters that ranges from one extreme – a downward spiral in which a natural resource-based community receives no external support and possesses relatively little internal financial resources – to another extreme in which a community does not have its important natural resources destroyed; also, at this extreme, the community does receive considerable external support for local efforts at recovery (see Figure 5.1).

Taking these continua as a framework, the objectives of this methodology are to help ascertain local dependence on natural resources and the degree to which external support (e.g., federal assistance, massive charity) is available and likely. This methodology need not be applied to disasters or hazards, but can be used to understand the degree to which major changes from whatever sector might play out for local communities, and/or why things play out the way they do in situations of environmental change and in contexts where communities depend on natural resources. Table 5.6 displays the kinds of data useful for this approach.

Another useful methodology – perhaps one that could be used in concert with the Dyer approach to arrive at more fine-tuned results regarding survival potential of natural-resource dependent communities – is provided by Nelson and Finan (2009) in their study of drought in northeastern Brazil. In two communities, they characterized each

Natural Resource dependent; outside support available. MODERATE VULNERABILITY	Not dependent on natural resources; outside support available. MINIMAL VULNERABILITY
Natural resource dependent; outside support not available. MAXIMUM VULNERABILITY	Not dependent on natural resources; outside support not available. MODERATE VULNERABILITY

Figure 5.1   Matrix of dependence on natural resources and availability of outside help (adapted from Dyer 2009).

household's non-farm income as primarily climate-neutral (e.g., jobs in government, commerce, and non-agricultural labor), climate-sensitive (e.g., agricultural labor) or coming from social transfers (e.g., pensions), in addition to relative household reliance on sales of crops and livestock.

Vulnerability to drought at the household level was measured by the degree to which the households would suffer if they lost all of their climate-sensitive income: the most vulnerable are those falling below the Brazilian indigence line if they lost all climate-sensitive income; the moderately vulnerable would fall below the poverty line; and the least vulnerable would remain above the poverty line even if losing all climate-sensitive income. Sale of crops and livestock plays the role of buffer for the short term for many families, but overexploitation and/ or significant depletion of herd sizes can result in greater vulnerability (i.e., smaller buffer for next time). Their study was longitudinal, and thus comparisons were made over time in terms of the degree of vulnerability, as well as in terms of the point at which the Brazilian government would step in to avoid disaster, i.e., irrevocable negative changes to households and livelihoods. While the Brazilian and state governments averted disaster and typically tend to do so for the case of drought, the methodology helps indicate how vulnerable certain sectors of the economy are to environmental fluctuation. Drought need not be the focus, but any climate-sensitive, weather-sensitive, or environmentally sensitive source of income can be evaluated for degree of vulnerability. The next approach similarly focuses on the

Table 5.6 *Data collection for dependence on natural resources methodology.*

Variable	Example measures
Dependence on natural resources	% employed in extractive/natural resource/agricultural industries;
	% value of economic product from extractive industries;
	% value of economic product from adding value to extractive products;
	# of extractive industries and distribution of employment and economic activity across those industries
	nature of alternatives to reliance on any specific extractive industry or extractive industries in general
Availability of outside help	# of local branches of regional/national/international not-for-profit organizations/agencies (e.g., Catholic Church, United Way, office of state Department of Fish and Game, Lion's Club) per capita;
	nature of involvement of branches and outside organizations in community/civic activities, particularly those related to either environment (e.g., tree planting, erosion control) or employment (e.g., job training programs, support of unions)

household for determining environmental vulnerability but also likely environmental behaviors.

HOUSEHOLD LIVELIHOOD STRATEGIES

Another political economic approach to understanding the vulnerability of households is to characterize the role of the household in the local economy. This general approach comes from Wallerstein and Smith (1992), who create a dynamic typology, similar to Nelson and Finan's (2009) above, in which households move up and down in the economy based on world and regional economic changes.[3] These groups

---

[3] Wallerstein and Smith (1992) argue that the role of households may be overemphasized in some contexts (especially pre- and proto-capitalist periods) but, rather, extended families or communities take on a majority of the activities involved in production and reproduction.

Table 5.7 *Core and periphery household activities in phases of economic expansion and contraction (Wallerstein and Smith 1992).*

	Basic household income/ subsistence activities	Activities under economic expansion	Activities under economic contraction
Core households	Combination of wages and do-it-yourself activities	Increased wages, decreased do-it-yourself purchases/ activities	Increased reliance on transfer payments, on do-it-yourself activities in short-term (long-term loss of tools/capacity to do so)
Peripheral households	Combination of wages, petty market operations, and subsistence activities; usually insufficient resources to acquire do-it-yourself equipment (e.g., tools, appliances)	Increased wages; transformation of subsistence activities into petty market operations (e.g., crops for sale); occasional acquisition of do-it-yourself resources	Reduction of wage-based income, increased reliance on non-agricultural petty market operations plus increased time spent on subsistence activities where possible

of households embrace predictable strategies as they face specific patterns of constraint and opportunity (see Table 5.7). Specifically, since wages are insufficient for providing all household needs for all but the most wealthy elite households – the true proletariat is able to cover all expenses with wages – worker households rely on self-provisioning/ subsistence activities (e.g., home garden, making own dresses), transfer payments (e.g., social security, welfare), do-it-yourself activities (e.g., washing clothes in own washer and dryer, installing own light fixtures), and petty market operations (e.g., making Christmas ornaments for sale, sale of contraband).

The utility of this political economic typology for human–environment research is that it shows how various subsets of the population change their behaviors under economic expansion and contraction and, thus, the nature of pressures that might be put on biophysical environments. Examples include major demands on non-sustainable lumber sourced by do-it-yourself home improvement stores, or increased purchases of pesticides for new home gardeners unfamiliar with non-chemical means of pest control. Table 5.8 presents potential measures for this methodology, and highlights environmental contexts in which it might be useful.

EVENT QUALITIES

Somewhat reminiscent in structure of the approach of the technique on societal response to major environmental change, this methodology is based on the concept that each non-human phenomenon can be measured in terms of duration, intensity and regularity. In other words, a drought or tornado or fish population decline are short/long, intense/mild, and predictable/unpredictable. As such, we expect that human interaction with such phenomena will vary in patterned ways.

Event quality has been conceived of in sociology as a relatively qualitative approach (Kroll-Smith and Couch 1991). However, this approach to general environmental conditions also builds conceptually on quantitative approaches from ecology (Colwell 1974).[4] An example of the latter is from Cohen (1999), who showed in an analysis of several dozen rain-fed agricultural societies that rainfall predictability and variability was associated with the degree to which vertical modes of information transition were utilized for teaching younger members of society about agriculture practices. Cohen's work does not discuss political economy per se, but does associate

---

[4] I should note that this approach is similar conceptually to the culture core of Steward (1955). However, rather than debating the utility of environmental determinism, it is important to clearly state the assumptions and concepts necessary to move forward: in this case, one assumption is that humans have a limited number of sufficiently efficient/sustainable and culturally relevant adaptations to any given suite of environmental parameters; the necessary concepts are contingency, constancy, and predictability.

Table 5.8 *Measures for household livelihood strategies in expanding/contracting economies.*

Household income/subsistence	Example measures	Potentially relevant environmental contexts, including interactions between multiple household strategies
Wages	Yearly income; monthly income; weekly income; predominance of salaries vs. hourly/daily vs. piece rate	Declining income may result in increased exploitation via petty market operations and potentially wasteful do-it-yourself efforts; type of wage indicates degree of centralization/decentralization regarding kind of extraction/exploitation
Petty market operations	Per capita yard sales; change in small-scale vegetable sales in open markets; homemade diapers on online auction sites	Increased/decreased local agricultural production; sourcing of cheap materials potentially containing toxins or produced unsustainably; sourcing of organic and chemical-free materials by petty market operators since larger companies will not fill niche
Subsistence activities/self-provisioning	Retail fabric sales for making own garments; per capita or % home gardens; decrease in restaurant visits	Overuse of pesticides and fertilizers in home gardens; use of contaminated soils for growing food; increased demand for organic retail fabrics; decrease in cultivation of specialty crops/animals
Do-it-yourself	Growth of home improvement stores per capita; decrease in use of contractors, plumbers, etc.	Increased sourcing of unsustainable timber; reuse of lumber or bricks from old houses/barns/buildings
Transfer payments	Welfare; pensions; charities	Demand for higher economic return on pensions, resulting in unsustainable practices aimed at profit; increase in welfare payments increases economic capability to make environmentally sound purchases; potential bias against environmental charities when social charities are more needed

cultural behaviors regarding food production with environmental constancy and contingency.

Colwell's (1974) formulas for examining constancy and contingency are derived as below. Time must be divided into equal increments (e.g., Cohen used 12 months in a year), and the number and range-values of states must be specified. For example, Cohen calculated evapotranspiration rates using Hargreaves' (Hargreaves and Samani 1982) method requiring day of year, latitude, and temperature; Cohen delineated three evapotranspiration states: insufficient rainfall; sufficient rainfall for plant growth but not soil moisture; and sufficient rainfall for plant growth and soil moisture. Table 5.9 presents data in a sample format (frequency matrix or contingency table) that can be plugged into the following formulas, where t is the number of columns (times within a cycle) and s is the number of rows (states of the observed phenomenon). The first three formulas provide results that are then used to derive the measures of uncertainty in the next three equations, which are then used to create measures of predictability, constancy and contingency in the last three of the following equations (Colwell 1974).

Column totals are defined as $X_j = \Sigma_{i=1}^{s} N_{ij}$,

row totals are defined as $Y_i = \Sigma_{j=1}^{t} N_{ij}$,

and the grand total is defined as,

$$Z = \Sigma_i \Sigma_j N_{ij} = \Sigma_j Y_j = \Sigma_i Y_i,$$

such that uncertainty with respect to time is

$$H(X) = -\Sigma_{j=1}^{t} X \frac{X_j}{Z} \log \frac{X_j}{Z}$$

and uncertainty with respect to state is

$$H(Y) = -\Sigma_{i=1}^{s} Y \frac{Y_j}{Z} \log \frac{Y_j}{Z}$$

and uncertainty under the interaction of time and state is

$$H(XY) = -\Sigma_i \Sigma_j \frac{N_{ij}}{Z} \log \frac{N_{ij}}{Z}.$$

Table 5.9 * Sample calculation table of predictability, constancy and contingency for a ten year period. Raw data are monthly totals for the years 1951–1960 taken from World Weather Records for the Luguru culture located at 8° S, 38° E; Station Dar Es Salaam, Tanzania (US Weather Bureau, Washington, DC).

Rain	Jan	Feb	Mar	Apr	May	Jun	Jul	Aug	Sep	Oct	Nov	Dec
1 (Inadequate)						1	1	1	1			
2 (Plant growth but no soil moisture)	2					1	1	2	1		1	
3 (Adequate)	8	10	10	10	10	8	8	7	8	10	9	10

* Table from Cohen (1999). Constancy = 0.19; contingency = 0.26; predictability = 0.45.

Finally, predictability $(P = C + M)$ is

$$P = 1 - \frac{H_x(Y)}{\log s} = 1 - \frac{H(XY) - H(X)}{\log s},$$

constancy is $C = 1 - \dfrac{H(Y)}{\log s}$,

and contingency is $M = \dfrac{H(X) + H(Y) - H(XY)}{\log s}$.

As shown above, Cohen (1999) used rainfall and temperature to produce evapotranspiration rates, but other examples of measures might include:

- Daily availability of irrigation water in the case of irrigated agriculture, where effectiveness and productivity of irrigation management is thought to be a function of regularity and variability of irrigation availability
- Monthly fish counts for different rivers, where variation within a region between local traditions of reciprocity, gifting, and in organization might be associated with regularity and variability in fish availability in addition, perhaps, to the degree or amount of fish available
- Weekly levels of pest infestation in the case that informal rules governing access to a resource are associated with other stresses on the resources.

Many non-political economy uses of this technique are imaginable, but the challenge is to apply this technique in ways that the dependent variable incorporates the control of production, the foci of allegiance, and the traditional modes of accessing prestige in a human ecosystem.

TECHNOLOGICAL UTOPIANISM

Perhaps the most important book in the last few decades on political economy of environment is Hornborg's (2001) *The Power of the Machine*. Although all the chapters had been published previously as peer-reviewed articles, the book carefully analyzes where Marx and H. T. Odum went wrong analytically in explaining the human condition, i.e., their insistence that the value/price of goods reflect the actual labor and environmental costs of producing those goods is normative theory, not predictive of how people behave. Hornborg proposes that human fetish for technology combined with all-purpose money (i.e., fetishized money, or Marx's D form of exchange, such as dollar bills, metal alloy coins, or credit cards) provides fertile ground for economic growth that at some point is unsustainable economically and environmentally due to the limits of human consumption and the limited ability of the biophysical environment to support exploitation and pollution. According to Hornborg, industrial capitalism's efforts toward growth and concomitant accumulation of wealth would not be sustained without the ubiquity of all-purpose money.

Leaving to one side *The Machine*'s broad claims about industrial capitalism, one objective here is to understand what forms of compensation are available in addition to the existence of wages paid with all-purpose money. Following this objective allows investigation of the extent to which local forms of reciprocity can be supported, and thus the degree to which local human–environment interactions are buffered against external forces or even rapid local rearrangement that may be unsustainable. However, since industrial capitalism must co-exist with other forms of exchange – in order to access surplus and make use of procedures for expropriating surplus – it is necessary to examine the relationship between the tendencies of capitalism and local modes of exchange and reciprocity.

Relatedly, a second objective of this methodology is to make sure that the human obsession with tools and new technology – the "fetishization of the machine" – is not ignored. Humans are toolmakers and tool fetishizers. Tools allow for concentration of productive activities and thus likely concentration of wealth and perhaps even transfer of wealth between sectors of society. Of course, this concentration of wealth potentiates greater tool production, and transfer of wealth from one part of society to another typically reduces local autonomy over exploitation and can compromise the appropriateness of exploitation for local needs.

At base, the process of economic development is typically one in which external factors have greater influence than a community on the flow of resources in that community. As a result of the lack of weight of local traditions of reciprocity, exchange, prestige, and social sanctions, the process of development typically forces communities to oppose one another and, within communities, for community groups to oppose one another as they seek external resources (e.g., charity, development money, publicity, investment).

This same process of intercommunity competition for resources is a factor in David Harvey's (1985) "spatial fix" in which the lowest costs of doing business (or development or charity) are sought geographically.

The net transfer of wealth from one sector of society is assured by people's evaluations that support a certain rate of exchange. Those who accumulate and those who produce surplus that is accumulated by others engage in a system of beliefs that support the process of accumulation. One common characteristic of belief systems associated with accumulation (and some other belief systems, as well) is the presence of hope or expectation about the "Power of the Machine" to solve the wide variety of problems faced by society. People with more and people with less do not always believe in the same use of tools, although often they do. For example, industrial capitalists and most farmers (even in developing countries) and even many farm laborers believe tractors to be an important part of a stable and productive agriculture. However, in a another example, while logging companies in Indonesia that do illegal logging (and their investors) want better skidders, delimbers, and harvesters, regulators want DNA testing of forests and lumber to show which trees are illegally harvested. Thus, local villages are caught in a battle of external forces over the promise of technology.

My indications for the application of this technique remain general. In studies of development, particularly of conservation and development, attention should be given to the following:

- Major tenets of the belief system ascribed to by various sectors of society – particularly have-mores and have-lesses – regarding the promise of technology, and where these tenets overlap and where they do not overlap
- Degree to which non-monetary compensation, exchange and reciprocity exist and ways in which they might remain viable vis-à-vis external forces
- Sources of tension between groups affected by impacts of or seeking the benefits of development, charity, publicity, etc.

REGIONAL ANALYSIS AND LOCAL-GLOBAL DYNAMICS

Many academic traditions of regional analysis exist, although the ideas for this technique are drawn from survey archaeology and landscape archaeology. My goal with the presentation of this methodology is to account for the dynamics of political economy across regions while accounting for both household/community activities as well as external pressures concerning food production and resource extraction. The focus on external pressures echoes the prior methodology on Technological Utopianism. Most of the ideas for regional analysis stem from a theoretical framework that assumes that centralized authority in the form of states or kingdoms is not necessary for sophisticated and widespread intensive agricultural practices to develop (Perez Rodriguez 2008), or for regional surpluses to be accumulated and thus considerable status differentiation to occur (Håkansson 2008).

In one sense, this begins as a bottom-up approach by initially assuming that states are not responsible for the initial development of wealth accumulation or intensive production practices in the archeological and ethnohistorical records. Nonetheless, it is useful to then start from the top down by studying how global or extraregional processes subsequently incorporate and alter local and regional practices. Application of the methodology need not be directed only at historic and prehistoric cases, but this method of describing local and regional dynamics of accumulation, prestige making, and allegiance, and then placing those in a broader context, can be applied to contemporary societies and populations that are undergoing change (or likely will undergo change) due to external forces. The building blocks of this approach are:

- The extent to which local leaders have access to local labor
- The mechanisms by which local labor is made accessible and reliable (e.g., prestige, offices, payment in money or gifts, access to land, water, and other resources, marriage)
- The degree to which intra-regional specialization exists such that several occupations (e.g., herding, crop growing, metal working, salt production; see Håkansson 2008) can accrue surplus through exchange/trading. In Håkansson's eighteenth century Tanzania case, all of these occupations ultimately are trying to increase wealth by acquiring cattle for prestige, productivity, and allegiance (i.e., lineage along with marriage and other ritual and allegiance-oriented activities)
- As with the Technological Utopianism methodology, there is a focus on the degree to which external forces push toward

exchange homogenization – Håkansson's example is the ivory trade in late precolonial and colonial Tanzania

- The degree to which households can realistically produce observed production without coercion by the state or without external demand
- The ways in which decrease in one area of exploitation (e.g., cattle herding) can be countered in another area of exploitation (e.g., agriculture) by incorporating those who left the former
- How local processes of prestige making, reciprocity, and exchange fit into a regional economic system
- How regional modes of accumulation (e.g., tribute, plunder, exchange, gift exchange of prestige goods) are incorporated into broader or global processes of accumulation.

DYNAMICS OF THE COMMONS

For the purpose of this research methodology, Trawick's (2008) research on irrigation management in Peru provides a very accessible set of variables. Many very good works are available on the commons and I necessarily omit them, including various works by Elinor Ostrom. Table 5.10 provides a list of the main variables along with explanations and example measures.

These variables should be couched in a larger framework that includes causal links, such as offered in Jones (2003; see Figure 5.2). Figure 5.2 presents a graphic model of the common pool resource use, but not solely using variables like those above. Rather, the Figure 5.2 model presents a larger context and a set of causal relationships provided by Ostrom's (1992) very concise and accessible presentation of commons dynamics and outcomes, specifically the origins, performance, and survival of common pool resource management activities. Thus, in addition to seeking greater clarity in linkages between commons variables from Table 5.10, the researcher also would benefit from carefully delineating the three main panels of Figure 5.2, which are resource users, resource management institution (however formal or informal), and external factors.

I have also studied environmental commons using network analysis in order to ascertain potential fissures in commons management (Jones 2004). Johnson (this volume) provides methodological guidance on the use of network methodologies for human-environment interactions.

Table 5.10 *Variables for understanding opportunities and constraints of commons (variables and explanations adapted from Trawick 2008).*

Variable	Explanation of ideal condition for effective commons management	Example consequences of variation in conditions
Scarcity	Moderately low per capita abundance of resource or good	Greater scarcity increases importance of compliance and transparency, as well as efficiency of distribution
Autonomy	Local users control access and maintenance	Greater autonomy provides congruency with local customs and ability to adapt system to local needs
Degree of hierarchy in access	Social status does not corfer greater access	Lack of social privilege for access decreases opportunities for free-riding, increases likelihood of fulfilling responsibilities, and increases general commitment due to perceived fairness
Proportionality/equitability in rights and duties	The more inputs by a person/group, the more access	Greatest overall fairness is perceived if a person with more resources both contributes proportionally more to the commons and has greater proportional access to the commons; greater efficiency is achieved this way, also, since likelihood of larger contributions to the commons is increased
Uniformity in frequency of access	All users expected to access resource at the established regular frequency	Decreased commitment to management plus increased conflict if frequency is chaotic or users not each given their regular turn
Regularity and stability of boundaries	User group, resource and rules are well defined and not frequently changing	Changing user group makes it difficult to use informal mechanisms of control; ill-defined boundaries make non-compliance difficult to detect and sanction
Transparency	High visibility of the frequency and amount of use by all users	Low transparency makes detection of cheats difficult
Justness, graduation and enforcement of sanctions	The existence and the will to enforce sanctions that are fair and that increase with gravity of offense	Lack of enforcement may decrease compliance; unfair sanctions usually punish those without power and cause defection

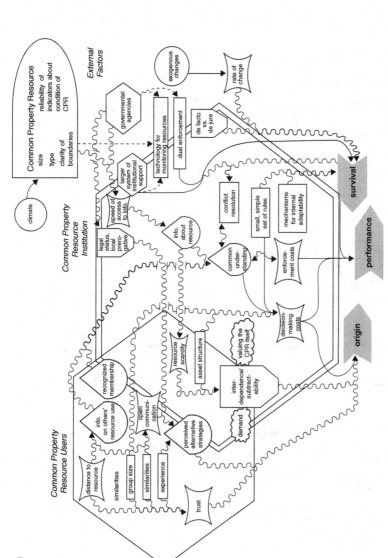

(a)

Figure 5.2 (a) A graphical model of Ostrom's (1992) origins, survival, and performance of common-property institutions (Jones 2003). Reproduced by permission of the Journal of Ecological Anthropology. (b) Key to human ecosystems models (1998 Georgia Journal of Ecological Anthropology, original publication of the key) is based on H. T. Odum (1983) and conventions established by the Information Ecology Group, Department of Anthropology, University of Georgia.

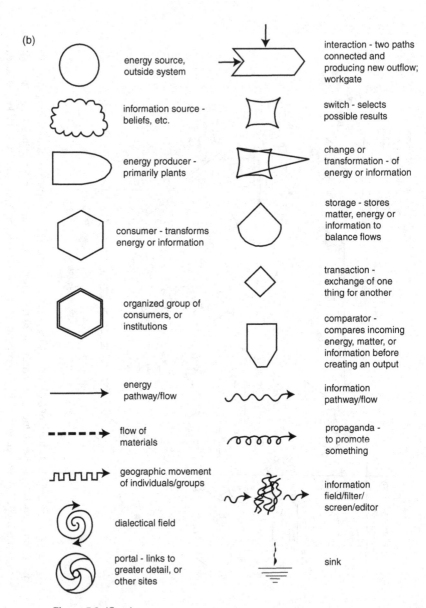

(b)

energy source, outside system

information source - beliefs, etc.

energy producer - primarily plants

consumer - transforms energy or information

organized group of consumers, or institutions

energy pathway/flow

flow of materials

geographic movement of individuals/groups

dialectical field

portal - links to greater detail, or other sites

interaction - two paths connected and producing new outflow; workgate

switch - selects possible results

change or transformation - of energy or information

storage - stores matter, energy or information to balance flows

transaction - exchange of one thing for another

comparator - compares incoming energy, matter, or information before creating an output

information pathway/flow

propaganda - to promote something

information field/filter/screen/editor

sink

Figure 5.2 (Cont.)

SUMMARY OF THE POLITICAL ECONOMIC METHOD
IN HUMAN–ENVIRONMENT STUDIES

The varied techniques for measuring and studying political economic factors in environmental research that account for daily life attempt to highlight the relationship between elite focus on production, expected mode of allegiance, and political style. Taken together, these factors provide insight into how both elites and commoners interact with the biophysical environment, whether as groups or individuals, in normal times or crises, or in the context of broader externally induced change.

As part of a suite of methods focused on ethnographic aspects of human ecosystems or human experience of the biophysical environment, the goal of the political economic method is to understand the social structuring of access to and use of elements in the biophysical environment. Additionally, an improved systematization of analytical techniques should help in addressing issues of sustainability, natural resource management, and development.

REFERENCES

Azar, D. and D. Rain 2007. Identifying population vulnerable to hydrological hazards in San Juan, Puerto Rico. *GeoJournal* **69**(1/2): 23–43.

Blaikie, P. T., I. D. Cannon, and B. Wisner 1994. *At Risk: Natural Hazards, People's Vulnerability, and Disasters*. London: Routledge.

Blanton, R. E., G. M. Feinman, S. A. Kowaleski, and P. N. Peregrine 1996. A dual-processual theory for the evolution of Mesoamerican civilization. *Current Anthropology* **37**: 1–14.

Cohen, M. 1999. Evaluating cross-cultural patterns in the transmission of information: an evolutionary approach. Unpublished MA thesis, University of California at Davis.

Colwell, R. K. 1974. Predictability, constancy and contingency of periodic phenomena. *Ecology* **55**: 1148–1153.

Cutter, S. L., 1996. Vulnerability to environmental hazards. *Progress in Human Geography* **20**(4): 529–539.

Cutter, S. L., B. J. Boruff, and W. L. Shirley 2003. Social vulnerability to environmental hazards. *Social Science Quarterly* **84**(2): 242–260.

Cutter, S. L., C. T. Emrich, J. T. Mitchell, *et al.* 2006. The long road home: race, class, and recovery from Hurricane Katrina. *Environment* **48**(2): 8–20.

Dyer, C. L. 2009. From the phoenix effect to punctuated entropy: the culture of response as a unifying paradigm of disaster mitigation and recovery. In E. C. Jones and A. D. Murphy, eds., *The Political Economy of Hazards and Disasters*. Lanham, MD: AltaMira Press, pp. 313–336.

Ember, C. R. and M. Ember 1992. Warfare, aggression, and resource problems: cross-cultural codes. *Cross-Cultural Research* **26**(1–4): 169–226.

Georgia Journal of Ecological Anthropology 1998. Key to ecosystem models. *Georgia Journal of Ecological Anthropology* **2**(1): 5.

Håkansson, N. T. 2008. The decentralized landscape: regional wealth and the expansion of production in Northern Tanzania before the eve of colonialism. In L. Cliggett and C. A. Pool, eds., *Economies and Transformation of Landscape.* Lanham, MD: AltaMira Press, pp. 239–265.

Hargreaves, G. H. and Z. A. Samani 1982. Estimating potential evapotranspiration. *Journal of Irrigation and Drainage Engineering* **108**(3): 225–230.

Harvey, D. 1985. The geopolitics of capitalism. In D. Gregory and J. Urry, eds., *Social Relations and Spatial Structures.* New York: St. Martin's Press, pp. 128–163.

Hornborg, A. 2001. *The Power of the Machine: Global Inequalities of Economy, Technology, and Environment.* Lanham, MD: AltaMira Press.

Jones, E. C. 2003. Building on Ostrom's 'The rudiments of a theory of the origins, survival, and performance of common-property institutions.' *Journal of Ecological Anthropology* **7**: 65–72.

Jones, E. C. 2004. Wealth-based trust and the development of collective action. *World Development* **32**(4): 691–711.

Jones, E. C., and A. D. Murphy, eds. 2009. *The Political Economy of Hazards and Disasters.* Lanham, MD: AltaMira Press.

Justinger, J. M. 1978. Reaction to change: a holocultural test of some theories of religious movements. Ann Arbor, University Microfilms, no 7817047. State University of New York at Buffalo, Dissertation, Anthropology.

Kroll-Smith, J. S. and S. R. Couch 1991. What is a disaster? An ecological–symbolic approach to resolving the definitional debate. *International Journal of Mass Emergencies and Disasters* **9**(3): 355–366.

Odum H. T. 1983. *Systems Ecology.* New York: John Wiley and Sons.

Oliver-Smith, A. 2009. Anthropology and the political economy of disasters. In E. C. Jones and A. D. Murphy, eds., *The Political Economy of Hazards and Disasters.* Lanham, MD: AltaMira Press, pp. 11–28.

Ostrom, E. 1992. The rudiments of a theory of the origins, survival, and performance of common-property institutions. In D. W. Bromley, D. Feeny, M. A. McKean, *et al.* eds., *Making the Commons Work: Theory, Practice, and Policy.* San Francisco, CA: Institute for Contemporary Studies Press, pp. 293–318.

Nelson, D. R. and T. J. Finan 2009. Weak winters: dynamic decision-making in the face of extended drought in Ceará, Northeast Brazil. In E. C. Jones and A. D. Murphy, eds., *The Political Economy of Hazards and Disasters.* Lanham, MD: AltaMira Press, pp. 107–132.

Pérez Rodríguez, V. 2008. Household labor and landscape transformation in Ancient Mixteca Alta, Oaxaca, Mexico. In L. Cliggett and C. A. Pool, eds., *Economies and Transformation of Landscape.* Lanham, MD. AltaMira Press, pp. 77–102.

Piegorsch, W. W., S. L. Cutter, and F. Hardisty 2007. Benchmark analysis for quantifying urban vulnerability to terrorist incidents. *Risk Analysis* **27**(6): 1411–1425.

Steward, J. H. 1955. *Theory of Culture Change: The Methodology of Multilinear Evolution.* Urbana, IL: University of Illinois Press.

Stonich, S. C. 1992. *I Am Destroying the Land: The Political Ecology of Poverty and Environmental Destruction in Honduras.* Boulder, CO: Westview.

Trawick. P. 2008. Reading history in an irrigated landscape: the drama of the commons in the Andes. In L. Cliggett and C. A. Pool, eds., *Economies and Transformation of Landscape.* Lanham, MD: AltaMira Press, pp. 47–76.

Wallerstein, I. and J. Smith 1992. Core-periphery and household structures. In J. Smith and I. Wallerstein, eds., *Creating and Transforming Households.* Cambridge, UK: Cambridge University Press, pp. 253–262.

Whiteford, L. M. and G. A. Tobin 2009. If the pyroclastic flow doesn't kill you, the recovery will: cascading effects of Mt. Tungurahua's Eruptions in rural Ecuador. In E. C. Jones and A. D. Murphy, eds., *The Political Economy of Hazards and Disasters*. Lanham, MD: AltaMira Press, pp. 155–176.

Winograd, M. 2009. From natural events to "natural" disasters: assessing environmental vulnerability in Honduras. In O. Ensor, ed., *The Legacy of Mitch: Lessons from Post-Disaster Reconstruction in Honduras*. Marisa Tempe, AZ: University of Arizona Press.

Wisner, B., P. Blaikie, T. Cannon, and I. Davis 2004. *At Risk: Natural Hazards, People's Vulnerability and Disasters, 2nd edn*. London: Routledge.

6

Local communities and natural resources: ethnobiology in practice

LAURA ZANOTTI, DENISE M. GLOVER, AND JENNIFER SEPEZ

INTRODUCTION

This chapter focuses on methods specific to the field of ethnobiology. Literally, ethnobiology is the study of the logic of life (the *logos* of *bios*) among a group of people (*ethnos*) (Glover 2005: 24). Ethnobiologists examine the knowledge systems that social and cultural communities have developed to explain the natural world. Ethnobiology is also a multidisciplinary field, which means that ethnobiologists use a variety of interdisciplinary methodologies and theories. Ethnobiologists often occupy multiple roles as social and natural scientists. Finally, ethnobiology is at the same time a positivist and interpretative field of inquiry. Scholars conducting ethnobiological research employ a wide range of quantitative and qualitative techniques.

The history of the field has been split into several phases to account for the different schools of thought that have dominated ethnobiology over the years (Ellen 2006; Nazarea 2006; Hunn 2007). The initial phase was a period where researchers were conducting "salvage" ethnobiology in an attempt to document local biological knowledge of economically and medically useful plant species (Ellen 2006: S2; Hunn 2007). Phase two began in the 1950s but peaked in the 1960s and 1970s with the rise of cognitive anthropology. Inspired by linguistic studies of the Prague School (circa 1920s), cognitive anthropologists sought to document and classify folk biological knowledge in order to understand how different cultural groups conceptualize their environment (Nazarea 2006). In this strand, ethnoscientists were

Environmental Social Sciences: Methods and Research Design, ed. I. Vaccaro, E. A. Smith and S. Aswani. Published by Cambridge University Press. © Cambridge University Press 2010.

primarily concerned with methodologies that could be utilized to elicit local categories while at the same time searching for non-local, cross-cultural grids with which to compare cultural groups. From a theoretical perspective, much of the work generated from this phase focused on demonstrating why it is "notable that nonliterates know so much about nature" (Berlin 1992: 5). Conklin's agroecological study (1954) of the Hanunóo (Philippines), and Hunn's (1977) and Berlin, Breedlove, and Raven's (1974) on Tzeltal Maya classification are all exemplary of this period.

In the late 1970s and 1980s ethnobiologists expanded the previous focus on economic botany and taxonomic research to incorporate traditional ecological knowledge and local research management practices (Alcorn 1990; Denevan 1992; Nazarea 2006). An interest in indigenous knowledge and management was a reaction to the delocalizing impacts of modernization (Appadurai 1996) and state-making policies (Dove 2006: 195). Ethnobiologists discussed the complexity of local classification systems, observing that gender, ethnicity, kinship, and other notions of hierarchy play a role in the acquisition and transmission of ethnobiological knowledge (Ellen 2006). Ethnobiological research has also moved toward more process-oriented approaches. For instance, ethnobiologists "now study the processes of cultivation and domestication; the management of useful plant and animal populations; the process of traditional knowledge acquisition and organization" and so on (Salick et al. 2003: 2). Furthermore, an applied, activist approach to ethnobiology brought ethnobiology research to the forefront of international discussions about indigenous rights, intellectual property rights, and community-conservation issues.

Since its early phases, ethnobiology has flourished and expanded. Ethnobiology currently encompasses many different strands of research ranging from its classic taxonomic focus to more interpretative approaches. This chapter details the methods that ethnobiologists have developed to examine ethnobiology in contemporary societies and their associated place-based environmental knowledge. The theoretical shifts in ethnobiological research have corresponded with methodological expansion. This chapter outlines some of the classic methodologies used by ethnobiologists since its nascent years as well as some more recent developments, including participatory strategies. The goal of the chapter is to give researchers an overview of the many methods ethnobiologists employ, and how to discern which method is appropriate for which research design. The methods are discussed more or less in the historical order in which they were developed.

METHODS

Collection of voucher specimens

Identification of flora and fauna and the preservation of specimens are important in ethnobiological studies to document and establish reference points. Such documentation makes scientific revisions and redefinitions possible, and generally acts to provide a permanent and material archive that can be accessed in future work (Bye 1986: v). For these purposes, the collection and construction of voucher specimens is necessary. Proper processing of specimens entails advanced planning and preparation, including careful selection of collection sites, appropriate handling and processing of specimens, and having proper permits to collect and transport materials (Martin 2004: 28–65). When obtaining specimens, a field notebook is essential allowing data-gathering information to be recorded, such as location coordinates, description of local habitat, description of organism, cultural uses if known, conditions under which collection took place (e.g., season), and other related information. Bye (1986) stresses that diagnostic features of identification (such as inflorescence in plants) must be included in any sample; if they are not present at the initial time of collection then an additional collection should be made when these characteristics are present. In addition to field collection data, biological identification, notation of local name(s), and collector's name and cataloguing number should be included with each specimen (Bye 1986; Martin 2004). Proper processing is essential so as to preserve the biological materials; see Martin (2004: 28–65) for a thorough description of these for botanical materials. Specimens should be deposited in appropriate institutions both within the country of research and in the researcher's country of residence (if different); these institutions usually handle the mounting or further preservation of materials according to standard protocols. If you are working in an international setting, you will need to coordinate with researchers (and preferably a reputable institution) about how to obtain the proper permits for collection and/or transfer of specimens between countries.

Flora and fauna identification and classification

Species identification establishes a point of reference and must be included with a voucher specimen. Generally ethnobiologists rely on Linnaean classification, since this is a *lingua franca* of the scientific community worldwide that also allows for cross-cultural comparisons.

Determination of such identity will usually need to be made by a trained biologist; this can be done on-site with a local biologist or through transporting specimens to taxonomic specialists. In addition, local systems of identification are often of particular interest to ethnobiologists, in large part because of what they can reveal about local conceptualizations of the natural world.

One of the more difficult aspects of identification can be making sense of the variety of terms used within a local community among informants (and between adjacent communities). In some cases, linguistic analysis is necessary to determine whether terms are mere phonological variations, linguistic borrowings, or related cognates (sharing linguistic heritage). If you are not trained in the skills needed to make these distinctions, you can enlist the expertise of a linguist. In any case, it is important to either work with specimens (live, dried, or stuffed) or photographs when inquiring about the correspondence between an actual organism and the name(s) for it, since assumptions of identification can be wrong without an objective reference point.

In some instances, the ethnotaxonomy of a sociolinguistic group may not be in line with taxonomic distinctions recognized in Western science. When there are more distinctions recognized in some part of an ethnotaxonomy than that in Western taxonomy, the term over-differentiation is used to describe the contrast; under-differentiation is used to describe the reverse situation (Berlin 1973: 267–8; Berlin 1992). Generally speaking, over-differentiation tends to occur among organisms that are culturally significant for utilitarian or cognitive reasons (although *size* may increase cultural salience among *faunal* taxa – see Hunn 1999). Berlin notes that there is particularly striking agreement (as high as 60 percent) in the taxonomies of folk systems and those recognized in Western science, especially at the level of folk generic (see Berlin 1992).

Largely, however, ethnobiological studies that focus on classification do rely on a variety of lexical elicitation methods (and analysis of the lexical data gathered). One useful method employed to elicit classificatory schema is the frames and slots approach, adopted from structural linguistics. This approach is based on the idea that "one can get at the meaning of items through the way items are distributed in different [linguistic] environments [or frames]" (D'Andrade 1995: 59). The "frame" generally constitutes a nearly complete phrase with a "slot" omitted that the respondent needs to fill in to make the phrase true. Hence in the construction "_____ is a kind of vegetable," the slot can be filled in by any number of items (broccoli, bean, etc.) to make the phrase/sentence culturally true. One can use this technique to generate a list of items in a cultural domain and examine the taxonomical relationship of set inclusion. Metzger and Williams (1966) pioneered an extension of this technique now known as free listing (described below), where the researcher simply asks "What kinds of vegetables are there?" or uses a similarly direct line of questioning to elicit a list of terms.

Cultural consensus analysis

In the 1980s cognitive anthropologists developed cultural consensus analysis to determine shared cultural beliefs and analyze amount of shared knowledge among informants (Romney and Weller 1984; Romney, Weller, and Batchelder 1986; Romney, Batchelder, and Weller 1987; Reyes-García et al. 2004; Weller 2007: 339). Romney, Weller, Batchelder, and other associates developed cultural consensus theory (CCT), cultural consensus models (CCM), and other aggregative analysis methods that anthropologists and other scholars use today (Romney and Weller 1984; Romney 1999; Reyes-García et al. 2004). Cultural consensus analysis is particular useful in ethnographic contexts since it "estimate[s] the culturally correct answers and the cultural knowledge or accuracy of informants" (Weller 2007: 340). This allows the researcher to aggregate the "culturally best" responses, estimate the culturally correct answers, and establish the amount of cultural competence an individual has in a certain domain or topic (Dressler et al. 2005: 335; Weller 2007). Cultural consensus analysis is an excellent method to ascertain shared cultural beliefs and determine informant reliability in a cultural domain or topic, and is used in ethnobiological research.

Cultural consensus analysis operates best with systematic data collection methods, such as open-ended questionnaires with a short or single response, dichotomous questions, multiple choice questions, and fill in the bank questions (see Bernard 2002: 280–97; Miller et al. 2004; Reyes-García et al. 2004; Weller 2007). Cultural consensus analysis has a formal and informal method for analyzing data (see Weller 2007: 343–348). The informal methods uses reliability analysis and the formal model relies on a mathematical model found only in ANTHROPAC and UCINET software. Cultural consensus models are "a family of formally derived mathematical models that simultaneously provide an estimate of the cultural competence or knowledge of each informant and an estimate of the correct answer to each question asked" (Romney et al. 1996: 4701).

In the formal and informal method, the researcher should collect the information on an individual basis (not in focus groups) so that responses from one individual are independent of those from other interviewees (Weller 2007: 341). In addition, the questions should cover just one topic or domain at a time (Weller 2007: 341). The analysis does not work unless there is a high degree of agreement in the responses so that a consultant's competence can be tested against the "consensus" (Weller 2007: 341). As such, during data collection it is best to sample at least thirty individuals for reliable results, although there are always exceptions to the rule (Weller 2007: 355).

Cultural consensus analysis can be applied to any type of question that deals with the relationships among plants, animals, and people. For often cited examples of cultural consensus analysis, see Boster's (1986) study of manioc varieties, Miller et al.'s (2004) analysis of yellow fin tuna fisheries, Reyes-García et al.'s (2004, 2005) work with Tsminane plant knowledge, Atran et al.'s (1999) examination of plant classification, Garro's (1986) work on folk medicine in Mexico and Romney et al.'s many other publications. Also, refer to Weller (2007) for an excellent overview of cultural consensus and frequently asked questions associated with working with cultural consensus theories and models.

Ethnosemantics

Ethnosemantics is the study of categories of meaning within a cultural group with a focus on lexical contrasts, particularly in systems of classification. This type of examination got its start in anthropological kinship studies (and linguistics before that) but quickly spread to other areas of ethnoscientific inquiry. The key in ethnosemantics is to identify a cultural domain, to elicit terms of identification and classification from within that domain, and then to discover the distinguishing features of each term. Terms are elicited using free listing as well as through careful observation of conversation and social interactions. Besides qualitative inquiry, where a researcher can inquire directly what the various features of categories are (by asking what the difference between an aunt and an uncle is, for example), a number of more quantitative methods can be utilized. These techniques include pile sorts and triads, which are explained below, followed by analytical tools such as multi-dimensional scaling (MDS), PROFIT analysis, QAP (matrix correlation analysis), and cluster analysis. The following subsections detail additional data collection methods that are common for ethnosemantics.

Free listing

As highlighted previously, a focus on eliciting explicit cultural information via lexicon is central to many of the methods employed in ethnobiological work. Free listing is a technique in which an informant is asked to freely list (that is, no specific order of listing is requested) terms for a cultural domain. The format of elicitation is along the lines of "Tell me [list] all the names of _____" where a particular domain is identified.[1] Lists can be elicited either orally or in written form, depending on circumstances and time constraints. Generally speaking, if one is trying to arrive at an understanding of larger cultural tendencies, it is wise to get as broad a sampling as possible and therefore elicit as many free lists as one can. The technique of successive free listing is a way of further fleshing out connections between items, informants, and related cultural domains not targeted in the initial free-listing tasks (Ryan, Nolan, and Yoder 2000). For example, after asking a respondent to list all the names of locally occurring medicinal plants, one could then ask for the uses, parts used, preparation, and healing properties of each plant listed.

After acquiring the lists, statistical techniques can be used to analyze the cultural consensus that exists between informants (Weller and Romney 1988) as well as salience levels for items listed (Smith 1993); such levels of salience calculate the rank order of items listed (those listed first have a higher ranking of salience, being the ones remembered first by informants) as well as how often items appear on informants' lists.

Potential drawbacks with free listing include a focus on lexical items where substantive information may be overlooked (see Ellen 1999). Relatedly, Quinlan (2005) remarks that other methods of extended interviewing may in fact yield more detailed and fuller inventories than those obtained through free listing. The fact that free lists can be quantified is helpful, although the statistical reliability of free lists is dubious (Weller and Romney 1988). Furthermore, Miranda *et al.* (2007) argue that visual stimuli present during the course of free listing can have an influence on the inventory of items obtained.

---

[1] Note that free listing technically does not entail constraining the respondent's time frame, although sometimes such a limit is used (responses are restricted to 3–4 minutes long, for example). In these cases, the term used to describe this technique is a restricted list task (Sutrop 2001: 264).

Pile sorts and triads

Pile sorting and triad comparisons are techniques that have had much longevity within ethnoscience and cognitive anthropology. Although quite different in execution, there is an underlying similarity between these techniques in the shared goal of assessing categorical or semantic relations between items within a cultural domain. With both procedures, items can be previously obtained either through free listing tasks or through other informed decisions made by ethnographer and/or informant. Similar statistical analyses are used for both techniques, such as MDS where relations between items are projected into Euclidian space. In order to be able to effectively process data obtained through pile sorting and triads, statistical software is usually necessary. ANTHROPAC and UCINET, developed by Steve Borgatti and produced by Analytic Technologies, are the software packages most widely used by ethnobiologists (see www.analytictech.com for further information on these products).

Pile Sorting

In pile sorting, the basic idea is to ask respondents to organize a set of items (actual specimens, photos of specimens, or names written down) into piles based on whatever criteria the respondent feels is relevant but so that the items in each pile "belong together." In a constrained form of pile sorting, the researcher would request that a particular number of piles be made. In an unrestricted task, the respondent can make as many or as few (although there needs to be more than one) piles as he/she wishes. A number of variations are possible in the basic pile sorting task, including allowing items to be sorted into more than one pile (this requires having "copies" of items available), and conducting successive piles sorts. The ethnographer can record the information (which items were sorted into which piles – and even when in the sorting process) and subsequently use MDS or other techniques to identify aspects that seem to be significant in the cognitive orientation of the respondent. The ethnographer also usually asks the respondent to explain why he/she made the piles as such (generally after all sorting tasks have been completed), so there is overt and direct discussion about the piles between the ethnographer and respondent.

Weller and Romney (1988) note that there can be significant differences between what are known as "single sort" and "multiple sort" tasks. With a single sort task, the respondent sorts only once, while with multiple sorting the respondent sorts and re-sorts as many times as desired, using a different criterion each time. In addition, successive pile sorts can be used to elicit taxonomies. In this procedure, respondents are asked to first make piles and then to either combine or split the piles (or both – but not at the same time) for as many times as is appropriate. The aim of this approach is to generate a taxonomic tree that shows the relations of set inclusion between groupings of items.

The advantages of pile sorting include being able to process many items simultaneously (over 100 items at once), the relative ease at which the task is understood, and the ability to use with non-literate subjects. Disadvantages include the difficulty of comparing across respondents, and the need for 20–30 respondents (unless you use an extensive number of items, in which case fewer respondents is fine). Finally, in successive pile sorts there may be an imposition of a taxonomic hierarchy that is not appropriate for the items being considered (although see Berlin 1992).

Triads

In the comparative/contrastive technique known as triads, items are presented to respondents in groups of three, with a request given either to choose the one that is the "most different" or to order the items from having the most to the least amount of a particular characteristic. Generally a number of iterations are randomly generated (most expediently with the use of a computer) to compare a list of items ($N < 12$) in sets of three. The basic idea of this technique is that one can identify salient aspects in making similarity judgments between the given items, especially after submitting the data to tools of analysis; by running the results through MDS, for example, one can discover which items cluster together into groups and how "cognitively distant or close" items may be.

Triads are most useful when dealing with small numbers of items and with few informants. The more items one has, the more triads will be generated. For example, a list of 21 items would produce 1330 triads (Weller and Romney 1988). One way to use more than 10–12 items and reduce the number of triads is to utilize a balanced, incomplete block (BIB) design (Weller and Romney 1988; Ross, Barrientos, and Esquit-Choy 2005). This type of design eliminates the number of times *pairs* of items are presented in triadic comparisons and significantly reduces the overall number of triads that informants have to compare. If adopting a BIB design, one may need to increase the number of informants in order to stabilize the results.

Generally speaking, triads are easy to explain and to administer. Additionally, one can use either an oral or a written format. The drawbacks include not being able to compare long lists of items, boring respondents with a repetitive task, and the possibility of missing or incomplete data (respondents not marking any item in a set of three as being different). This last point may be mitigated by allowing for a "no judgment" option (cited in Ross, Barrientos, and Esquit-Choy 2005), but too many of such choices may have an adverse effect on the overall results of comparison (see Case Studies).

Situated knowledge: interviews, surveys, and questionnaires

Several different types of qualitative and quantitative interview techniques exist to situate traditional and local environmental knowledge within the sociocultural context. These range from structured to more unstructured data collection methods. This section, therefore, offers a brief overview of the techniques that an ethnobiologist might consider.

Interviews are divided into three categories: unstructured, semi-structured, and structured. Unstructured interviews can take place anywhere and are unscheduled, open-ended interviews where the researcher engages in informal conversation with the interviewee (Bernard 2002: 204). These types of interviews are useful at the beginning of a project in order to gain rapport, build friendships, and learn about the complexities of community life (Johnson 1992; Bernard 2002: 206). Informal interviews are also valid as a primary method to explore human–environment relationships, natural resource management techniques, and other topics of interest to ethnobiologists.

On the other hand, semi-structured interviews have "much of the freewheeling quality of unstructured interviewing and requires the same skills" but are based on an "interview guide" (Bernard 2002: 205). For example, Hunn et al. (2003) used informal, guided interviews to discuss gull egg harvests with the Huna Tlingit to document local harvest techniques and knowledge about gull populations in Glacier Bay National Park and Reserve, Alaska. The project members "encouraged interviewees to elaborate on their experiences, perspectives, and opinions" (Hunn et al. 2003: S85). The result was a rich dataset from 43 community members, which was used to help with sustainable resource management in Glacier Bay National Park and Reserve.

Structured interviews utilize a standardized list of questions that "control the input that triggers people's responses so that their output can be reliably compared" (Bernard 2002: 240). Structured interviews include survey instruments, such as questionnaires. These methods are best when the researcher has "clear and circumscribed" objectives (Johannes, Freeman, and Hamilton 2000: 266). Structured interviews contain open-ended questions, forced-choice (fixed response) questions, a combination of the two types of questions, or multiple types of one or the other (Bernard 2002: 254). Forced-choice questionnaires are extremely common in cultural consensus analysis. For example, Reyes-García et al. (2004) used three different types of forced-choice questionnaires accompanied by an initial free listing exercise to test adult Tsminane ethnobotanical knowledge. In the multiple choice component of their questionnaire, Reyes-García et al. (2004: 140) generated a list of plants and asked each Tsminane consultant about each one in a multiple-choice format: "For example, we asked, 'Can you tell me if X [name of plant] can be used as firewood?'(yes/no), 'to build a house?' (yes/no), 'to eat?' (yes/no), 'to cure?' (yes/no), 'to make a canoe?' (yes/no), and 'to make a tool?' (yes/no)." The researcher should pay close attention to word choice and what type of questionnaire is most appropriate for the subject in order to reduce response error (Bernard 2002: 256). See Bernard (2002: 256–265) and Fowler (2002) for excellent discussions on writing questionnaires.

Each unstructured and structured method has benefits and drawbacks. For instance, Ferguson and Messier (1997) drafted and then used a questionnaire in their preliminary research with a Baffin Island Inuit community. The researchers were documenting indigenous knowledge about caribou populations and initially thought that a questionnaire would be the best interview technique. However, the questionnaire was abandoned "in favor of a standard, yet flexible interview protocol" (Ferguson and Messier 1997: 18) after pre-testing revealed it was an inadequate survey tool. On the other hand, questionnaires are imperative for cultural consensus analysis and gathering specific types of standardized quantitative ethnobiological data that can not otherwise be collected. Many researchers chose to employ both structured and unstructured methods to improve informant reliability, sampling techniques, and the quality of the dataset.

Photo elicitation and interpretation

One very specific form of interviewing is photo elicitation. Harper (2002: 14) defines photo elicitation as, "the simple idea of inserting a photograph into a research interview." The premise of this research method is that visual images (e.g., photos, drawings, graphics, etc.) elicit different types of memories, sensations and information than verbal ones (Whyte 1984; Johnson and Griffith 1998; Harper 2002: 14; Stewart, Liebert, and Larkin 2004). Photo elicitation arguably reduces fatigue in longer, non-photo based interviews and often evokes more substantive and comprehensive material from the informant (Collier 1967; Collier and Collier 1986; Ziller 1990: 36). This method is common in visual sociology, leisure studies, cognitive psychology, and cognitive anthropology (Taylor *et al.* 1995; Banks 2001; Stewart, Liebert, and Larkin 2004). Photo elicitation is also a method used for analyzing human–environmental relationships in visual mediums, and can also be employed in consensus analysis for communities that are illiterate or have low literacy levels (Johnson and Griffith 1998: 215; Atran *et al.* 2002: 428).

Photo elicitation techniques offer ethnobiologists a "bridge between worlds that are more culturally distinct" (Harper 2002: 21). This method: (1) helps to identify local classifications of the biophysical environment; (2) determines different attitudes and values about the landscape; and (3) elicits stories about the landscape. The first step to photo elicitation is to determine what photos to use that best suit the research objective. The researcher can bring photos from the research site, historical photos, aerial photos, photos of scanned biotic material, or other types of graphic materials depending on the research task at hand. For example, Aswani and Lauer (2006: 267) used aerial photo interpretation as one method to identify the local "hierarchical cognition of the seascape" in the Solomon Islands.

Alternatively, researchers can also distribute cameras and ask community members to record their own experiences of a specific task or event and bring these photos to the interview, or ask the interviewee to bring photos that they might already have on hand. The same technique applies to videos (Worth and Adair 1972). This approach to photo elicitation can empower the consultant since they are providing the content for the interview (Clark-Ibáñez 2004: 1512). Once the photos are displayed, an "interview guide approach" (Stewart, Liebert, and Larkin 2004: 319) helps lead the interviewees through the photo-elicitation process. Photo elicitation functions best when combined with other methodologies that have a longer-standing history in ethnobiological studies.

Participatory mapping and plant trails

Participatory mapping is a method where a researcher actively collaborates with a local community to map different parts of the community's landscape (Brody 1981; Feld and Basso 1996). This method is an effective tool for: (1) analyzing community based resource management practices; (2) documenting key features, ecotypes, and subsistence areas within and surrounding a community; (3) documenting cultural sites (Chapin and Threlkeld 2001); (4) attributing stories, names, emotions and memories to contemporary, historical, and ancestral locations; (5) documenting political claims to land rights; and (6) "reaffirming historical and cultural links" (Smith *et al.* 2003: 357). This method is particularly useful to analyze how a community perceives, thinks about, and interacts within a landscape. In addition, mapping biographies are special types of interviews that solicit information on plants used and known within living memory of community members (Freeman 1976; Berkes *et al.* 1995). The researcher can employ this type of interviewing technique before, during or after the participatory mapping exercises.

Participation can take many forms in participatory mapping. For instance, a community may determine the context and content of research, guiding researchers to collect information according to the community's needs (Herlihy and Knapp 2003: 303). This is a common practice when a community is interested in mapping their lands for legal reasons, but also applies in other cases as well (Chapin, Lamb, and Threlkeld 2005). The researcher and community might jointly select community members as field assistants and train them in specific mapping techniques (Smith 2003: 334). On the other hand, individuals within the community might volunteer as consultants for the proposed project. In each case, the researcher should consult with the local community to determine the extent to which the community wishes to participate.

Several different mapping techniques exist to "transform cognitive spatial knowledge into map and descriptive forms" (Herlihy and Knapp 2003: 303). These techniques range from the simple to the highly technical. Hand-drawn or sketch mapping is a simple activity that the researcher can use to elicit knowledge or generate cognitive maps to uncover what features and areas are salient to the community (e.g., see Brody 1981; D'Antona, Cak, and Vanwey 2008). This technique is often the first step to identify what other mapping procedures to use, but also can stand on its own as a method (Chapin and Threlkeld 2001: 9). Remotely sensed data, such as aerial photography and satellite sensor imagery are other mapping options (Aplin 2003: 295). Aerial photographs taken from different time periods, if available and accessible, can elicit stories about changes in the landscape. Satellite images, digital terrain maps, 3-D maps and GIS technologies are newer forms of spatial analysis but some of the most prevalent in participatory mapping techniques (Chapin, Lamb, and Threlkeld 2005; Fox *et al.* 2008; Rhoades and Nazarea 2009). In this scenario, researchers and consultants use hand-held GPS devices to mark key features and points of interest to create participatory community maps of the designated area.

Finally, plant trails are a mapping method where a researcher marks specific plants on a predetermined route in the village. This marked trail is a representative sample of plants in the village and serves to measure an individual's ethnobiological knowledge (Stross 1970; Zarger and Stepp 2004; Wyndham 2004; Voeks 2007; Hunn 2008). On the trail, the researcher is careful to intentionally mark plants that have "cultural significance and abundance" (Zarger and Stepp 2004: 415) to the community, however, the composition and emphasis of the plant trail can vary depending on the research question at hand (e.g., Voeks 2007: 9). A number of consultants are asked to identify the marked plants on the trail and, often, to discuss other knowledge associated with the identified plants (Zarger and Stepp 2004). For another application of the plant trail methodology please refer to the vast literature on household garden surveys and suite of associated methodologies (Stoler 1975; Boster 1986; Vogl, Vogl-Lukasser, and Purl 2004)

In all cases, maps can be dangerous and contain within them sensitive cultural information so make sure to take into consideration the implications of the work (Fox *et al.* 2008: 204).

ETHNOBIOLOGY IN PRACTICE: THREE CASE STUDIES

This section presents three case studies where in each instance the researchers decided to implement one or more aspects of ethnobiological research in their project design.

Medicinal plant classifications and Tibetan doctors

Glover's focus on classification and ethnosemantics (2005) highlights the way in which a variety of classificatory schema were utilized, for varying purposes, by doctors of Tibetan medicine in Rgyalthang, Yunnan Province, PRC. Some of these schema have important textual precedent, which led Glover to investigate the relationships between categories of *materia medica* in various medical texts and in relation to the larger system of Tibetan medicine (Glover 2005; Glover forthcoming). Glover used a variety of interview techniques (open-ended, semi-structured and structured) as well as free listing and pile sorting tasks (with some modifications). Semi-structured interviews often focused on explanation of a particular topic of relevance – how names and characteristics of medicinal plants are learned throughout the course of a doctor's education, for example. Structured interviews with pre-determined list of questions could be especially helpful when time constraints were an issue.

Restraints were put on the free listing tasks, where Glover asked five area doctors to list the top 30 most useful or most important plants in their practice. She next utilized photographs to confirm with each doctor the identity of all names given in each list. Glover then chose the plants that occurred in all lists ($N = 19$) and asked respondents to sort these plant names, written in Tibetan on pieces of paper, together in whatever manner they thought the plants should be grouped. Glover explained that more than one pile was needed, names could be sorted into multiple piles and provided blank slips of paper for the purpose of copying names if needed. One doctor performed successive pile sorts, while the others did not. While statistically too small a sample size for consensus analysis, patterns did emerge from the pile sorts that were easily discernable. There was some variation of placement within each pile and some of the piles highlighted different aspects of categorization. The most common type of pile was one that grouped plants according to the disorder(s) that they treat. Free listing and pile sorting did not appear to be an arduous or troublesome task for the doctors, although it did seem a bit strange at first. The abstraction of using chits of paper (rather than actual specimens) may have in fact been the oddest part of the task, but did not seem especially problematic.

Finally, Glover deposited voucher specimens from her fieldwork at the Kunming Institute of Botany in China, the University of Washington, and the Missouri Botanical Garden.

Makah, ethnobiology, and present-day subsistence practices

The Makah Tribe is a Northwest Native American group on the Makah reservation in Neah Bay, Washington State. The Makah tribe has a long tradition of subsisting on the local terrestrial and marine resources, and community members have strong place-attachments to the eco-scape around Neah Bay (Sepez 2001: 1). From 1997 to 1999 Sepez (2001) conducted an analysis of the present-day subsistence practice of the Makah, focusing on the impact political histories have had on Makah foraging strategies, traditional environmental knowledge associated with these practices, and the sociocultural and economic valuation attributed to the subsistence complex. Sepez decided to constrain her research to the subsistence practices of hunting, fishing, and shell-fish collecting and document local ethnobiological knowledge associated with harvesting animal resources. She combined more customary qualitative ethnographic methods with statistical analysis of a random sample survey administered to 15 percent of the households.

In this instance, qualitative methods and quantitative methods complemented one another to cross-check data and generated a portrait of hunting, fishing, and shellfish collecting practices. Participant observation afforded Sepez (2001: 35) the opportunity, for example, to "participate in and observe river and ocean fishing, clam digging and other shellfish gathering ... and my favorite activity of all, octopus hunting" along with other subsistence activities. Coinciding with these observations and events, Sepez also collected statistical data on subsistence harvesting. The survey, a structured interview technique, was initially tested and then approved by the Makah Cultural and Research Center. The survey included questions about household composition, subsistence harvests for specific animal resources, resource-sharing practices, and other questions associated with local natural resource management and use.

At the time of research, 99 percent of households surveyed participated in subsistence activities, indicating the continued importance, and preference, the Makah have for subsistence foods despite access to non-native food (Sepez 2001: 327). In addition, the social and cultural interactions that resulted from subsistence activities placed added value on foraging practices beyond merely a dietary need. In this case, the local perception of and preference for subsistence activities would have been difficult to document without a combined quantitative and qualitative approach to ethnobiological knowledge.

Place-making, ethnoecology, and the Kayapó

The Kayapó are a central Brazilian indigenous group who live in a series of federally demarcated protected areas, which are located in the states of Mato Grosso and Pará, Brazil. The Kayapó were able to successfully demarcate most of their territory in the latter half of the twentieth century, and their protected area network was further consolidated in the twenty-first century. In her 2007 study, Zanotti examined the impact that protected area status had on Kayapó livelihoods in Aukre village. Zanotti incorporated an ethnoecological component into the research design to examine Aukre's place-making strategies, place-attachments, and local understandings of the landscape. In this case, ethnoecological methods provided an analytical framework for collecting and analyzing local knowledge and place-attachments.

Zanotti employed two methodologies in the ethnoecology portion of her research. First, she drew upon participatory mapping techniques and mapping biographies to better understand the local use of the landscape. Zanotti asked consultants to guide her to places in the landscape that were important to them and their community. On foot and by canoe, community members pointed out fishing spots, old wasp ritual areas, hunting trails, fruit trees, seasonal bridges, and other areas of interest. Zanotti recorded these areas with a GPS unit, hand-sketched maps, and jotted down notes as she went. She followed the informal participatory walks with semi-structured interviews with different consultants. In these interviews, Zanotti questioned about the different parts of the landscape that the community members had pointed out to her, why they were important to the interviewee, and what meaning they had for the community in general. The combination of these methods provided a suite of cartographic data, visual materials, and verbal responses. To conclude the study, Zanotti analyzed the data to identify the salient aspects of the landscape that were critical for the Kayapó (see Zanotti 2008).

CONCLUSION

This chapter outlines the methods a researcher can choose from when undertaking ethnobiological research. Because ethnobiology is a multi- and interdisciplinary field, the methods ethnobiologists use include both qualitative and quantitative approaches. Ethnobiology has emerged as a complex field within anthropology, and arguably environmental sciences, that is well equipped to answer several different types of research questions. Ethnobiology offers several valuable methodologies to analyze the human dimensions of natural resource management (Ellen 2006), and also has the explanatory potential to evaluate the impact of rapid change in socioenvironmental systems. Finally, this chapter is merely the first step to understanding the several rich methodologies available to ethnobiologists. We urge those interested in pursuing ethnobiological research to consult the references we have cited to continue to build their research design.

REFERENCES

Alcorn, J. B. 1990. Indigenous agroforestry systems in the Latin American tropics. In M. A. Altieri and S. B. Hecht, eds., *Agroecology and Small Farm Development*. Boca Raton, FL: CRC Press, pp. 203–213.

Aplin, P. 2003. Using remotely sensed data. In N. J. Clifford and G. Valentine, eds., *Key Methods in Geography*. Thousand Oaks, CA: Sage Publications, pp. 291–308.

Appadurai, A. 1996. *Modernity at Large: Cultural Dimensions of Globalization*. Minneapolis, MN: University of Minnesota Press.

Aswani, S. and M. Lauer 2006. Benthic mapping using local aerial photo interpretation and resident taxa inventories for designing marine protected areas. *Environmental Conservation* **33**(3): 263–273.

Atran, S., D. Medin, N. Ross, *et al.* 1999. Folkecology and commons management in the Maya Lowlands. *PNAS* **96**: 7598–7603.

Atran, S., D. Medin, N. Ross, *et al.* 2002. Folkecology, cultural epidemiology, and the spirit of the commons. *Current Anthropology* **43**(3): 421–450.

Banks, M. 2001. *Visual Methods in Social Research*. London: Sage Publications.

Berkes, F., A. Hughes, P. J. George, *et al* 1995. The persistence of Aboriginal land use: fish and wildlife harvest areas in the Hudson and James Bay Lowland, Ontario. *Arctic* **48**(1): 81–93.

Berlin, B. 1973. Folk systematics in relation to biological classification and nomenclature. *Annual Review of Ecology and Systematics* **4**: 259–271.

Berlin, B. 1992. *Ethnobiological Classification: Principles of Categorization of Plants and Animals in Traditional Societies*. Princeton, NJ: Princeton University Press.

Berlin, B., D. E. Breedlove, and P. H. Raven. 1974. *Principles of Tzeltal Plant Classification: An Introduction to The Botanical Ethnography of a Mayan-speaking People of the Highlands of Chiapas*. New York: Academic Press.

Bernard, H. R. 2002. *Research Methods in Anthropology: Qualitative and Quantitative Approaches*. 3rd edn. Walnut Creek, CA: Altamira Press.

Boster, J. S. 1986. Exchange of varieties and information between Aruaruna manioc cultivators. *American Anthropologist* **88**: 429–436.

Brody, H. 1981. *Maps and Dreams: Indians and the British Columbian Frontier*. London: J. Norman and Hobhouse.

Bye, R. 1986. Voucher specimens in ethnobiological studies and publications. *Journal of Ethnobiology* **6**(1): 1–8.

Chapin, M., Z. Lamb, and B. Threlkeld 2005. Mapping indigenous lands. *Annual Review of Anthropology* **34**: 619–638.

Chapin, M. and B. Threlkeld 2001. *Indigenous Landscapes: A Study of Ethnocartography*. Arlington, VA: Center for the Support of Native Lands.

Clark-Ibáñez, M. 2004. Framing the social world with photo-elicitation interviews. *American Behavioral Scientist* **47**: 1507–1527.

Collier, J. 1967. *Visual Anthropology: Photography as a Research Method*. Austin, TX: Holt, Rinehart and Winston.

Collier, J. and M. Collier 1986. *Visual Anthropology: Photography as a Research Method*. Albuquerque, NM: University of Mexico Press.

Conklin, H. 1954. The relation of Hanunóo culture to the plant world. Ph.D. dissertation. Yale University, New Haven.

D'Andrade, R. 1995. *The Development of Cognitive Anthropology*. Cambridge, UK: Cambridge University Press.

D'Antona, Á. de O., Cak, D. A., L. K. VanWey, et al. 2008. Collecting sketch maps to understand property land use and land cover in large surveys. *Field Methods* **20**: 66–84.

Denevan, W. 1992. The pristine myth: the landscape of the Americas in 1492. *Annals of the Association of American Geographers* **82**(3): 369–385.

Dove, M. R. 2006. Indigenous people and environmental politics. *Annual Review of Anthropology* **35**: 191–208.

Dressler, W. W., C. D. Borges, M. C. Balieiro, et al. 2005. Measuring cultural consonance: Examples with special reference to measurement theory in anthropology. *Field Methods* **17**: 331–355.

Ellen, R. 1999. Modes of subsistence and ethnobiological knowledge: Between extraction and cultivation in Southeast Asia. In D. Medin and S. Atran, eds., *Folkbiology*. Cambridge, MA: MIT Press, pp. 91–118.

Ellen, R. 2006. Introduction. *Journal of the Royal Anthropological Institute* N.S.: S1-S22.

Feld, S. and K. H. Basso, eds. 1996. *Sense of Place*. Santa Fe, NM: School of American Research Press.

Ferguson, M. A. D. and F. Messier 1997. Collection and analysis of traditional ecological knowledge about a population of arctic tundra caribou. *Arctic* **50**(1): 17–28.

Fowler, F. 2002. *Survey Research Methods*, 3rd edn. Thousand Oaks, CA: Sage Publications.

Fox, J., K. Suryanata, P. Hershock, and A. H. Pramono 2008. Mapping boundaries, shifting power: the socio-ethical dimensions of participatory mapping. In M. K. Goodman, M. Boykoff, and K. Evered, eds., *Contentious Geographies: Environmental Knowledge, Meaning, Scale*. Burlington, VT: Ashgate Publishing, pp. 203–218.

Freeman, M. M. R., ed. 1976. *Report on the Inuit Land Use and Occupancy Project*. Ottawa: Department of Indian and Northern Affairs.

Garro, L. C. 1986. Intracultural variation in folk medical knowledge: a comparison between curers and noncurers. *American Anthropologist* **88**(2): 351–370.

Glover, D. M. 2005. *Up from the roots: Contextualizing medicinal plant classifications of Tibetan doctors in Rgyalthang, PRC*. Ph.D. Dissertation, University of Washington.

Glover, D. M. Forthcoming. Classes in the classics: Historical changes in plant classifications in two Tibetan medical texts. In M. Schrempf, S. Craig, F. Garrett, and M. Tsomo, eds., *Medicine, Health, and Modernity: Proceedings from the XIth International Association for Tibetan Studies Meetings*. Bonn: International Institute for Tibetan and Buddhist Studies, Contributions to Research on Central Asia Series.

Harper, D. 2002. Talking about pictures: a case for photo elicitation. *Visual Studies* **17**(1): 13–26.

Herlihy, P. H. and G. Knapp 2003. Maps of, by, and for the Peoples of Latin America. *Human Organization* **62**(4): 303–314.

Hunn, E. S. 1977. *Tzeltal Folk Zoology: The Classification of Discontinuities in Nature.* New York: Academic Press.

Hunn, E. S. 1999. Size as limiting the recognition of biodiversity in folkbiological classifications: One of four factors governing the cultural recognition of biological taxa. In D. Medin and S. Atran, eds., *Folkbiology.* Cambridge: MIT Press, pp. 47–69.

Hunn, E. S. 2007. Four phases of ethnobiology. *Journal of Ethnobiology* **27**(1): 1–10.

Hunn, E. S. 2008. *A Zapotec Natural History: Trees, Herbs, and Flowers, Birds, Beasts, and Bugs in the Life of San Juan Gbëë.* Tucson, AZ: University of Arizona Press.

Hunn, E., D. R. Johnson, P. N. Russell, *et al.* 2003. Huna Tlingit traditional environmental knowledge, conservation, and the management of a "wilderness" park. *Current Anthropology* **44**: S79-S103.

Johannes, R. E., M. M. R. Freeman, and R. J. Hamilton 2000. Ignore fishers' knowledge and miss the boat. *Fish and Fisheries* **1**: 257–271.

Johnson, J. and D. C. Griffith 1998. Visual data: collection, analysis and representation. In V. C. de Munck and E. J. Sobo, eds., *Using Methods in the Field: A Practical Introduction and Casebook.* Walnut Creek, CA: AltaMira, pp. 211–228.

Johnson, M., ed. 1992. *Lore: Capturing Traditional Environmental Knowledge.* Ottawa: Dene Cultural Institute and International Development Research Centre.

Martin, G. J. 2004. *Ethnobotany: A Methods Manual.* Sterling, VA: Earthscan.

Metzger, D. and G. Williams. 1966. Some procedures and results in the study of native categories: Tzeltal "Firewood." *American Anthropologist* **68**: 389–407.

Miller, M., J. Kaneko, P. Bartram, *et al.* 2004. Cultural consensus analysis and environmental anthropology: yellowfin tuna fishery management in Hawaii. *Cross-Cultural Research* **38**(3): 289–314.

Miranda, T. M., M. Christina de Mello Amorozo, J. Sílvio Govone, *et al.* 2007. The influence of visual stimuli in ethnobotanical data collection using the listing task method. *Field Methods* **19**: 76–86.

Nazarea, V. 2006. Local knowledge and memory in biodiversity conservation. *Annual Review of Anthropology* **35**: 317–335.

Quinlan, M. 2005. Considerations for collecting freelists in the field: examples from ethnobotany. *Field Methods* **17**: 219–34.

Reyes-García, V., E. Byron, V. Vadez, *et al.* 2004. Measuring culture as shared knowledge: do data collection formats matter? Cultural knowledge of plant uses among Tsimane' Amerindians, Bolivia. *Field Methods* **16**(2): 135–156.

Reyes-García, V., V. Vadez, E. Byron, *et al.* 2005. Market economy and the loss of folk knowledge of plant uses: estimates from the Tsimane' of the Bolivian Amazon. *Current Anthropology* **46**: 651–656.

Rhoades, R. E., and V. Nazarea 2009. Forgotten futures: scientific models vs. local visions of land use change. In P. Sillitoe, ed., *Local Science Versus Global Science.* New York: Berghahn Books, pp. 231–256.

Romney, A. K. 1999. Cultural consensus as a statistical model. *Current Anthropology* **40**: S103–115.

Romney, A. K., and S. Weller 1984. Predicting informant accuracy from patterns of recall among informants. *Social Networks* **6**(1): 59–77.

Romney, A. K., W. Batchelder, and S. Weller 1987. Recent applications of cultural consensus theory. *American Behavioral Scientist* **31**(2): 163–177.

Romney, A. K., J. P. Boyd, C. C. Moore, *et al.* 1996. Culture as shared cognitive representations. *PNAS* **93**(10): 4699–4705.

Romney, A. K., S. Weller, and W. Batchelder 1986. Culture as consensus: a theory of culture and informant accuracy. *American Anthropologist* **88**(2): 313–338.

Ross, N., T. Barrientos, and A. Esquit-Choy 2005. Triad tasks, a multipurpose tool to elicit similarity judgments: the case of Tzotzil Maya plant taxonomy. *Field Methods* **17**: 269–282.

Ryan, G. W., J. M. Nolan, and P. S. Yoder 2000. Successive free listing: using multiple free lists to generate explanatory models. *Field Methods* **12**: 83–107.

Salick, J., J. Alcorn, E. Anderson, *et al.* 2003. Intellectual Imperatives in Ethnobiology NSF Biocomplexity Workshop Report. St. Louis, Missouri Botanical Garden.

Sepez, J. 2001. *Political and social ecology of contemporary Makah subsistence: hunting, fishing, and shellfish collecting practices.* Ph.D. Dissertation, University of Washington.

Smith, D. A. 2003. Participatory mapping of community lands and hunting yields among the Buglé of Western Panama. *Human Organization* **62**(4): 332–343.

Smith, J. J. 1993. Using ANTHROPAC 3.5 and a spreadsheet to compute a free-list salience index. *Cultural Anthropology Methods Journal* **5**(3): 1–3.

Smith, R. C., M. Benavides, M. Pariona, and E. Tuesta 2003. Mapping the past and the future: geomatics and indigenous territories in the Peruvian Amazon. *Human Organization* **62**(4): 357–368.

Stewart, W. R., D. Liebert, and K. W. Larkin 2004. Community identities as visions for landscape change. *Landscape and Urban Planning* **69**: 315–334.

Stoler, A. 1975. Garden use and household consumption pattern in a Javanese village. Ph.D. dissertation, Columbia University, New York.

Stross, B. 1970. Aspects of language acquisition by Tzeltal children. Ph.D. dissertation. University of California, Berkeley, California.

Sutrop, U. 2001. List task and a cognitive salience index. *Field Methods* **13**(3): 263–276.

Taylor, J., K. Czarnowski, N. Sexton, *et al.* 1995. The importance of water to Rocky Mountain National Park visitors: an adaptation of visitor-employed photography to natural resources management. *Journal of Applied Recreation Research* **20**: 61–85.

Voeks, R. A. 2007. Are women reservoirs of traditional plant knowledge? Gender, ethnobotany and globalization in northeast Brazil. *Singapore Journal of Tropical Geography* **28**:7–20.

Vogl, C. R., B. Vogl-Lukasser, R. K. Purl 2004. Tools and methods for data collection in ethnobotanical studies of homegardens. *Field Methods* **16**(3): 285–306.

Weller, S. C. 2007. Cultural consensus theory: applications and frequently asked questions. *Field Methods* **19**: 339–368.

Weller, S. C. and A. K. Romney 1988. *Systematic Data Collection.* Qualitative Research Methods Series (Vol. 10). Newbury Park, CA: Sage Publications.

Whyte, W. F. 1984. *Learning From the Field: A Guide from Experience.* Beverly Hills, CA: Sage Publications.

Worth, S. and J. Adair 1972. *Through Navajo Eyes: An Exploration in Film Communication and Anthropology.* Bloomington, IN: Indiana University Press.

Wyndham, F. S. 2004. Learning ecology: ethnobotany in the Sierra Tarahumara, Mexico. Ph.D. dissertation, University of Georgia, Athens.

Zanotti, L. 2008. *Re-envisioning indigenous territoriality: nature, place, and space in the Kayapó reserve*. Ph.D. Dissertation, University of Washington, Seattle.

Zarger, R. K. and J. R. Stepp 2004. Persistence of botanical knowledge among Tzeltal Maya children. *Current Anthropology* **45**: 413–418.

Ziller, R. 1990. *Photographing the Self: Methods for Observing Personal Orientations*. London: Sage Publications.

7

Mapping histories: cultural landscapes and walkabout methods

VERONICA STRANG

INTRODUCTION

This chapter considers "cultural mapping" as an ethnographic method. Like many anthropological ideas (and indeed the concept of "culture" itself), this methodology has achieved wider utility. UNESCO (2009) makes use of it, as do many local community projects. There are now cultural mapping "toolkits" available, and newsletters and websites designed to assist people in employing these. Here, however, we are concerned with cultural mapping as a scientific method for the systematic collection of social data.

Cultural mapping explores people's historical and contemporary relationships with local environments. It entails "going walkabout" with informants in the places that they consider to be important, and collecting social, historical and ecological data *in situ*. It observes that places not only reflect the physical materialization of cultural beliefs and values, they are also a repository and a practical mnemonic of information. Thus the process is simultaneously an exercise allowing the collection of basic site and area-specific data; a participatory and observational exercise focused on people's interactions with places; a process of elicitation, enabling informants to articulate the cultural landscapes and territorially situated ethnohistories embedded in a physical topography; and a collaborative process through which cultural representations of the area are composed. Interviewing informants "in place" draws on both experiential and abstract forms

Environmental Social Sciences: Methods and Research Design, ed. I. Vaccaro, E. A. Smith and S. Aswani. Published by Cambridge University Press. © Cambridge University Press 2010.

of knowledge, and the use of "walkabouts" provides a relaxed and productive context for interviews.

The process is systematic and comprehensive and collects both visual and textual material. Places are literally "mapped," sometimes informally, using and adapting existing maps and sketches, or more formally, using GIS technology, satellite imagery and related technologies. Interviewing is generally a mix of informal and more structured approaches. A range of datasets can be sought including, for example, topographic and ecological information; local histories; socio-spatial information; ownership and rights of access; local ecological knowledge; religious and secular understandings of the environment; economic practices, and resource use and management. The major objective is to gain an in-depth, holistic view of people's engagements with the places that they inhabit, and to illuminate particular cultural and ethnohistorical landscapes. In addition to providing comparative data for analytic questions about human–environmental interactions, this methodology is helpful in resolving conflicts over land and resources, and in considering issues of environmental management (and co-management) (see Sillitoe 1998). Cultural mapping exercises often intersect with related methods such as "counter-mapping" and Participatory Action Research (PAR).[1]

Any ethnographic or ethnohistorical research can gain from employing these methods, but this chapter suggests that cultural mapping is an especially valuable approach for environmental anthropology. Why should this be so? It is intuitively obvious that a spatially oriented approach would fit well in an area focused on human–environmental interactions. But cultural mapping can also illuminate some core theoretical issues. How do people inhabit and make sense of places? How do their sensory experiences and cognitive processes articulate with the material environments that they encounter? How do they represent notions of space and time?

Map-making is fundamental to human–environmental relationships. Cognitive and sensory engagement with the world entails a process of creative "mapping." Inhabiting a particular ecological context, human groups are confronted with a practical necessity to organize themselves spatially; to map resources and to manage their economic use of these. They act creatively upon their physical surroundings, producing cultural landscapes composed of ideas, categories, knowledges

---

[1] These terms are sometimes conflated as Participatory Action Research Mapping (PARM) (see Herlihy and Knapp 2003; McIntyre 2008).

and values; social and spatial arrangements; economic and political practices; and religious and scientific cosmologies. As Benjamin's influential work illustrated (1970), there are complex linkages between spatialities, histories and the production of cultural identity (see also Carter 1987).

This suggests three major dimensions of human–environmental relationships to consider in relation to cultural mapping. First, the basic processes of engagement, in which map-making and story-telling are central to people's capacities to "make sense" of their place (and emplacement) in the world; second, the mutually constitutive formations of material and ideational cultural landscapes – places formed by human activities and spatialities imbued with memories, meaning and identity; and, third, the representational forms that express particular relationships with place. The latter are also recursive: Foucault's observation that words, stories, narratives, discourses and texts "form the objects of which they speak" (1972: 54) is readily applied to the making of places through both narrative and graphic representations.

Cultural landscapes also reflect political relations. Cosgrove (1989) observed that they reproduce the norms and values of dominant groups, and Keith and Pile suggest that "all spatialities are political because they are the (covert) medium and (disguised) expression of asymmetrical relations of power" (1993: 38). Around the world there are many longstanding contests for social, economic, and political dominance, and for the ownership and control of land and resources. The representations that people make of their particular cultural landscapes are central to these contests, forming vital discursive objects in political negotiations (see Bender 1998; Orlove 1991, 1993).

A map can be composed in many ways: with a dot painting; a song; a story; a dance; a series of knots; a drawing in the sand; and, of course, with cartographic techniques. All function to reduce complex spatial information to a manageable, communicable form, and many encapsulate temporal elements through the inclusion of narrative. Indeed, in approaching the analysis of maps, it may be best to discard conventional distinctions between graphic and narrative forms of representation, as they are generally intertwined, with spatial imagery appearing in even the most linear of narratives, and – though it is more challenging to explicate – temporal change embedded in purportedly "spatial" representations.

Some forms of mapping are particularly successful in articulating temporal information, and these can inform the design of cultural mapping projects focused on ethnohistorical issues. Examples include the "itinerary maps" that described early journeys across Europe; the "diary maps" of explorers; and Australian Aboriginal song lines, which conflate topographical information with narratives of ancestral journeys and creative activities. As well as providing representational models encompassing temporality, these draw attention to the use of a physical landscape as a repository for memory (see Kuchler 1993; Morphy 1993; Schama 1996; Stewart and Strathern 2003). Such mnemonic use of a physical environment for the location of social data is particularly evident in non-literate societies, where Henige (1982) suggests "remembering" is a more vital skill,[2] but it is plain that all human societies locate memories and meanings in place.

Cultural mapping produces representations that can be interrogated in a variety of ways, and it can also be considered reflexively, as a process of collaboration. In this sense it may involve all three of the activities that Banks and Morphy define as "visual research methods": making visual representations; the analysis of existing representations; and the collaborative production of visual representations (1997: 14). Visual media have become an increasingly important part of ethnographic research (Pink 2001, 2006). As well as producing spatial representations, cultural mapping is often supplemented by photography, video and film, GIS databases, digital, and hypermedia.

Because of its capacity to represent specifically cultural perspectives, mapping exercises are often used in Participatory Action Research (PAR) or "counter-mapping," in which researchers assist communities' efforts to protect or regain land ownership and access to resources, to prevent environmental degradation and social disruption, or simply to uphold a particular cultural identity (see Reason and Bradbury 2008). This more egalitarian collaborative approach, initiated by the reflexive critiques of feminist scholars in the 1960s and 70s, often involves direct advocacy, which some writers argue is a predictable outcome of long-term ethnographic relationships (see Ramos 2004). Even when this is not the case, the ethical codes governing contemporary ethnographic

---

[2] As he notes:

> Members of literate societies can be selective or careless in retaining memories, yet still be able indefinitely to retrieve some of what they have forgotten.
>
> Because members of oral societies do not have this opportunity, the past necessarily assumes a very different role for them. The vague collective memory is formalized, systematized, replenished with details, and shaped into formal traditions time and time again...without effective mnemonic devices forgetting is a disease without a cure. (Henige 1982: 5)

research have encouraged researchers to give closer consideration to the equality of relationships with informants and the benefits of their research for all of the people involved.

Thus projects are often co-designed with host communities; data collection is undertaken in partnership; and research outputs – textual and visual – are co-produced. Typically this shapes projects more closely in accord with community needs (see Durington 2004). In making cultural maps, researchers either work directly with members of a community, or facilitate the process by suggesting methodological approaches and providing training, technology, and advice.

Such collaborations create what Flores describes as "hybrid products" (2004).[3] They also raise a set of ethical issues about ownership. Who owns the research process? Who makes the decisions about its aims and methods? And, most particularly, who owns the outputs of the research? All of these issues need to be considered and negotiated. With claims for land and resources increasingly involving adversarial legal contests, maps can be a particularly sensitive form of representation, and careful thought therefore needs to be given to the possible ramifications of producing outputs that may be used by all parties in a legal process. To provide an illustrative anecdote: a few years ago, the head of Australia's Native Title Tribunal visited the Pitt Rivers Museum in Oxford. As a local Australianist, I was sent to meet him. "Oh yes," he said, "I know your name: your book landed on my desk recently as Exhibit Number 11."

Exhibit Number 11 was a comparative ethnography which considered the very different cultural landscapes of Aboriginal groups and graziers[4] in the Mitchell River area in North Queensland (Strang 1997). I had subsequently produced several cultural mapping reports for the Aboriginal community in Kowanyama. These and later research with groups in the Brisbane River catchment provide case studies through which we can explore the cultural mapping process.

---

[3] The notion of hybridity, as I have argued elsewhere (Strang 2006), suggests that anthropological knowledge itself is the product of long-term intellectual exchanges across cultural boundaries. On this basis, it has been argued that all ethnographic representations are hybrid products (Arce and Fisher 2003; Clifford and Marcus 1986; Lassiter 2005), although there are wide variations in the way that working relationships with informants are constructed; in the degree of equality involved; and in the level of host communities' participation in the research.

[4] This term is used in Australia to describe cattle ranchers.

MAPPING ALONG THE MITCHELL

The Aboriginal community in Kowanyama, composed of approximately 1200 people belonging to Kunjen, Kokobera, and Yir Yoront language groups,[5] is located on the west coast of Cape York, near the mouth of the Mitchell River. The ex-mission reserve area encompasses some of the traditional land of each of these groups, but this also extends into neighboring cattle stations and the Mitchell-Alice River National Park. Being remote, the area was only visited sporadically by Europeans until the early 1900s. Early exploratory meetings with indigenous people were generally marred by violence, which continued in the early days of settlement of the area. By the mid 1900s, Aboriginal people were either living in the Anglican mission reserve area established in 1903, or providing unpaid labor on neighboring cattle stations in order to remain on their traditional "country." Legislation in the 1960s requiring wages to be paid for this work saw them expelled from the stations into the mission, which was then handed to the State following a major hurricane in 1964. The reserve area was given to the community under a Deed of Grant in Trust in 1987, and some degree of self-governance was achieved with the establishment of an Aboriginal council, and – presciently – an office for the management of Aboriginal land and resources.

In the early 1990s the Aboriginal elders asked me to assist them in mapping their traditional "story places"[6] in the Mitchell-Alice River National Park. They were hopeful that new legislation would enable them to reclaim their traditional country, or at least gain some voice in the management and use of it.[7] They were equally concerned that, under contemporary social, economic and educational pressures, traditional knowledge was not being passed on to younger generations

---

[5] The Kunjen group is also described as Olkol language speakers. The Yir Yoront group was famously studied by Lauriston Sharp in the 1930s. Sharp compiled detailed maps, ethnographic, and genealogical records, which have proved to be an invaluable historical resource for the community.

[6] In north Queensland, sacred sites are called Story Places and the ancestral era from which Aboriginal Law has been passed down is called the Story Time. In other parts of Australia this has been described as the Dreamtime.

[7] The Native Title Act (1993) was passed shortly afterwards. This was a landmark act which, after 200 years of denial, admitted that Aboriginal Australians had had a system of land ownership, and could claim land where this title had not been extinguished. The political furore that followed led to the fall of the Keating Government and to the election of John Howard, who set about "revising" the Act substantially.

effectively. They wanted this knowledge recorded systematically "for future generations." Many of the most knowledgeable members of the community were aging and increasingly frail. There was an urgent need for this work to be done, and a great deal of it to do – as one Kunjen elder said: "All year you got to travel, to show you the country." (Paddy Yam 1992).[8]

Working with the Land Office and the Aboriginal Rangers, I therefore organized a number of trips out to the National Park with key groups. These were planned in accord with the community's priorities about where we should go, and which sites should be visited. They were keen to be as systematic and comprehensive as possible, encompassing all of the culturally important sites within the park area, and focusing especially on the "story places." This cohered readily with a scientific approach to cultural mapping, in which such planning generally entails gathering information about all relevant sites, while also getting a sense of which are particularly significant.

Given the distance from the settlement, and the logistical realities, it was then necessary to negotiate who should be included in the process. There was more divergence in aims here. In general, ethnographers hope to engage with a diverse cross-section of informants in any cultural group: a representative sample of each generation, gender, class, and so forth. However, Aboriginal societies are gerontocratic, with people (both men and women) gaining restricted – often sacred – knowledge as they pass through each stage of life. The community's elders are firmly positioned as the authoritative holders of cultural information and are therefore seen as the "proper" experts in a cultural mapping process. This control of cultural information, and of the collaborative research itself, both reflected and upheld their political authority.

Our achievement of a useful compromise was assisted by the reality that, at that time, organizing cultural mapping expeditions was quite logistically challenging. It entailed getting hold of several reliable vehicles (it being essential to have more than one in an area where getting bogged is a regular occurrence); gathering sufficient camp gear and equipment for the exercise; and ensuring that we had

---

[8] All of the language groups in Kowanyama were keen to work with anthropologists and archaeologists in this regard: John Taylor had done useful mapping work in the 1970s in the adjoining Aboriginal community at Pormpurraw (see Taylor 1975), and the Kowanyama community also persuaded Bruno David and John Cordell to assist them with this kind of work in the early 1990s (see David and Cordell 1993). I collaborated with Bruno David in some of this work.

sufficient recording equipment, films, and tapes (the latter having to be sent from Cairns). There were other practical challenges in taking a number of elderly people far from the settlement and its support facilities; carrying sufficient food and fuel; and getting around sites in areas that sometimes degenerate into "packhorse country."[9] On our first mapping foray I did all the camp cooking myself, which was detrimental not only to the data collection, but doubtless to the health of the group as well. On subsequent trips the Land Office was persuaded to employ a couple of my adoptive "aunties" as camp cooks. Not only was this more manageable (and edible), it served to bring more women into the project, thus equalizing the gender representation within the group. With a need for several drivers it was also possible to include rangers from the Land Office and their families, which brought a number of younger people into the process. Nevertheless, the formal responsibility for the provision of cultural information at each site remained with the elders, and information from the younger people had to be sought less formally and with some diplomacy, as they shared the view that the elders were the proper people to speak about cultural knowledge.

There were other logistical challenges with implications for the process of data collection. GPS devices were relatively new technology at the time, and reception in the area was not always reliable. However, we were able to triangulate our site markings subsequently with OS maps and aerial photographs, which helped iron out some of the anomalies in the readings. I used a range of methods of data collection, taking photographs everywhere we went, and recording video interviews with the elders (and occasionally others) at each site. I also audiotaped many longer interviews, beginning with a series of formal questions and then expanding the discussion with more open queries. I did many opportunistic informal interviews; employed standard participant observation techniques to observe how people engaged with each place; and made copious notes and sketches (see Figure 7.1). Over time, I also found it useful to use the photographs and sketches as elicitative tools for discussing the landscape with a wider range of people.

---

[9] Most of this area is impassable in the wet season, and, even in the dry, the roads can be very rough. It was necessary to ford sizeable rivers and creeks, large dry creek beds, and to push through much dense scrub. My Aboriginal collaborators apparently believed that a vehicle could be taken anywhere that one could take a horse – thus, over time, our expeditions ventured further and further into roadless, trackless "packhorse country."

THE ALICE-CROSBIE JUNCTION

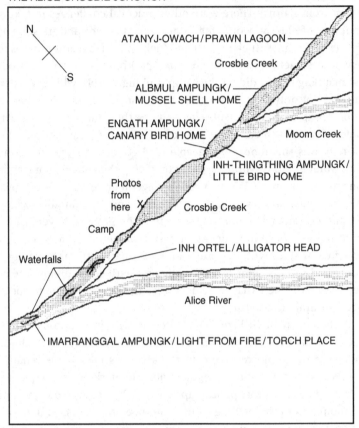

Figure 7.1   Sketch map of story places at the junction of the Alice River and Crosbie Creek, Cape York, made with Kunjen elders.

The hot, dusty environment of northern Australia can be fairly unkind to recording equipment, requiring a willingness to fall back on notes and sketches at times. However, this had some major compensations: a discursive collaboration involving sketching is invariably productive, particularly when informants can be persuaded to produce their own sketches.[10] As Afonso says, this often produces useful iterative material: "By offering local interlocutors the possibility of actively participating in creating, codifying and suggesting corrections to the

[10] Many of these were done on the ground with a sharp stick – a classic Queensland mapmaking method for both Aboriginal people and graziers.

sketches, it involved them in further constructing their discourses and reinterpreting their memories" (2004: 87).

The mix of formal and informal recording methods produced different kinds of information. For example, video recording encouraged some of the elders to give rich performative renditions of the ancestral stories at each site, providing the sounds and movements of the totemic ancestors, the calls of birds, and the histrionics of the *dramatis personae*. This produced a terrific record for the community archives. But less formal interviewing permitted more rambling flows of information and questioning, which opened up other areas of enquiry. Thus the mapping process gained from employing a range of data recording techniques, which not only provided a practical "Plan B" when equipment succumbed to environmental stresses, but also increased the diversity of form and content in the data collected.

So, what kinds of data should be collected in a cultural mapping project? We might consider two levels here: the contextual and the particular. From an ethnographic or ethnohistorical perspective, cultural mapping data, like any social data, are best considered in relation to a contextualizing "background" comprehensively encompassing all of the key aspects of cultural life: historical information; social and spatial organization; economic activities; cosmological beliefs; political arrangements; and laws and moral principles. These various dimensions of human life provide a basic set of questions about places. Who owns, lives here, or uses this place? How do they use it? How do they understand and think about it? How do they make decisions about it? What events have shaped their interactions with it over time? What do the features of the place mean to them? Social data also require a material context, which leads to complementary questions about the sites themselves. Where is this place? What does it look like? What features and resources does it contain? How has it changed over time? What are the local ecological opportunities and constraints?

But each cultural mapping project has its own aims, and it is these that define the areas of enquiry that are approached more intensively. In this case, the holistic nature of Aboriginal worldviews meant that the elders' aims were very compatible with the "contextualizing" ethnographic process - they were keen to record everything about each place. However, they foregrounded in particular the importance of recording the "stories": the ancestral myths located in the landscape, and the way that these defined who owned and had rights to each tract of land and its resources. And they were equally clear that they wanted to record the Aboriginal history of the area, which had previously been subsumed by European historical accounts.

From my perspective, these emphases were fine, since my research was focused on cultural landscapes and environmental values, and I was therefore happy (both intellectually and politically), to have the project shaped in accord with what my Kunjen collaborators thought was most important: accepting their direction was clearly a useful way to allow their particular values to emerge. This raises a useful point. In an academic environment requiring formalized grant proposals and subjecting researchers to constant auditing, ethnographers and historians often go into the field with a clear-cut list of the kinds of data deemed necessary for answering a particular research question. It is easy for this to become quite prescriptive and thus constraining. However, in terms of producing good ethnography or ethnohistory (i.e., effective representations of an emic perspective) it is vital to ensure that there are plentiful opportunities for informants to foreground what *they* think is important, not just in the co-design of the research, but also throughout the research process.

With this in mind, I had a number of meetings with key groups. These were composed primarily of the Kunjen clans for whom the park area was "country." In such a small community it was plain which families could "speak for that country," but working in larger research contexts I have made use of focus groups or social and professional networks. Similarly, in Kowanyama, arriving at a consensus about the project was also unproblematic, and did not require consensus analysis, or the kinds of negotiated design steps that might be needed in a less cohesive context. Following discussions about the kinds of data that were needed, I prepared a *pro forma* for mapping the sites. This included fields for the following information:

- date of the site visit;
- audio and/or video tape number;
- photographic film number (with a subset of numbers for photographs);
- GPS coordinates;
- site language name, and a translation;
- clan tract language name, and a translation;
- notes on language (some sites in the park also having non-Kunjen/Olkol names or names in the "respect language" Uw-Ilbmbanhdhiy);
- non-Aboriginal name of site;

- physical features of the site;
- totemic association for the site;
- synopsis of the related ancestral story(s);
- description of any related rituals and prohibitions;
- past and contemporary usages of the site;
- "bosses" for that place;
- associated clan names;
- related family names;
- historical data;
- "other information."

It will be apparent that the *pro forma* was intended as a system of data management as well as a checklist of key questions and areas of enquiry. Effective information management was vital, as the time available for each trip was limited and the mapping process commensurately intense. At the time, I made use of a computerized database I had designed prior to going into the field: a customized (one might say bastardized) Hypercard indexing system, with key areas relating to the information on the *pro forma*. There are now many "off the shelf" and doubtless vastly superior data management systems available, any of which are usable: the main requirement is that researchers can lay out a detailed landscape of data and find their way around it easily. But this basic necessity reminds us, of course, that data collection is in itself a process of virtual map making.

Many researchers add a further level of detail to basic index categories with a set of keywords or codes, which they insert as they collect data or take notes, so that they can search, find, and extract subthemes readily. I used quite a few of these, adding them, for example, where material related to issues such as "values," or "identity," which were the focus of my own research, or where people covered specialized topics, such as "legal" or "economic" issues. I also collected language terms and coded these too.[11]

There is no doubt that designing an organizational database and set of keywords is an excellent exercise prior to going into the field, but this is largely because it requires a thorough assessment of the aims of the research, and the kinds of data that are needed, and thus serves to clarify the project. However, in the field, considerable iterative adaptation and simplification of this system is often necessary,

---

[11] The *lingua franca* in Kowanyama is Aboriginal English, but at the time there were still some fluent Kunjen speakers, and I tried to record as much of the orthography as possible.

and it is probably a good idea to anticipate this.[12] And, as noted above, it is also critical to leave the door open to what the host community thinks is important.

In the Mitchell-Alice area, the actual mapping process was straightforward: the elders had a comprehensive and precise mental map of the park, and directed us from one key site to another. Most of these were water sources: creeks, waterholes and lagoons. At each, the elders who were "bosses" for that place would "tell the story." Although we had discussed the sites when planning the trip back in Kowanyama, this on-site process produced a set of data that was a quantum leap forward in terms of depth and detail, clearly tapping into a fountain of information held mnemonically in the landscape. Ancestral stories, histories, genealogies, key events, patterns of use, rituals, prohibitions, and a whole set of connections with related people and places would pour forth. The elders pointed out the key resources at each site, naming trees and plants, and discussing their uses, and recalling the kinds of fish and game to be found.[13] They noted many physical signs of use: scars in trees where shields, boomerangs, or burial bark had been cut; creeks where fish weirs had been built; stands of timber where they had collected spears or cabbage palm leaves for string; and the domiculture clustered around regular camp sites.

There was a constant flow of historical data about "early days": accounts of massacres and poisonings of local clans; the capture of women for enforced concubinage, and other events of the early colonial era. The elders noted the establishment of Koolatah Station nearby, and the pros and cons of the various sites at which the homestead had been located. Most had been stock workers for the station, and places therefore contained memories of events that had occurred during this time: where one man had been thrown from his horse and injured; where a bull had bailed up and had to be shot; where the stock team had had its "dinner camps."

The most important material was concerned with the ancestral story places and their tracks (or songlines) linking sites in the park and beyond. These sites are also known as "poison places," referring

[12] I suspect that most of us, flushed with early career-stage enthusiasm, tend to produce over-elaborate database management systems at first, and then, finding that these are too unwieldy or constraining, adopt simpler, more flexible approaches later on.

[13] In many places people had fishing lines in the water almost before I had turned off the truck engine, and this and other food gathering allowed us to extend the time that we could spend away from the settlement.

to the powerful concentration of ancestral forces that they contain. The elders systematically recounted the ancestral stories for each site and noted the related tracks. On arriving at each place, they called out to the ancestral beings. Like other newcomers, I had been formally "baptized" into that country previously, so that the ancestors would "know" me and not be malevolent (as they are reported to be to trespassers). Even so, at each site the elders explained our purpose to the ancestral beings: "We have come here with Ronnie, she is going to take photographs and write things down for us." Some of the more powerful places had traditionally demanded very respectful rituals. Thus at Stormbird Story place, where collective "fish poisoning" used to take place,[14] it was necessary for young boys to pull branches from the overhanging trees using a hooked stick, but without looking up, going only by the trees' shadows on the ground.

> See here, I gotta go like that. I can't look up, there's the story here. Break that limb, next feller come along. Head down, I can't look up ... cut him, tie 'em up in a bundle, right, go. Keep on walk ... This really story ground here ... he very good Law this feller. (Lefty Yam, Kunjen elder)

Other places had strict prohibitions: for example, Darkness Story Place links several important creation myths involving rainmaking and the bringing of fire to humankind. Even though the elders noted that, like other story places, it has unusually large and productive fruit trees due to the focus of ancestral power, it is forbidden to camp at the site, to collect any bush medicine, food, or materials, or to hunt there. It is a dangerous place, with any transgression resulting in illness or injury, and it has been known to try to take things, including horses:

> And that's where we lost one horse, right here. Right here, see that big tree there – they bin hold him. They [the ancestors] won't let go. Lot of us bin try, try to get him, you know, chase him back to the yard there ... He stand there, he not be dead ... "Come on, you better come with us," we bin sing out [to the ancestors], "Oy, don't hold that horse here! I want to go home!" (Lefty Yam, Ronnie Smiler, and Victor Highbury, 1992)

The ancestral stories provide a rich narrative of creative place-making. In them, totemic beings – usually in the form of birds and animals – hunt, gather, cook and fish, fight, fornicate, but above all make

---

[14] This entailed a large social gathering around a waterhole. Fish poisoning involves the use of bundles of sticks from a particular tree whose sap stuns fish, causing them to float to the surface. Having been collected they would be made into "fish cakes" for storage.

the features of the landscape. They bring rain, fire, wind, floods and storms; they push up sand ridges; wriggle through the land as snakes making rivers and creeks; they stick their spears in the ground making trees, or chop logs causing chips to fly everywhere and make plants; they release whole species of animals into the world. They define morals and social behavior; detail the ecological knowledge necessary for a successful hunter–gatherer economy; perform systems of trade and exchange. They also develop rituals and magic; generate "spirit children," and provide an entire cosmology of life and death, space and time. At the end of the creative era, they "sat down" into the land to provide clan ancestors, thus distributing people both socially and spatially in the landscape, and providing a permanent link between each individual and her or his "home" place.[15] They are visible as particular features of the landscape: for example, two date palms at Two Girls Story Place "stand for" the two women swallowed by a rainbow catfish at the site. At Emu Story Place, a creek bears the shape of the emu that, in a fight with Brolga, fell from the sky. More generally, though, the ancestral beings remain in the land as immanent, sentient forces, taking responsibility for the care of that landscape in partnership with their human descendents.

The ancestral stories are therefore not just a body of knowledge which informs every aspect of Aboriginal life, but also an indigenous narrative for the process through which cultural landscapes are made. In this sense, the narratives of place offered by the Kunjen elders are, in themselves, a vernacular process of mapping, demonstrating that people do this all the time, as a way of "being in the world." This is amply demonstrated, for example, by the ethnohistorical material that emerged relating to their relatively recent involvement in stockwork. A map of dinner camps, mustering yards, and community history was overlaid on that of the ancestral story places. By articulating and representing this information formally, our mapping project simply made this process and its cultural particularity more visible and explicit, which is, after all, the major purpose of ethnographic research. In effect, the elders were "reading the country" to me, drawing out the knowledge and history embedded in it, and pointing to the meanings of each local feature – which is how cultural mapping functions to enable anthropologists and historians to understand people's interactions with places.

---

[15] This is the site from which a person's spirit emerges, and to which it must be ritually returned upon their death.

When the data collection for the cultural mapping was complete, my task for the community was to create a report that laid out the information in a coherent way.[16] Following an introduction giving some ethnographic background and explaining the hybridity of the methods used, this was primarily composed of detailed site descriptions (in accord with the *pro forma*) and maps overlaying ancestral sites and tracks onto existing Ordnance Survey maps of the area. The oral material was transcribed and included *verbatim*, but, as Aboriginal narratives are often intensely circular and so confusing in written form, I also summarized the stories in a more readable linear form. This highlights the way in which representational forms themselves constrain or direct narrative style. The written reports were accompanied by photographs and by video and audio tapes, recording not only the stories and site visits from the park area, but also songs and dances relating these, sung and performed at other times during the fieldwork.

My own research had a different set of needs, requiring the analysis of the data, and the elucidation of findings. Here it was useful to consider Banks' comments about the analysis of visual material:

> In broad terms, social research about pictures involves three sets of questions (i) what is the image of, what is its content? (ii) who took it or made it, when and why? and (iii) how do other people come to have it, how do they read it, what do they do with it? (Banks 2001: 7)

Thus, in considering maps (collaborative or otherwise), it is useful to consider what elements people have chosen to include or exclude; what is prioritized; how the images express relations between things; and how places, people and events are formally represented. Researchers should consider which members of a community are given responsibility for making maps (and why); and how other people within the community and elsewhere engage with these representations.

But cultural mapping produces far more than visual images. As will be apparent from the case study, it makes use of discursive representational forms, eliciting oral histories and narrative accounts of places and events. Various approaches have been developed for parsing and analyzing narrative representations, building on early work, such as Barthes' structural analysis of narrative (1977). Derrida's deconstructive approach has also been influential, with Boje recommending

---

[16] I produced several reports following this format between 1994 and 2002. These remain confidential to the community and can only be accessed with the Kunjen elders' permission.

a series of steps considering the dichotomies or bipolarities in a narrative, its hierarchies, and its subaltern or excluded voices and issues (2001).

> Narrative analysis takes as its object of investigation the story itself ... Interpretation is inevitable because narratives are representations ... Human agency and imagination determine what gets included and excluded in narrativization, how events are plotted, and what they are supposed to mean. Individuals construct past events and actions in personal narratives to claim identities and construct lives. (Huberman and Miles 2002: 218)

Such analyses can be close-grained, particularly when interviews are recorded and transcribed *verbatim*. As van Maanen says: "crunching text requires text to be first put in crunchable form" (1988: 13). "Crunching" increasingly entails critical discourse analysis, which considers the relationships between language, ideology and power: "Power is conceptualised both in terms of asymmetries between participants in discourse events, and in terms of unequal capacity to control how texts are produced, distributed and consumed" (Fairclough 1995: 1).

There is obvious resonance between these approaches to narrative and Banks' recommendations regarding visual media. Both visual and textual media are amenable to analyses that consider their semiotic and symbolic structures, as well as the social and political relationships that they encapsulate. Maps employ specific graphic forms ranging from the multivalent symbols of Aboriginal dot paintings (see Morphy 1991) to the much more generic and explicit "universal" symbols of ordnance and survey maps. In this sense they may be said to have their own visual languages which are highly revealing of particular cultural worldviews.

The range of methods of collecting data in the National Park therefore produced material that could be interrogated in a number of ways. As well as enabling the cross-checking and triangulation of information for factual consistencies,[17] it allowed for a close-grained analysis of both textual and visual material to reveal recurrent themes

---

[17] Over time it revealed an enormous consistency in the ancestral stories and their location in place. About a decade later I did some cultural mapping in an area contiguous to the park, which was also crossed by some of the ancestral tracks running across the park area. The elder being interviewed recounted the whole story of each track, including the sections situated in the park. I compared it to the recording I had made in the earlier mapping expedition, and it was almost

and patterns. This provided a firm foundation for an ethnographic analysis, and also became part of the community archive.

The outcome was thus, as Flores described it, several hybrid products which fulfilled the goals of all parties (2004). For the elders, it created a resource which has been intensively used to educate younger members of the community, and to provide legal evidence for the community's efforts to reclaim its traditional land. It has assisted negotiations with the Queensland Parks and Wildlife Service, gaining the community special use rights and a co-managerial role in the Mitchell-Alice National Park. It has provided translatory material for the education of outsiders about Aboriginal culture, and supported the community's efforts to gain self-determination and a role in the wider management of the Mitchell River catchment. It led to my own involvement in further collaborative mapping expeditions, which over time have broadened into being training exercises for younger people, designed to establish more independent cultural mapping activities in the community.

This work was also invaluable in advancing my understanding of Aboriginal cultural landscapes. It provided useful experience of a methodology which could be applied elsewhere, and I have regularly employed similar methods in research with cattle graziers in the Mitchell River area, visiting the sites that they define as being important, and recording a wealth of data about their own uses of these; their perceptions about local ecology and landscape; their historical accounts; and their current engagements with places. Often, because both Aboriginal and non-Aboriginal land uses require reliable water sources, these are the same sites that I have visited with Aboriginal elders, but as I have noted previously (1997), they are very different cultural landscapes.

In recent years I have made extensive use of cultural mapping techniques, for example, in the UK with water users along the River Stour in Dorset. This research involved collaboration with an Arts and Environment group, Common Ground, whose project *Confluence* produced a cultural map unusual in European terms (though familiar to Aboriginal people) – a series of stories and musical compositions about places along the river. In Australia I have continued to do cultural

> 100% consistent with the version recorded then. I mention this in particular, because in the increasingly bitter contests over land ownership in Australia, those opposed to Aboriginal claims often accuse indigenous people of "making things up." Evidence of such consistency is therefore critical in the legal arena, emphasizing the potential legal utility (and risks) of cultural mapping.

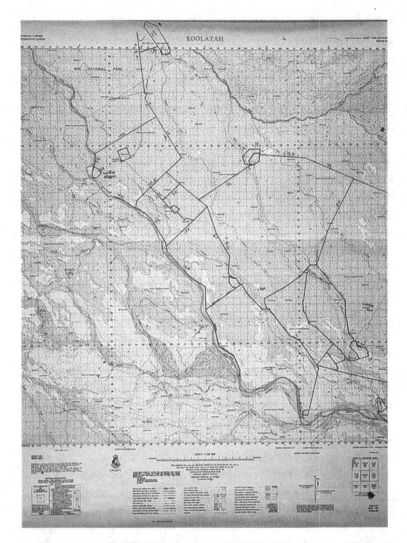

Figure 7.2   Map of paddocks and yards, Koolatah cattle station, Cape York.

mapping in the Mitchell and Brisbane River catchments, exploring the environmental engagements and territorially situated histories not only of Aboriginal people and graziers, but also of local farmers, miners, industries, catchment management groups, and recreational water users (Strang 2009).

I also give close consideration to the maps that informants use in their daily lives. For example, Australian graziers generally use standard OS maps, but superimpose upon them the things that they consider vital. Thus their additions focus on the roads, fencelines, dams, bores and paddocks they have constructed; the names that they have given to places; and information relating to water and fodder supplies (see Figure 7.2). They use the maps to describe and organize an annual cycle of movement of stockworkers, horses, cattle, and maintenance activities. Miners' maps similarly provide insights into a wholly different perspective, in which the landscape is seen in both spatial and temporal strata of soil and mineral deposition. For recreational water users, the focus is on fish or wildlife distributions, and aesthetic and sensory experiences of place (Strang 1996). Each mapping process therefore illuminates each group's particular engagements with place.

CONCLUSION

I have described above a quite detailed and formal process of cultural mapping: one that gives substantial depth to a research process. But this kind of methodology can be conducted much less formally too. Perhaps the most important element of cultural mapping is that it entails movement through places. This movement creates a very different kind of ethnographic interview. Even the simplest walkabout with a farmer on his or her land is vastly more informative than a static interview in the kitchen. A stroll down to the field to see how the carrots or melons are growing opens up discussions about access to water, and changes in rural life over time. A meander through the garden highlights the careful efforts that people make to create green oases in a dry country. In motion, people are more relaxed and forthcoming, and some of the most productive interviews I have had have been on long musters on horseback, where traditionally taciturn stock workers become more willing to open up and chat (see Figure 7.3). There are some technical challenges that come with this approach! It makes audio recording difficult (though not impossible), and photography somewhat risky to both person and equipment. Similarly, canoe trips with recreational water users, while wonderful in unfolding their experiences of river environs, does present some risk to expensive equipment.

However, even allowing for less than ideal recording quality (and at times transcription hell), cultural mapping and interviewing people *in situ* does, I believe, have significant advantages in terms of data quality. As well as providing opportunities to draw on the mnemonic value

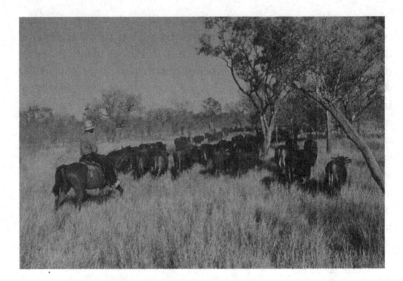

Figure 7.3   Mapping in motion: long cattle drives offer useful
opportunities for interviews.

of the physical landscape to elicit a wide range of data, cultural mapping
provides participatory and observational opportunities to consider the
places themselves, and the everyday engagements that people have
with them. As a collaborative and active exercise, it builds productive
relationships between researchers and informants. It produces representational objects that can be further interrogated analytically, and
which have multiple use values for host communities. I would therefore suggest that, as an approach to ethnographic and ethnohistorical
data collection and analysis, cultural mapping offers one of the most
useful and informative methods available to researchers.

There is considerable potential for the expansion of cultural
mapping into a wider range of representational forms. Pink observes
that "visual and digital technologies are becoming more economically accessible and 'user friendly'" (2006: 19). Computer programs are
increasingly interactive, enabling highly dynamic representations that
readily encompass both spatial and temporal change: "Besides being
able to draw a new map literally in the blink of an eye, the computer
is capable of displaying time dynamically ... These capabilities have
allowed the easy generation of 'map movies', and cartography in general has become an interactive tool" (Peuquet 2002: 155).

Researchers are now producing cultural maps that involve the
combination of digital photography, video, and audio recordings with

satellite imagery, GPS data, and other spatial representations. They also draw on other datasets, such as demographic information, land ownership and use data, and ecological information (see Vassilopoulos *et al.* 2008). Such projects are often directed towards widening access: thus Vanclay, Wills, and Lane (2008) report on a museum outreach program using web-based technologies and giving digital cameras to participating communities in the Murray-Darling river basin. "'Basin Bytes' was a digital photography, storytelling and collecting project [which] asked a range of participants in regional communities to reflect on their local landscape and sense of place through images and stories" (2008: 282).

The Centre for Research and Information Outreach (CRIO) at the Australian National University has produced a range of interactive web sites using a range of digital media to explicate and further develop cross-cultural research projects. This body of work highlights the utility of more flexible representational forms that, by encompassing multiple dimensions of spatial and temporal information dynamically, can assist theoretical and analytical developments in anthropology. These also have useful potential application in interdisciplinary research, bringing together diverse datasets, such as hydrological, ecological and social data. In recent years I have been working with some UNESCO colleagues to bring cultural mapping techniques into interdisciplinary water management. Such work presents significant technical and epistemological challenges, but promises much in terms of integrating concepts across disciplinary boundaries.

There are some cautionary considerations too. Every form of representation has a recursive life of its own, and researchers need to consider the cultural effects of collaborations directed towards hybrid representational forms. As Andrew Lattas notes (pers. comm. 2009), "landscapes are mapped onto people," and the representations that are produced therefore have meaningful implications for them. Even with more flexible technical methods for incorporating dynamic change over time, there is a tendency for cultural maps to fix boundaries and lifeways. This can be potentially positive and/or negative, enabling the preservation of cultural knowledge and assisting people's efforts to maintain continuities, but also inhibiting movement and underemphasizing the fluidity of cultural processes and environmental change. The reduction necessary to create comprehensible maps can obscure issues such as the contestation of spaces, intergenerational differences in engagements with places, and subaltern perspectives. And, even in the most apparently uncontroversial social environments, map-making almost always has a political dimension which needs careful consideration. Nevertheless, conducted ethically, and with scientific rigor, it has a great deal to offer researchers and the communities with whom they work.

ACKNOWLEDGMENTS

This chapter has had much useful input from colleagues at various stages. I would like to thank in particular my own colleagues in Auckland, as well as those in departments of anthropology in Oslo, Bergen, Belfast, and Durham. I am grateful to the editors of the volume for their advice, and I am, as always, indebted to the Kunjen people in Kowanyama and to the many other people who have participated in this research. The completion of this chapter was also enabled by a Fellowship at the Institute of Advanced Study at Durham University.

REFERENCES

Afonso, A. 2004. New graphics for old stories: representation of local memories through drawings. In S. Pink, L. Kurti, and A. Afonso, eds., *Working Images: Visual Research and Representation in Ethnography*. London and New York: Routledge, pp. 72–89

Arce, A. and E. Fisher 2003. Knowledge interfaces and practices of negotiation: cases from a women's group in Bolivia and an oil refinery in Wales. In J. Pottier, A. Bicker, and P. Sillitoe, eds., *Negotiating Local Knowledge: Power and Identity in Development*. London, Sterling, and Virginia: Pluto Press, pp. 74–97.

Banks, M. 2001. *Visual Methods in Social Research*, London: Sage.

Banks, M. and H. Morphy 1997. *Rethinking Visual Anthropology*. New Haven, CT: Yale University Press.

Barthes, R. 1977. Introduction to the structural analysis of narratives. In R. Barthes *Image–Music–Text*. London: Fontana Collins, pp. 79–124.

Bender, B. 1998. Subverting the Western gaze: mapping alternative worlds. In R. Layton and P. Ucko, eds., *The Archaeology and Anthropology of Landscape: Shaping your Landscape*. London: Routledge, pp. 31–45.

Benjamin, W. 1979. *One Way Street and Other Essays*, London and New York: Verso.

Boje, D. 2001. *Narrative Methods for Organizational and Communication Research*. London: Sage.

Carter, P. 1987. *The Road to Botany Bay: An Essay in Spatial History*. Boston, MA: Faber and Faber.

Clifford, J. and G. Marcus 1986. *Writing Culture: The Poetics and the Politics of Ethnography*. Berkeley, CA: University of California Press.

Cosgrove, D. 1989. Geography is everywhere: culture and symbolism in human landscapes. In D. Gregory and R. Walford, eds., *Horizons in Human Geography*. Basingstoke: Palgrave, pp. 118–135.

David, B. and J. Cordell 1993. Cultural site mapping in the Mitchell River Delta. Unpublished report to the Kowanyama Aboriginal Land and Resources Management Office, Kowanyama.

Durington, M. 2004. The hunters redux: participatory and applied visual anthropology with the Botswana San. In S. Pink, L. Kurti, and A. Afonso, eds., *Working Images: Visual Research and Representation in Ethnography*. London and New York: Routledge, pp. 191–208.

Fairclough, N. 1995. *Discourse Analysis: The Critical Study of Language*. London and New York: Longman.

Flores, C. 2004. Sharing anthropology: collaborative video experiences among Maya film-makers in post-war Guatemala. In S. Pink, L. Kurti and A. Afonso, eds., *Working Images: Visual Research and Representation in Ethnography*. London and New York: Routledge, pp. 209–224.

Foucault, M. 1972. *The Archaeology of Knowledge*. transl. A. Sheridan Smith. New York: Pantheon Books.

Henige, D. 1982. *Oral Historiography*. New York: Longman.

Herlihy, P. and G. Knapp 2003. Maps of, by, and for the peoples of Latin America. In P. Herlihy and G. Knapp, eds., Participatory Mapping of Indigenous Lands in Latin America, Special Issue. *Human Organization* **62**(4): 303–314.

Huberman, M. and M. Miles, eds. 2002. *The Qualitative Researcher's Companion*, Thousand Oaks, CA: Sage Publications.

Keith, M. and S. Pile, eds. 1993. *Place and the Politics of Identity*, London and New York: Routledge.

Kuchler, S. 1993. Landscape as memory: the mapping of process and its representation in a Melanesian society. In B. Bender, ed., *Landscape, Politics and Perspectives*. Oxford, UK: Berg, pp. 85–106.

Lassiter, L. 2005. Collaborative ethnography and public anthropology. *Current Anthropology* **46**(1): 83–106.

McIntyre, A. 2008 *Participatory Action Research*, Los Angeles, CA: Sage Publications.

Morphy, H. 1991. *Ancestral Connections: Art and an Aboriginal System of Knowledge*. Chicago, IL: Chicago University Press.

Morphy, H. 1993. Colonialism, history and the construction of place: the politics of landscape in Northern Australia. In B. Bender, ed., *Landscape, Politics and Perspectives*. Oxford, UK: Berg, pp. 205–243.

Orlove, B. 1991. Mapping reeds and reading maps: the politics of representation in Lake Titicaca. *American Ethnologist*, **18**(1): 3–40.

Orlove, B. 1993. The ethnography of maps: cultural and social contexts of cartographic representation in Peru. *Cartographica* **30**(1): 29–46.

Peuquet, D. 2002. *Representations of Space and Time*. London: The Guilford Press.

Pink, S. 2001. *Doing Visual Ethnography: Images, Media and Representation in Research*. Thousand Oaks, CA: Sage Publications.

Pink, S. 2006. *The Future of Visual Anthropology: Engaging the Senses*. New York: Routledge.

Ramos, A. 2004. Advocacy rhymes with anthropology. In B. Morris and R. Bastin, eds., *Expert Knowledge: First World Peoples, Consultancy, and Anthropology*. New York: Berghahn Books, pp. 56–66.

Reason, P. and H. Bradbury, eds. 2008. *The SAGE Handbook of Action Research: Participative Inquiry and Practice*. Los Angeles, CA: SAGE.

Schama, S. 1996. *Landscape and Memory*. London: Fontana Press.

Sillitoe, P. 1998. The development of indigenous knowledge: a new applied anthropology. *Current Anthropology*, **39**(2): 223–252.

Stewart, P. and A. Strathern, eds. 2003. *Landscape, Memory and History*. Cambridge, UK: Cambridge University Press.

Strang, V. 1996. Sustaining tourism in far north Queensland. In M. Price, ed., *People and Tourism in Fragile Environments*. London: John Wiley, pp. 51–67.

Strang, V. 1997. *Uncommon Ground: Cultural Landscapes and Environmental Values*. New York: Berg.

Strang, V. 2006. A happy coincidence? Symbiosis and synthesis in anthropological and indigenous knowledges. *Current Anthropology* **47**(6): 981–1008.

Strang, V. 2009. *Gardening the World: Agency, Identity, and the Ownership of Water*. New York: Berghahn Publishers.

Taylor, J. 1975. Mapping techniques and the reconstruction of aspects of traditional Aboriginal culture. Unpublished m.s., AIATSIS.

Vanclay, F., J. Wills, and R. Lane 2008. Museum outreach programs promoting a sense of place. In F. Vanclay, M. Higgins and A. Blackshaw, eds., *Making Sense of Place: Exploring Concepts and Expressions of Place Through Different Senses and Lenses*. Canberra: National Museum of Australia Press, pp. 278–287.

Van Maanen, J. 1988. *Tales of the Field: On Writing Ethnography*. Chicago, IL: University of Chicago Press.

Vassilopoulos, A., N. Evelpidou, O. Bender, and A. Krek, eds. 2008. *Geoinformation Technologies for Geo-Cultural Landscapes: European Perspectives*. London: Taylor and Francis.

UNESCO web site http://www.unescobkk.org/culture/our-projects/protection-of-endangered-and-minority-cultures/cultural-mapping/. Accessed April 20, 2009.

8

Metaphors and myths in news reports of an Amazonian "Lost Tribe": society, environment and literary analysis

CANDACE SLATER

INTRODUCTION

In the last days of May 2008, striking photos and accompanying stories of an Amazonian "Lost Tribe" found their way into an array of international news sources. One particularly arresting image of this previously "uncontacted" group – three natives in red and black body paint firing arrows from longbows at a low-flying aircraft – was beamed around the world (see Figure 8.1).[1] By the end of June, however, a number of news organizations had dismissed accounts of the Lost Tribe as a hoax. Although others continued to energetically defend the story's basic outlines – which were, indeed, true – it was now clear to all that the group in question had first been contacted a full century earlier and that the leader of the photographic mission had been fully aware of the "lost" tribe's existence for some time.

---

[1] See Survival International's initial press release "Uncontacted tribe photographed near Brazil-Peru border," Survival International, May 29, 2008, http://www.survivalinternational.org/news/3340. The release clearly mentions other uncontacted tribes "whose homes have been photographed from the air," but not all news sources do. The image bears an uncanny similarity to the reproduction of a photo of Xavánte men shooting arrows and hurling clubs at a low-flying airplane originally published in a 1944 edition of the magazine *O Cruzeiro* and reproduced in Coimbra *et al.* (2002: 76).

Environmental Social Sciences: Methods and Research Design, ed. I. Vaccaro, E. A. Smith and S. Aswani. Published by Cambridge University Press. © Cambridge University Press 2010.

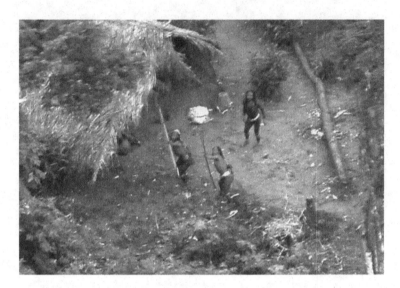

Figure 8.1   A much-disseminated photo of the people who became
known as the "Lost Tribe." Image © GLEISON MIRANDA/FUNAI. The
complete photo archive is available at www.survivalinternational.org.

The mission leader's assertions that he had taken the photos
expressly to rally worldwide opposition to illegal logging on the Brazil–
Peru border made it easy for some news sources to write off the story
as one more cautionary tale about news-hungry journalists and easily
swayed publics. However, it is also possible to see the case as proof of
the ongoing power of long-existing metaphors and myths that acquire
new meanings within contemporary political and economic contexts.
By "myths," I do not mean fallacies, but rather symbolic expressions
of collective beliefs and deep concerns that affect the perception and
presentation of apparent facts. The often complex ways in which different groups of environmental actors use these tropes for different
ends is both the focus of this chapter and the true moral of this story
of a not-all-that-Lost Tribe.

Whatever one's final understanding of the Lost Tribe narrative,
its analysis begins with the recognition of the deep importance of such
apparently straightforward stories to far larger perceptions of nature
and society. It is these narratives – which are always simplifications of
extremely complex cultural and environmental issues – that prompt
policies and actions. It is our task as scholars and political actors to
understand what gets distorted or ignored in these accounts of an at
once human and non-human world. Since this mission is impossible

without a comprehension of how these stories work, this chapter provides an initial framework for this crucial form of analysis.

Narrative analysis requires the use of a set of literary and linguistic tools customarily trained on clearly artistic objects (novels, poems, plays, new forms of digital expression). However, their rhetorical possibilities extend far beyond "creative writing." They permit the identification and interpretation of those larger metaphors and myths that lie close beneath the surface of what may initially look like straightforward journalistic accounts of one small group of Amazonian natives. Although this interpretive process does not directly indicate which policies work best in cases involving environmental problems that affect indigenous peoples, it leaves no doubt about the sorts of cultural desires and broader narrative expectations that even the most careful readers are apt to bring to accounts of isolated native peoples. This knowledge makes possible more clear-eyed and appropriate responses to environmental issues.

LITERARY ANALYSIS AS APPLIED TO ENVIRONMENTAL STUDIES

The last four decades of the twentieth century saw an explosion of new literary approaches linked to social discourse theories.[2] It would be hard to overestimate the importance of Marxist, feminist, psychoanalytical, semiological, post-colonial, and various other post-structural currents in present-day literary analysis.[3] The emergence of ecocriticism – "a term used primarily by scholars trained in literary studies to describe an interdisciplinary approach to the study of nature, environment, and culture" – has particular interest for researchers in the environmental field (Levin 2002:171).[4] All of these perspectives, however, depend to some degree on such fundamental elements of literary inquiry as plot, point of view, and verbal imagery.[5] The analysis that occurs in the following pages therefore

---

[2] There is a vast bibliography on literary criticism and theory. Useful overviews include Bressler (2003), Culler (1997), Selden, Widdowson, and Brooker (1997), and Waugh (2006). For specific links between literary and social discourse theories, see Hawkes (2003).

[3] For definitions of these approaches, see relevant entries in Groden, Kreiswirth, and Szeman (2005) and Waugh (2006). Classic texts include Culler (2003), Eagleton (2006), Elliott (1994), Moi (1985), and Said (1978).

[4] See Buell (2001, 2005), Glotfelty and Fromm (1996), and Levin (2002).

[5] Classic introductions to these sorts of devices include Strunk and White (2007) and Wellek and Warren (1947).

does not constitute an end in itself. Instead, it represents a requisite beginning capable of opening out into a number of successive literary and social questions that have generated an ample bibliography.

Scholars of environment-related issues have become increasingly attuned to issues of narrative in the last two decades and some have provided exemplary models of their use.[6] However, the field as a whole often continues to treat narrative as a more or less transparent vehicle for communication rather than a force that inevitably helps to shape ideas and behavior. My goal here is to further encourage "literary" readings of non-literary texts by scholars in a wide range of fields. Because of their insertion into a larger cultural framework all of these texts – even the most seemingly "factual" and straightforward – invite this sort of analysis.[7]

Individuals trained in literary criticism have much to gain from the creation of a broader context and extended audience for the texts that interest them. They can do this by broadening their focus to include narrative objects such as UN initiatives and research reports on global warming, as well as the sorts of mass media presentations that concern me here.[8] Likewise, the work of researchers in the social and environmental sciences can only profit from more systematic attention to the ways that words work in a wide array of texts.

The benefits of these sorts of "literary" readings will seem obvious to some readers. The "text" metaphor has been central to interpretive traditions in anthropology ever since Clifford Geertz's comparison of the practice of ethnography to the deciphering of a manuscript.[9] However, contemporary researchers' frequent emphasis on critical discourse analyses that stress political–economic histories and histories of difference tends to downplay the longstanding links between cultural anthropology and basic methodologies of textual analysis.

The reiteration of these links can do much to ease the still marked divide between primarily policy-oriented and more interpretive

[6] Diverse examples come from the fields of history (Cronon 1996), sociology (Guha 2000), economics (Guha and Martínez-Alier 1998), geography (Kosek 2006), anthropology (Lutz and Collins 1993), political science (Dryzek 1997), and literature (Handley 2007; Heise 2008; Outka 2008). See also a number of the essays in Cronon (1996). A notable attempt to apply narrative policy analysis to a concrete case (the Greater Yellowstone Coalition) is available in McBeth et al. (2007).

[7] Roman Jakobson makes the point that there is no such thing as pure information and that "all verbal behavior is goal-directed" in Jakobson (1960: 351).

[8] See, for instance, David Mazel's work on the discursive regime of the National Park Service in Mazel (2000).

[9] Geertz (1973: 10).

approaches to environmental issues. Instances of the policy/interpretative divide that come to mind include a long succession of TV documentaries on topics such as toxic waste or desertification that begin with a poem or snippet from a classic nature essay before quickly veering off into an avalanche of statistics. Another example would be academic conferences in which a single panel devoted to literary texts or similarly artistic forms is sandwiched into a long line of other presentations about climate change or indigenous rights as these emerge in environmental laws.

The incorporation of literary analyses and various forms of artistic expression into considerations of urgent, concrete problems is unquestionably useful. However, ongoing treatment of the two domains as largely separate suggests potential obstacles to problem-solving. The complexity of the issues facing researchers in the environmental field today makes it crucial to employ all methods that can produce clearer understandings, and therefore more effective policies. Basic literary analysis is one such approach.

A CAPSULE INTRODUCTION TO LITERARY METHODS

How then does one begin to engage in textual analyses linked to environmental problems? Here, I outline eight initial questions essential to approaching environment and society through the lens of narrative. No inviolable formula, the relevance and order of the steps outlined here will vary in accord with particular research frameworks. The questions should be seen as a kind of fluid menu meant to remind the researcher that even the most seemingly objective descriptions of the environment and environmental problems are never totally transparent. Though their degree of transparency may vary, they are always cultural texts.

The analytic process begins with the *recognition that images and stories of nature and society are always multiple and reflective of broader cultural preoccupations*. We will see, for instance, that the Lost Tribe story is often less about indigenous peoples than it is about the losses that a contemporary civilization sees itself as suffering. The very term "tribe" (as opposed to, say, "native group" or "indigenous community") conjures up a kind of close-knit intimacy hard to find in a globalizing world.

The second question involves *decisions regarding the collection of relevant narrative materials*. How many newspaper accounts constitute a representative sample in a given case, for instance? What kinds of visual sources are important? The collection process also requires the identification of the often multiple origins of images and stories. In the case of the Lost Tribe, these origins are often much older literary sources.

The *enumeration of the social, political, and economic interests most crucial to the story and its supporting images* constitutes the third step. Some of the major players who influence the particular presentation of the Lost Tribe story will be the Brazilian government, the National Indian Foundation, and a British non-governmental organization (NGO).

The fourth question concerns *changes over time through the incorporation of new developments and interests*. Partial answers to this question lie in shifts in vocabulary, choice of narrative focus (which personages or events), and plot as the story unfolds in the mass media. One such development in the case of the Lost Tribe is the later flurry of accusations that recast the original story as a hoax.

This focus on changes raises a fifth and crucial question regarding *the identity of key myths and metaphors used to describe the land and the people*. These key tropes – an "endangered paradise" versus a "savage wilderness" in accounts of the Lost Tribe, for instance – are not just multiple, but often, contradictory.

The sixth question hinges on *the ways in which tensions among these myths and metaphors become manifest within the story*. Accounts of the Lost Tribe are full of verbal claims and graphic images that do not entirely mesh. The spectacular and symbolically potent nature of the photographs of the Lost Tribe, for instance, casts at least a modicum of doubt on the idea of a child-like people entirely innocent of civilization.

The next question focuses on *ideas within the stories that would appear to challenge the prevailing narratives about this place and people*. Alternative accounts of the Lost Tribe as a group long known to scientists, for instance, challenge staunch assurances of their novel status.

The eighth and final question concerns *the relation of these alternative ideas to contemporary social, political, and economic concerns* that impact the people and the environment as a whole. What, one must ask in the case of the Lost Tribe, would be the policy implications of a new vision of the group as full-fledged actors with a special role within a larger, contemporary world? How does the publicity surrounding the existence of uncontacted Indians impact on a particular territory's legal status in regard to land use and tenure? Who are the primary participants' stakeholders in this representational project and how would particular images advance some projects and not others?

All of these questions, to be sure, suggest the importance of theory for analysis. The questions themselves constitute a kind of requisite beginning that establishes directions to be developed in accord with the particular narrative material. In the case of the Lost Tribe, one such thread might be a detailed analysis of the "smooth objects" in which complex relationships between humans and non-human environmental entities are polished in a way that removes from view the rough spots of disjuncture.[10] Another might be the identification within the stories of various "assemblages" or interacting constellations of disparate elements (Indians, oil, ideas about rain forests).[11] Yet another thread would entail detailed examination of the varied yearnings that revolve about particular environmental entities in different times and places.[12]

DISCOVERING THE LOST TRIBE: BACKGROUND
AND RESEARCH QUESTIONS

The Brazilian government National Indian Foundation, FUNAI, was the initial source of the account of the photographing of a remote Amazonian tribe. The release was then swiftly disseminated by Survival International, an NGO headquartered in Great Britain and devoted to ensuring the continued existence of tribal peoples around the world. The report was also taken up by worldwide news services including the Associated Press, the BBC, Al-Jazeera, and Reuters. Individual newspapers and broadcasting corporations, as well as a host of internet blogs in Brazil, went on to spread the story to many other corners of the globe. Although the heaviest coverage occurred in late May and throughout June, accounts of the "Lost Tribe" continued to appear well into August 2008.

Reports of an uncontacted native group triggered a certain degree of skepticism within Brazil from the outset. Although the word "uncontacted" can mean "living in isolation" in some contexts, a scattering of persons noted that the tribe's existence had been known for some time. This skepticism also reflected a more general wariness towards FUNAI, a government agency with tutelary responsibilities for native peoples, who are considered legal wards of the Brazilian State.[13] FUNAI, however, has moved away from older policies based on

[10] For a definition of the concept of "smooth objects," see Latour (2004: 22).

[11] The basic idea of an assemblage is that elements take on new identities through interaction. A "biker dude," for instance, is clearly more than just a man on a motorcycle. For more on assemblages, see Deleuze and Guattari (1987: 3–4).

[12] Here, I am thinking of a twenty-first century version of Stephen Greenblatt's (1992) meditation on the place of marvels in the Age of Discovery.

[13] The legal justification for guardianship is to defend the rights of those incapable of defending themselves. For an introduction to the modern history

"pacification" or the sorts of relations of exchange with governmental agents that have been calamitous to native peoples. The mass media, in contrast, still often fail to grasp the important practical implications inherent in seemingly synonymous terms such as "isolated," "uncontacted," and "undiscovered."

The story engendered fewer questions in an international context, where "uncontacted" was generally interpreted as having had no previous contact with a larger world. As we shall see, José Carlos dos Reis Meirelles Júnior, a FUNAI employee, played a central role in many news accounts. Although subsequent clarifications that he had already known about the tribe for some time prompted angry denunciations in some cases, it did not necessarily put an end to the story. Indeed, it often gave the tale new life.

Even this brief summary suggests a number of promising research questions. Two of these seem particularly fundamental to the case. First, in what sense was this tribe initially "lost" and what made its story so compelling to some readers even after it became clear that the group had long been known to "civilization"? Second, how was this story read within and outside Brazil? What parallels to other "Lost Tribe" narratives does it suggest and whose interests do they serve?

Both of these questions demand an understanding of what is old about the story (its larger literary underpinnings) and also of what is new about the particular social and environmental context that made the news reports compelling to a large and varied public. I argue that the narrative as disseminated in a hundred different variants drawn from the print and online versions of large and small newspapers as well as news blogs from throughout the world draws on elements of three time-honored myths or larger stories.

The first myth depicts Amazonian nature as both "Jungle" and "Rain Forest," two frequently competing concepts of tropical nature. (I use capital letters here and elsewhere to indicate the mythic construct.) The second myth portrays native peoples as "Noble Savages" or foils to civilization. The final myth asserts the existence of a rich but elusive realm whose name, El Dorado (literally "the Golden One"), suggests a close congruence between humans and non-human nature. Part of the task at hand is to demonstrate these stories' presence in accounts of the Lost Tribe. However, the real goal is to ascertain precisely which aspects of these time-honored tales have been

of indigenous peoples in Brazil, see Hemming (2003). For the roots of FUNAI (Fundação Nacional do Índio) in the earlier Indian Protection Service (SPI) see Diacon (2004: 101–130).

transformed to fit present-day environmental questions, and to suggest how and why. Through the use of rhetorical and stylistic tools associated with literary analysis one can tease out the mythic narrative structure that underscores contemporary depictions of these issues. Understanding the degree to which these mythic patterns underlie "objective" accounts makes researchers alert to unspoken biases that might otherwise escape them.

RESEARCH DESIGN

The three larger stories on which I focus are among the most common myths – a term already defined as symbolic expressions of collective beliefs – about New World nature and native peoples.[14] However, they are not the only such narratives. Rather than starting out by searching for particular tropes in the news accounts at my disposal, I was led to them by an initial analysis of basic literary traits.

Indeed, these seemingly straightforward accounts of the Lost Tribe held a number of surprises. The reports' insistence on the Amazonian natives' defense of their endangered forest home alerted me to elements of the idealized Noble Savage and the Rain Forest. However, I was less prepared for the additional presence of a more belligerent and enticingly dangerous Jungle.

Likewise, while some of the stories mention the dangers to the Lost Tribe posed by gold miners as well as loggers, gold, as such, is definitely not a major presence in these stories. It was therefore more than a bit startling to note the extremely powerful presence of El Dorado in many news reports. Although the precious minerals so important to Cortez and Columbus are in short supply here, the idea of a passionately desired, and yet unfailingly elusive nature turns out to be central. The related notion of people who embody a rich land – a cornerstone of the earliest El Dorado stories – is equally alive and well within contemporary narratives. These mythic roots will help to explain not only why the Tribe should be described as "lost," but why some reporters were outraged to learn of its previous discovery.

My analysis begins with a discussion of how the three sets of older myths and metaphors emerge through a close reading of the Lost Tribe reports. After showing how these recurring stories shape the news accounts, I reflect on the ways that they respond to contemporary social pressures. The examination then concludes with a brief

---

[14] For more on a number of these myths, see Slater (2002) and Stepan (2001).

consideration of how these myths can cast light not just on this story of a Lost Tribe, but also many other contemporary concerns including the ongoing yearning for wonder in a globalizing, high-tech era.[15] In the end, the Lost Tribe story is less about native peoples than the search for re-enchantment in a world where much that seemed most marvelous about non-human nature has either been destroyed or made to seem mundane (the once-surprising storms that are now the stuff of TV weather updates).

THE JUNGLE VERSUS THE RAIN FOREST: VOCABULARY AND RELATED LITERARY IMAGERY

The presence of a larger tension between the image of the Amazon as a nightmarish jungle and the Amazon as an Eden-like realm of nature (later to be known as "the rain forest") shows up in literary and non-literary sources ranging from multi-volume scientific studies to orange juice containers.[16] Although the two labels often refer to the same territory, the jungle is a much older word that retains connotations of savagery and tortuous complexity, as well as of adventure. The rain forest, in contrast, is a newer, more scientific designation for "a woodland with an annual rainfall of at least one hundred inches."[17] The term favored by environmental activists, it has acquired strong connotations of mystery, fragility, and magic which co-exist – sometimes uneasily – with this more scientific bent.

Contemporary divergences between the two concepts have deep roots.[18] An ongoing pull between an earthly heaven and an earthly hell within descriptions of New World forests is as old as the first colonial chronicles. Gaspar de Carvajal's sixteenth-century *Descubrimiento del Río de las Amazonas* (literally, "The Discovery of the River of the Amazon Women"), for instance, regularly flips between passages that describe impossibly forbidding vegetation and others that evoke an earthly paradise.[19]

---

[15] For a description of this sense of loss and the active search for re-enchantment, see Landy and Saler (2009).

[16] While Rain Forest ads in the 1980s and 90s stressed the need for biodiversity, more recent versions, such as the Rescue the Rainforest ad on Tropicana® juice containers during summer 2009, link the disappearance of rain forests to climate change.

[17] Webster's Third New International Dictionary, 1986 edn., s.v. "Rainforest." Not all authors agree on the hundred-inch criterion.

[18] For a detailed discussion of these, see Slater (1996).

[19] For an English translation, see Carvajal (1934).

While some accounts of the Lost Tribe favor one image over the other, the two often co-exist. The Jungle and the Rain Forest signal their pervasiveness through the use of vocabulary that can be divided into a half-dozen thematic clusters apparent in even the most cursory survey of news reports.

Words and phrases that convey intense sensation are particularly evident. Over and over, photos and accompanying stories about the Lost Tribe are described as "dramatic," "remarkable," "striking," and "extraordinary" – all terms that convey not just an intellectual judgment, but a visceral response.[20] If the appearance of the tribe is "like a scene from an Indiana Jones blockbuster," it is also a "stunning" and even "thrilling" discovery that is tinged with palpable excitement.[21] This astonishment reflects a digitalized, high-tech world's excitement at suddenly stumbling upon a people for whom a direct relationship with a still wonder-inspiring nature appears to be a fact of life.

This sense of surprise spills over into a second verbal cluster that deals directly with adventure and a kind of titillating danger. References to paths hacked through a nearly impenetrable forest and descriptions of "defiant" natives smeared in "vivid" body paint are good examples of this grouping. "Skin painted bright red, heads partially shaved, arrows drawn back in the longbows and aimed square at the aircraft buzzing overhead. The gesture is unmistakable: 'Stay Away'," declares the *Daily Mail*.[22] ABC News describes "nearly-naked Indians painted head to toe and brandishing bows and arrows."[23]

Often, these sorts of action-oriented terms are combined with long lists of unfamiliar objects whose presence on the page helps to create or deepen an existing aura of the exotic. Hard-to-pronounce fruits (acaí, uxi, patoá) and palm oils (copaíba, andiroba) are good examples. This third grouping also includes references to a number of animals

[20] See, for instance, Stuart Grudgings, "Amazon tribe sighting raises dilemma," *Reuters*, May 30, 2008, http://www.reuters.com/article/scienceNews/idUSN2938303320080530

[21] Jeremy Watson, "A tribe is discovered in a clearing of the Brazilian rainforest: should we leave them alone or prepare them for the 21st century?" *Scotland on Sunday*, June 1, 2008, http://news.scotsman.com/opinion/A-tribe-is-discovered-in.4139868.jp.

[22] Michael Hanlon, "Incredible pictures of one of Earth's last contacted tribes firing bows and arrows," *Mail Online*, May 30, 2008, http://www.dailymail.co.uk/sciencetech/article-1022822.

[23] Ashley Phillips, "Protection group knew about 'Lost' Tribe," *ABC News*, June 24, 2008, http://abcnews.go.com/Technology/story?id=5233627&page=1.

(lazy river turtles and colorful birds, but also frightening insects) that evoke a world very different from São Paulo or Manhattan.

A fourth vocabulary cluster includes a host of scientific and environment-related terms such as "habitat" and "fauna." References to "environmental heterogeneity," "isolated and unique ecosystems," and "anthropic transfers occasioned by sinkholes caused by greenhouse gases" signal a shift in register or level of discourse.[24] In contrast to the words in the first three groups, which often trigger colloquial, almost breezy descriptions, this fourth cluster is more apt to be associated with formal, sometimes, openly academic language that bespeaks authority.

These sorts of more scientific-sounding references may be allied to other terms that signal the presence of modern technologies such as GPS systems, reconnaissance aircraft, video cameras, and heat sensing devices. These words, which comprise a special subset of the fourth cluster, are regularly juxtaposed to other terms that conjure up a more elemental way of life. While references to thatched huts and dyes made from crushed seeds may suggest an element of the exotic, they are intended above all as lyrical contrasts with the world of machines and documentation or surveillance techniques.

This modern-versus-elemental theme only intensifies the sense of struggle suggested by a fifth category of words and images focused on encounters between unequal forces. Time and again, reporters speak of the "battle" (and, sometimes, the *batalha perdida* or lost cause) in which the Lost Tribe finds itself engaged. If its members are "warlike," this is because they have no choice but to do combat with monolithic forces – federal development programs, illegal loggers, and exploration by oil and gas companies – against which they have scant defense.[25]

A final group of words linked to fragility and the peril of extinction intensifies the aura of vulnerability surrounding the natives. Just as their immune systems are no match against imported diseases, so the encroaching shadow of deforestation threatens their wellbeing.[26] The Lost Tribe's apparently imminent disappearance coincides with the extinction of rare animal species – indeed, it is often described in terms ("habitat," for instance) that suggest

[24] "Governo anuncia novas medidas de proteção ao meio ambiente," *JB Online*, June 6, 2008, http://jbonline.terra.com.br/extra/2008/06/06/e06062769.html.

[25] See note 47 above.

[26] Daniel Howden, "The Amazonian tribe that hid from the rest of the world – until now," *The Independent*, May 30, 2008, http://www.independent.co.uk/news/world/americas/the-amazonian-tribe-that-hid-from-the-rest-of-the-world-ndash-until-now-836774.html.

its species-like identity. At the same time, the very fragility of the natives – and of that nature they defend so energetically – engenders an overriding sense of wonder reflected in words such as "surprise," "mystery," and "marvel."

It would be easy at first glance to see the first three vocabulary clusters as relating to the Jungle, the second three as relating to the Rain Forest, and accordingly to break the articles into two separate groups. This sort of division is readily visible in even very early news reports about the tropics. It also shows up in classic literary texts such as W. H. Hudson's 1904 *Green Mansions*, in which Rima the Bird Girl embodies the shimmering Forest while the brutal natives who pursue her stand in for the Jungle.

Sharp splits between the Jungle and Rain Forest continue into the present in mass market films such as *Anaconda* versus *The Emerald Forest*.[27] However, the distribution of the six vocabulary clusters throughout the Lost Tribe stories suggests that the concept of tropical nature in these accounts is far more intermingled. Although some news reports favor one vision of tropical nature over the other, the great majority combine elements from both. As a result, the world that emerges from these reports is neither an impossibly fierce Jungle nor a present-day Eden, but rather a kind of hybrid entity. Rarely perceived as a flaw by readers, the partial merger of these dissonant natures in reports of the Lost Tribe actually contributes to the story's appeal.

THE NOBLE SAVAGE: SUBPLOTS, CHARACTER ANALYSIS, AND POINT OF VIEW

Much in the way that an examination of vocabulary and primary images reveals underlying tensions between the Lost Tribe's home as Jungle and as Rain Forest, a look at other key literary devices suggests the presence of elements of a second myth – that of the Noble Savage. The term is often mistakenly associated with the Swiss Enlightenment philosopher Jean-Jacques Rousseau and those Romantic artists who celebrated the ideal of an unfettered humanity in harmony with nature and natural law. However, the Noble Savage actually began emerging with sixteenth century writers such as Michel de Montaigne who used

---

[27] *Anaconda*, directed by Luís Llosa, is a 1997 thriller involving a series of monstrous river snakes. *The Emerald Forest*, directed by John Boorman (1985), portrays a wondrous forest peopled by an aboriginal group besieged by civilization.

the figure of the socially wise, pacific savage to attack the more brutal aspects of civilization.[28]

Although the label "Noble Savage" is today often dismissed as racist and derogatory it is hard to ignore continuing elements of the concept within accounts of the Lost Tribe. The point is not so much that the natives are necessarily depicted as "savages" (though they are uncomfortably close to this stereotype in some reports), but rather that they inevitably serve as a foil to the modern world.

The lingering presence of the Noble Savage in a number of the Lost Tribe narratives emerges through examination of these stories' plots, their use of character development, and their point of view. The plot in virtually all of the initial stories is that of civilization's intrusion upon a group of Amazonian natives who seek to repel it. The tendency of character analyses to focus on Meirelles as a primary personage rather than on the natives, who are often depicted as too close to nature to have complex motivations, is highly revealing. So is the emphasis upon the ills of a jaded civilization from whose point of view these reports almost always speak.

We have already seen that the natives in Lost Tribe reports may reveal traits customarily associated with the Jungle: aggressiveness, defiance, wildness. The basic plot or story line nonetheless reveals civilization to be the true aggressor. This is clear from the very beginning when Meirelles declares that "what is happening in this region [of Peru] is a monumental crime against the natural world, the tribes, the fauna, and is further testimony to the complete irrationality with which we, the 'civilized' ones, treat the world."[29] His efforts to protect a group that has long lived in harmony with their surroundings underscores the story's debts to a long line of prior depictions of Amazonian Indians as guardians of nature in the fight against its would-be destroyers.

Today, "savage" usually has extremely negative connotations of brutality and barbarism. To the extent, however, that the term retains something of its initial Latin meaning of "pertaining to the forest; remote from human abodes and cultivation; in a state of nature;

---

[28] See "On cannibals" in Montaigne (1948). Montaigne's deeply ironic essay is sometimes said to be a partial response to the brutal three-day Saint Bartholomew Massacre eight years earlier. The term "Noble Savage" appears to have been coined by John Dryden in a 1672 poem. For a history of the concept, see Ellingson (2001).

[29] See note 1 above. The quote also appears in various Associated Press releases.

wild; as, a *savage* wilderness" most of the Indians who appear in these reports are definitely savages.[30]

The Lost Tribe's essential otherness finds expression in its resistance to the usual methods of character analysis. The "Amazonian natives" in these dispatches are not individual actors who invite speculation in regard to motives. Rather, they are embodiments – indeed, emanations – of that fluid nature (now Jungle, now Rain Forest) that is itself an idealized personage.

As embodiments of nature, the tribe's members do not offer much in terms of dialogue. Reporters must therefore seek out others who can speak for them. These persons include the head of FUNAI's Isolated Indians Department, the director of Survival International, the head of the Peruvian National Institute of Natural Resources (INRENA), and various Brazilian and Peruvian anthropologists and environmental activists. However, as noted from the outset, it is Meirelles who dominates a number of international reports.

Meirelles' identity as the initial eye witness to the Lost Tribe story, as well as the head of FUNAI's Environmental Protection Unit makes him an essential presence. His knowledge of the geographic area and his contacts with similar tribes makes him the source of a host of vivid details. He also regularly furnishes the sorts of statistics that inject a tone of authority into news reports based heavily on information gleaned from websites and the usual news services rather than primary resources.[31] His key role in the action and his colorful, often folksy quotations initially make him the perfect middle man or culture broker between two worlds. It is therefore not surprising to find him serving as a lead character in many news reports.

New media attention to Meirelles' assertions that he had known for some time about the Indians' existence causes what had been a single plot to fork into three separate narrative options. The first of these options is characterized by anger at his perceived misrepresentation of the tribe. The second involves a widening of the story into a more general report of environmental abuses. The third sees a shift in focus away from the discovery of the Lost Tribe to examinations of Meirelles' motives. All three options, however, permit reporters to

---

[30] Webster's Third New International Dictionary, 1986, s.v. "Savage." The Latin root is *silvaticus*.

[31] For an example, see Associated Press. "One of last remaining 'uncontacted' tribes spotted in Brazil," *CBC News*, May 30, 2008, http://www.cbc.ca/world/story/2008/05/30/brazil-tribe.html.

go on telling the story of a nature-focused tribe from a civilization-oriented point of view.

It is worth examining each of these variations with an eye to how they affirm this viewpoint. The first option – the denunciation of Meirelles' supposed misrepresentation of the Indians as previously uncontacted – is at once readily comprehensible and curiously excessive. Although no journalist likes being fed false information, irritation at Meirelles' attempts to generate publicity does not fully explain the outright fury that pervades some reports of the "deception." While Meirelles appears to have allowed, if not encouraged, ambiguous understandings of the word "uncontacted" (which many reporters took to mean "undiscovered" and not simply "isolated from civilization"), he did not invent them from thin air like some sort of Big Foot figure.[32] As a result, while it remains easy to question his actions and opinions, words such as "fraud," "scam," "trickery," and "PR joke" seem more than a bit harsh.

The frequent vehemence of these reactions underscores the degree to which these stories speak from the viewpoint of a civilization eager to believe in the continuing existence of human groups inseparable from nature. Meirelles' revelations represent an affront not just to journalists' professional pride but above all to the power of ideas concerning native peoples as guarantors of an uncorrupted natural law. Although some reporters do express concern for the fate of the Lost Tribe, this Tribe clearly represents an antidote to the imperfect modern world that is their readers' true concern.

The second narrative option – a diminution of the role of the Lost Tribe following Meirelles' clarifications – maintains a civilization-oriented point of view by shifting the story's focus away from the contacted tribe towards an overarching battle between nature's allies and its destroyers. This option often takes the form of detailed comparisons of Peruvian with Brazilian indigenous policies in which Peru is seen to turn a blind eye to environmental devastation while Brazil valiantly protects the natives' rights. These comparisons, which spur any number of charges and counter-charges, can be read as the continuation of a struggle over Amazonian territories between the two nations that dates back to the late nineteenth and early twentieth

---

[32] Several news sources actually compare the Lost Tribe to the Loch Ness monster. See, for instance, Cédric Gouverneur, "Les Indiscrets: La tribu perdue d'Amazonie n'était pas vraiment," *VSD*, June 25, 2008, http://www.vsd.fr/contenu-editorial/l-actualite/les-indiscrets/652-la-tribu-perdue-d-amazonie-ne-l-etait-pas-vraiment.

centuries.[33] However, to the extent that Brazil emerges as the guardian of a Lost Tribe inseparable from a beleaguered nature, the story moves from history towards myth.

The final narrative option – the transformation of Meirelles from sympathetic bureaucrat to complex "tribal guardian" – looks very different on the surface from the first two possibilities. In the end, however, it reveals the most clearly civilization-oriented point of view. This is because this transformation converts Meirelles into the subject of intense psychological interest while the members of the Lost Tribe become more or less supporting actors.

It would be possible to do an entire study of the literary tropes present in newspaper profiles of this *sertanista* or "wilderness explorer" as a sort of more racially sensitive, GPS-toting Davy Crockett.[34] For our purposes, however, the real point is less reporters' insistent probing of Meirelles' psyche than their treatment of the Lost Tribe's actions as wholly transparent

After Meirelles speaks of having purposefully arranged the flight over the natives' settlement in an aircraft provided by the state of Acre, reporters quickly zero in on the details of the "hoax."[35] Very few news sources of the many I encountered, however, take the trouble to explain that the plane made various passes over the area at different times thereby giving the Indians time to mount a response.[36] All of the other reports leave the reader to conclude that some members of the tribe normally stroll about in war paint and that they happened by chance to be assembling their longbows precisely in that moment that the aircraft appeared.

My point here is not that the Lost Tribe willingly cooperated on some level in a publicity venture. Rather, it is the almost complete

---

[33] These conflicts are the subject of a series of essays by the celebrated author Euclides da Cunha during the height of the Rubber Boom. See da Cunha (1986).

[34] See Hemming (2003) for more information on *sertanistas*.

[35] For the initial "hoax" story, see Peter Beaumont, "Secret of the 'lost' tribe that wasn't," *The Observer*, June 22, 2008. Survival International later brought a complaint before the British Press Complaints Commission which was decided in its favor. For the apology, see Stephen Pritchard, "How a tribal people's charity was misrepresented," *The Observer*, August 31, 2008, http://www.guardian.co.uk/commentisfree/ 2008/aug/31/voluntarysector. The *Observer* story nonetheless triggered any number of yet more indignant reports.

[36] Those few articles that describe various aircraft passes generally quote CNN. See, for example, "'Uncontacted tribes' sighted in Amazon," *Modern Ghana News*, May 30, 2008, http://www.modernghana.com/news/167637/1/uncontacted-tribes-sighted-in-amazon.html.

silence of the media regarding any possibility that the group consciously chose to make full use of the opportunity provided by Meirelles. That the natives expressly chose to show themselves instead of hiding in the forest suggests that the aircraft's repeated flights over the village may have struck them as an opportunity to send a message to a larger world.

The majority of the reports, however, read as if the Indians acted with the literal intention of scaring away the aircraft rather than a desire to take full advantage of its presence. As such, these stories suggest a perceived innocence on the natives' part that ultimately sets them apart from other humans. It also makes them minor characters within a drama in which they should, by all rights, star.

Why do reporters seem uninterested in the remotest possibility of some sort of impromptu collaboration between the natives and Meirelles? One possible answer has to do with the news organizations' strong sense of the Lost Tribe's physical distance from the rest of the world. This sense reflects in part material conditions including harsh terrain and dense vegetation. However, it also reveals a symbolic dimension that underscores the "noble" rather than the "savage" in the term "Noble Savage." The surety that the tribe acted spontaneously (rather than in calculated fashion) centers on perceptions of psychological as much as physical distance from civilization. The slightest hint that the Lost Tribe might have been involved in a publicity effort would place in question the very qualities that made them newsworthy in the first place. It would also create doubts about their status as useful foils to a modern world whose interest in the tribe's purity suggests its own need to find solace in the continuing existence of an unsullied nature.[37]

EL DORADO: PHYSICAL SETTING AND BROADER SOCIAL AND ENVIRONMENTAL CONTEXT

Ongoing depictions of the Lost Tribe as a group of contemporary Noble Savages "alarmed" about (but not yet corrupted by) an encroaching civilization are hard to separate from portrayals of their territory as one of the last patches of a wonderfully mysterious, if vulnerable Virgin Rain Forest. Close examination of the physical setting of these news

---

[37] It would put them in the category of tribes seen as having "sold out" to civilization such as the politically adept, but much-criticized Kayapó analyzed in Conklin and Graham (1995).

reports, however, suggests the presence of a world that goes beyond the dazzling array of rare and wondrous plants and animals that has become synonymous with rain forests. This world is a modern variant on the colonial El Dorado.

The lands described in reports of the Lost Tribe are as rich as any conventional representation of Amazonian nature. They contain a host of saleable commodities (gas and oil, as well as those tropical hardwoods that prompt loggers' invasions). They are also home to those more diffuse resources (species diversity, pharmaceutical potential, that moisture-retaining biomass seen to temper global warming) regularly associated with rain forests. And yet, while these riches unquestionably enhance the appeal of the Lost Tribe's lands to outsiders, the elusiveness that remains at the very heart of El Dorado is their prime attraction Although the iconic Rain Forest is often counter-posed to cities, it lacks the tenacious remoteness that distinguishes the Golden City. As a result, while El Dorado conceals itself at every juncture, even the most virginal Rain Forest invites scientific investigation.

Elusiveness demands the kind of physical and psychic distance we have already described in examinations of Noble Savage imagery in the Lost Tribe stories. The importance of the natives' uncontacted status to readers and reporters suggests the tribe's association with a contemporary shining realm boundless enough to shelter all sorts of undiscovered peoples, and yet, shrinking by the second. Although the natives' lands are described in ways that suggest elements of the Rain Forest and the Jungle, they are first and foremost an El Dorado in their promise of a world apart.

El Dorado is one of the most enduring myths to shape the exploration of the New World. For a number of the first explorers, gold was not just a precious object, but often a living thing. It evoked echoes of both medieval alchemy and a classical Golden Race or Golden Age in which all humans lived in perfect harmony with a bountiful nature. This tale often merged with other, native accounts of a Land without Evil.[38] This bounty found expression in stories of a king so rich that he would wash off every evening in a lake the thick golden coating applied to his skin at dawn.[39] With time, belief in an actual sovereign

---

[38] This Tupi-Guarani Land without Evil is described at length in Clastres (1975).

[39] For an introduction to the El Dorado myth see Ainsa (1992). In some versions of the story, the Golden King sets out on a raft to deposit offerings of gold, pearls, emeralds and other precious metals into the center of a lake.

who resembled a living golden ornament and of a shining lake at the heart of an unknown continent grew less common. However, the idea of a precious nature that remains just out of reach continues to find expression in a host of new forms.

In Latin America, the treasure trove that is El Dorado is inextricably linked to ideas about Lost Tribes through narratives about the Amazons – the warrior women of classic mythology known for their gold and silver armaments (and, later, their silver tears). The belief that these women could be found among the New World tribes had much to do with an initial conceptual meshing of the Indies and the Americas. Some Iberian explorers' contracts actually included a clause that enjoined them to look for the Amazons because where these warrior women were, treasure must abound. As a result, the search for El Dorado was never simply the search for gold, but also, the yearning to witness firsthand the marvelous secrets of the past.[40] This imaginative pull is nowhere more evident than in the contemporary geographical designation "Amazon," for not just an immense river, but all of a sprawling region.

The presence within the Lost Tribe stories of the far older idea of an El Dorado distinguished by its tenacious elusiveness (and thus, perennial novelty to a weary civilization) helps explain otherwise puzzling facets of these narratives. Chief among these is an open-ended, porous quality that makes the story of the Lost Tribe paradoxically familiar in its insistence on the natives' strangeness.

A quick internet search for "Lost Tribe" brings up a host of references to this and other tribes in a variety of times and places dating back to the very beginning of the twentieth century. A few of these stories contain unique details that distinguish the native group in question from various others. Many, however, are so similar as to be all but interchangeable. At one point, I found myself puzzling over an aspect of the story that seemed oddly out of place before realizing that I had pulled up an article about another "uncontacted" tribe from 2007.[41] The same thing happened with a case from 2001.[42] Moreover,

[40] A classic description of the scholarly literature on the New World Amazons appears in Gandia (1929: 71–101). The Dominican friar Gaspar de Carvajal describes an actual battle between Spanish explorers and what he believes to be these warrior women that took place in 1541–42.

[41] The 2007 articles are about the remarkably similar Mashco Piro tribe in Peru. See "'Unknown' Peru Amazon tribe seen," BBC News, October 4, 2007, http://news.bbc.co.uk/2/hi/americas/7027254.stm.

[42] The 2001 articles relate an encounter with the Tsohon Djapa. See "Brazilian lost tribe discovered," BBC News, April 9, 2001, http://news.bbc.co.uk/2/hi/americas/1267845.stm.

new, profoundly "isolated," if not actually "uncontacted" tribes continue to surface, as is clear in a report from October 2009.[43]

This parade of similar reports suggests that the larger story of a rich but ultimately elusive place of riches may have multiple beginnings and middles, but no visible end. Significantly, when Meirelles' Lost Tribe turned out to have been contacted, talk of other, yet more isolated tribes in even more remote locations quickly filled the gap.[44] The proliferation of assurances about these other groups once more suggests that the outside world's concern is less for the welfare of the tribe than for the preservation of its own irresistible fantasies. In this case the fantasies involve the continued existence of a group of people who had ignored their own extinction in order to suddenly waltz out into the world like human dinosaurs.

Another central facet of the El Dorado story – its equation of the golden monarch with his shining kingdom – lives on in more recent narratives such as that of the Lost Tribe. We have already noted the close association between the natives and the natural world of which they appear at times to be a mere extension. To the extent that this natural world appears to be a remote, elusive El Dorado, then, by definition, its residents cannot have been previously contacted.

The use of the word "lost" as a translation for "previously unknown" or "not yet contacted" in Portuguese seems curious at first glance. ("Perdido," the direct translation is never used in news reports, probably in part because of its negative moral connotations in Portuguese.) How could something or someone be lost if this word always signifies prior possession or control? If the tribe was "unknown to civilization" before its "discovery" by Meirelles, then how could it be deemed "unable to be found or recovered?" The idea that the Lost Tribe is known through reports and yet undiscovered links it to the story of an El Dorado that evades possession but whose existence is nonetheless assumed true thanks to widely circulated claims.

---

[43] Leonardo Guandeline, "Expedição vai passar dois meses na selva em busca de índios isolados da Amazônia, 23 October, 2009, http:oglobo.com/cidades/mat/2009/expedição-vai-passar-doismeses.

[44] FUNAI believes there to be up to 68 "uncontacted" tribes in other parts of Brazil – a fact quoted in many news articles. See, for instance, Associated Press. "Brazil reveals uncontacted Amazon tribe," Welt Online, May 31, 2008, http://www.welt.de/english-news/article2052327/Brazil_reveals_uncontacted_Amazon_Tribe.html. These "official estimates" are generally based on rumor, vestiges of former habitation sites, the discovery of outsiders' corpses, and occupation sites observed through aerial reconnaissance.

Countless prior attempts to locate El Dorado provide a kind of proof of its existence. Although Sir Walter Ralegh's early seventeenth-century quest for the golden realm of Manoa is probably the most famous of these searches, it is hardly unique.[45] Over and over, early European explorers set out to find the lake or king or city that others had only partially described in legends. The idea that this tantalizing destination was once known to someone, somewhere, made it possible for others to perceive the kingdom as only temporarily lost and thus waiting to be found by persons just like them. The notion of a wondrously attractive, if evanescent refuge lives on in celebrated mid-twentieth-century texts such as Claude Lévi-Strauss's *Tristes Tropiques* (1973) and Alejo Carpentier's *The Lost Steps* (1956). Although these narratives (one a piece of academic travel writing, the other a novel) are marked by a rueful irony alien to colonial writings, they too are quests for a rich and staunchly inviolate nature. As such, they provide a bridge between these colonial depictions and twenty-first-century reports of the Lost Tribe.

I have already suggested that the cherished notion of an undiscovered world of indescribable abundance together with a more general yearning for marvel and a lost sense of wonder helps explain much of the furious reaction to the news that the Lost Tribe had long been known to civilization. The real source of this seemingly disproportionate anger at Meirelles is almost certainly his perceived betrayal of a much older dream about the continuing reality of a virgin nature that lives on apart from civilization. Although it is the Lost Tribe that is in danger of losing its way of life, the blow to abiding hopes of an Edenic refuge yet to be discovered or rediscovered, along with the more general hunger for nature's re-enchantment, is the real source of the deep disappointment obvious in headlines from around the globe. "Photos of lost Amazon tribe are fakes," one says glumly.[46] "A savage hoax: the cave men who never existed," another indignantly laments.[47]

---

[45] See Ralegh (1997).

[46] Gareth Dodd, "Photographer: photos of lost Amazon tribe are fakes," *Xinhuanet*, June 24, 2008, http://news.xinhuanet.com/english/2008–06/24/content_8429135.htm.

[47] Benjamin Radford, "A savage hoax: the cave men who never existed," *LiveScience*, June 25, 2008, http://www.livescience.com/strangenews/080625-tasaday-hoax.html.

DIFFERENCES IN INTERPRETATIONS OF THE LOST TRIBE
STORIES WITHIN AND BEYOND BRAZIL

Although many news articles portray the Lost Tribe's lands as an El Dorado, they do so in a way suggesting different social and political contexts and varying perspectives towards key environmental problems and debates. While any hard-and-fast division between reports from Brazil and international coverage would be misleading, it is nonetheless both possible and useful to compare the two types of reports in terms of their reworking of centuries-old myths.

In general, international reports of the Lost Tribe are ultimately most concerned with much larger issues such as species extinction and, above all, climate change. They are particularly likely to register ambivalence about a tropical nature that contains elements of both Jungle and Rain Forest. They are also customarily focused on the ills of a civilization from which readers, like reporters, seek escape through the fantasy of a group of people who have never seen a cell phone, an overflowing email inbox, or a tax return.

Although a number of the Brazilian articles reveal similar tendencies, they are more apt as a whole to address specifically national concerns. Many of these stories focus on the relationship between economic development and environmental preservation. Despite their frequent reliance on the same sources, Brazilian reports are also likelier than their international counterparts to touch directly on practical problems. They are, for instance, generally more interested than reports from abroad in what exactly should be done about illegal logging. As a result, their larger context is strongly shaped by contemporary political events and economic interests.

In contrast to the event-oriented reports in many Brazilian news sources, international versions of the Lost Tribe story tend to express more diffuse environmental fears. References to rain forests as a hedge against global warming underscore the Lost Tribe's perceived importance as a fragile bulwark against the sorts of irremediable climatic changes that anxious readers and reporters rue.

If tropical nature in the form of the imperiled Rain Forest makes an ongoing appearance in international newspaper stories of the Lost Tribe, so does a Jungle that excites ongoing ambivalence. A number of later articles about the Lost Tribe appear on the same page as news reports regarding the experiences of former French-Colombian presidential candidate Ingrid Betancourt, whom Marxist guerrilla forces held prisoner in the Amazonian interior for more than six years.

It would be hard to prove that Betancourt's descriptions of her captivity in a conventionally horrific Jungle directly color accounts of the struggles between loggers and Indians in later Lost Tribe stories. Nonetheless, these descriptions, which begin with Betancourt's release on July 2, 2008, definitely utilize the sorts of more fearsome images of tropical nature that creep at times into the Lost Tribe reports.[48] These reports suggest the existence of new-style monsters (guerrilla fighters, outlaws, international terrorists) within forests once reserved for native peoples and wild beasts. These distinctly frightening elements may, however, co-exist with expressions of concern for a Jungle ultimately no less fragile than the shimmering Rain Forest.

International articles also tend to register a strong sense of disenchantment with a world in which economic worries were beginning to cloud the horizon. Over and over, online comments express the hope that the Lost Tribe can remain immune from the sorts of ever greater pressures that the authors of these postings experience in their own lives.

The Brazilian articles' generally more practical, specifically national perspective is clear in the debates about Peruvian versus domestic indigenous and environmental policies that I have already mentioned. A number of these articles openly declare that Brazil cares more about native peoples than does Peru. Other articles sharply criticize FUNAI's actions in regard to the Lost Tribe. Fairly often, bits and pieces of far-reaching debates about the environmental policies backed by the ruling Workers' Party and President Luís Ignácio da Silva ("Lula") find their way into descriptions of the tribe.

It is almost impossible to read Brazilian news accounts from May and June 2008 without positing some sort of connection between the Lost Tribe and the very public resignation of then-Minister for Environmental Affairs, Marina da Silva – a figure who first achieved prominence through her association with the celebrated rubber tapper Chico Mendes and whom international organizations continued

---

[48] "Everything in the jungle bites, each time you try to grab onto something so that you don't fall, you've put your hand on a tarantula, you've put your hand on a thorn, a leaf that bites, it's an absolutely hostile world, dangerous with dangerous animals. But the most dangerous of all was man, those who were behind me with their big guns," Betancourt says in a report by Steven Erlanger and Alan Cowell, "Betancourt, in Joyous Return to France, Details Her Suffering in Colombia," *New York Times*, July 5, 2008.

to hold in high esteem.[49] Her resignation – interpreted as a sharply negative judgment on Lula's environmental policies – occurred at a particularly awkward moment. Not only was Brazil hosting German chancellor Angela Merkel but a bevy of BBC reporters was busy filming a documentary about the Amazon – both facts that placed the region squarely in the European public eye.

There is no proof that the barrage of angry commentaries about Brazil's lack of commitment to environmental concerns that greeted this high-profile resignation directly triggered stories in which FUNAI comes across as a concerned guardian of native peoples. Nonetheless, it would be hard not to find the story's appearance so close on the heels of Marina da Silva's exit politically significant. As a result, while some Brazilian accounts closely resemble stories in other countries, many others are clearly colored by the particular moment in which the Lost Tribe reports arose.

Finally, the implications of the Lost Tribe's existence for the Amazon's extraction-oriented economy, while rarely spelled out in these articles, almost certainly influences portrayals of this native group. Much like the developers in the United States who dread the discovery of archaeological sites or endangered species on public lands, large economic interests in Brazil have little sympathy for the native peoples whose presence converts what was formerly "free space" into protected Federal Land. While the Workers' Party government had no alternative in this case but to support the Indians, the would-be developers – often linked to media empires – must have delighted in the media accusations of a hoax. The ties between symbols and land use in the case of the Lost Tribe are a sobering reminder of the power of myths and metaphors.

THE LOST TRIBE: A SUMMING UP

The analysis laid out in the preceding pages allows us to return to the eight basic questions outlined at the beginning of this chapter. The *broader cultural preoccupations* that run through the stories leave no doubt that news sources' concern for the members of the Tribe is often really a concern for lost origins and a supposedly "virgin"

---

[49] See, for example, the assessment of da Silva in "Welcome to our Shrinking Jungle," *The Economist*, June 5, 2008, http://www.economist.com/displayStory. cfm?story_id=11496950. See also Kennedy Alencar, "Ação de Dilma junto a Lula foi decisive para queda de Marina," *FolhaOnline*, May 18, 2008, http://www1.folha. uol.com.br/folha/colunas/brasiliaonline/ult2307u402986.shtml.

nature in whose surprising and marvelous existence the members of modern consumer societies deeply want to believe. As a result, the relevant narrative materials are not simply these news sources, but rather that long line of literary texts regarding lost paradises and Noble Savages on which so many of these contemporary sources unconsciously draw.

The *social, political, and economic interests central to these stories* turn out to be key forces within a globalizing world. They include national governments (Brazil and Peru), government agencies (not just the FUNAI, but the Ministry of the Environment), and NGOs (Survival International, in particular). They also encompass any number of information agencies, news publications, internet sites, and TV and radio stations – each with their own particular perspectives and needs. We have seen how the addition of other social actors as well as the accusations that the story is a "hoax" changes perceptions of the Lost Tribe vis-à-vis a larger world.

The search for the *key myths and metaphors used to describe the land and the people* within the narrative materials we have examined reveals not just considerable thematic multiplicity but fundamental contradictions. Newspaper and television reporters' desire to see the members of the Lost Tribe as both hopelessly wild and marvelously in accord with nature produce ongoing *tensions among and between those basic elements around which the stories are constructed*. So do dissonant insistences upon the Amazon as boundless forest and as an ever smaller and despoiled terrain.

Certain interpretations of the story that reject a number of these basic elements (the fundamental myths and metaphors) constitute *challenges to the prevailing narrative of a particular people and place*. An alternative insistence on the Lost Tribe's historical nature and its humanity – in opposition to its supposed novelty and not-quite-human identity – is present from the moment that the story breaks. These sorts of alternative readings have the benefit of fruitfully complicating a very old and highly formulaic narrative.

Finally, the *relation of these new ideas to contemporary, social, political, and economic concerns* raise important questions about policy. These take on a new urgency with Marina da Silva's resignation as Minister of the Environment as a stinging protest against development-oriented interests. The notion that the members of the Lost Tribe should be seen as citizens of a contemporary nation that has an obligation to defend both them and the lands that they inhabit creates pressure for a re-examination of customary tropes and, with them, existing policies.

SOCIETY, ENVIRONMENT, AND LITERARY ANALYSIS:
BROADER IMPLICATIONS AND CONCLUSION

The sort of basic textual analysis in which we have engaged here works best in cases where there are multiple variants on a theme. An array of vivid images also facilitates analysis. However, this sort of approach can be employed wherever one has words or allied expressive forms (films, architecture, rituals) with which to work.

As already noted, this type of examination represents a highly effective starting point. Not only can it be used in conjunction with other methods, but it actively invites them. The case of the Lost Tribe provides a useful introduction to larger discussions of environmental policies involving indigenous peoples around the world. It also offers a launching pad for more detailed considerations of the Amazon's role in international environmental campaigns.

Anthropologists and environmental researchers in general do not have to go far from academic home to see why this type of analysis is important. The sorts of myths and metaphors present in our exam-ination of the Lost Tribe are every bit as central to a controversy that shook Anthropology in 2000–2001 and that still has resounding impli-cations for the discipline.[50] This debate followed damning accusations about professional ethics made by investigative journalist Patrick Tierney (2000) in his *Darkness in El Dorado: How Scientists and Journalists Devastated the Amazon* – a book billed as "an explosive account of how ruthless journalists, self-serving anthropologists, and obsessed scien-tists placed one of the Amazon basin's oldest tribes on the cusp of extinction."[51]

Tierney's primary targets were anthropologist Napoleon Chagnon, author of the widely read *Yanomamö: The Fierce People* (1983 [1968]), which served as the basis for several ethnographic films,[52] and the geneticist James V. Neel. There is no room here to go into the actual texts and it should be noted that the accusations which Tierney levels at Chagnon and Neel have triggered multiple chal-lenges. However, there is no denying that the titles chosen by both

---

[50] For an introduction to the debate see Douglas Hume, "Darkness in El Dorado," http://www.nku.edu/~humed1/index.php/darkness-in-el-dorado. See also Borofsky (2005) and Coronil *et al.* (2001).

[51] Quoted in "New book, article accuses scientists of disrupting Yanomami tribes," CNN, October 2, 2002, http://archives.cnn.com/2000/books/news/10/02/anthro.controversy/.

[52] One of the best known of these is *The Ax Fight*, produced by Timothy Asch and Napoleon Chagnon in 1975 and available on CD-ROM.

Tierney and Chagnon suggest the sorts of myths and metaphors that permeate accounts of the Lost Tribe.[53] The presence of these by-now familiar literary devices within this absolutely crucial and intensely argued debate underscores the importance of the types of narrative considerations in which we have engaged. While one can find these sorts of myths and metaphors in short-lived mass media sources, they may also pervade accounts that play deeply critical roles within the academic world.

The El Dorado controversy leaves no doubt about the relevance of literary analysis for narratives that normally would be seen as largely transparent, documentary writing. In so doing, it reaffirms the fundamental place of tropes in studies of environment-related issues – a central point throughout this chapter. Although it is possible to pull apart texts simply for the pleasure of seeing how they were put together, the sort of basic examination we have outlined has decidedly practical implications.

The furor that arose around the Lost Tribe story, for instance, makes clear the ways in which a single word – in this case "uncontacted" – may cause problems due to fuzzy or competing interpretations. This furor underscores the importance of defining key terms so that they are immediately intelligible not just in newspaper reports, but above all in official policies that are then carefully explained and widely disseminated in schools and community organizations as well as governmental institutions.

Clear definitions, however, are only the beginning. Our examinations also suggest an undiminished need to portray native peoples as full-fledged human beings whose unique cultures need not vanish or undergo devaluation at the moment of supposed discovery. The El Dorado myth, for instance, can be transformed from an impossible and far too simple dream of untouched nature into programs of action that speak to the ongoing human thirst for wonder in a marvelously complex world. The idea that careful planning can help individual El Dorados to live on in their own way following "discovery" offers a far more useful starting point for thinking about environmental preservation than does the notion of a single, always distant answer to destruction.

---

[53] The question of tropes is mentioned, though not developed by several of the writers in Coronil *et al.* (2001) – Peter Pels, Charles L. Briggs and Clara E. Mantini-Briggs, and Alcida Rita Ramos.

No one entirely escapes the sorts of images that have appeared here; they are a cornerstone of language that can and should be used in conscious fashion to positive effect. Environmental researchers have no obligation to engage in literary acrobatics; they *do*, however, need to be alert to their own most cherished stories as well as others' words.

ACKNOWLEDGMENTS

I thank Lawrence Buell, Kathryn Freitas-Seitz, Laura Graham, Daniel Hoffmann, and Laura Ogden for their helpful comments on a draft version of this piece. I also thank Kathryn Freitas-Seitz for her editorial assistance.

REFERENCES

Ainsa, F. 1992. *De la edad de oro a El Dorado: génesis del discurso utópico americano.* Mexico: Fondo de Cultura Económica.

Borofsky, R. 2005. *Yanomami: The Fierce Controversy and What We Can Learn From It.* Berkeley, CA: University of California Press.

Bressler, C. E. 2003. *Literary Criticism: An Introduction to Theory and Practice.* Upper Saddle River, NJ: Prentice Hall.

Buell, L. 2001. *Writing for an Endangered World: Literature, Culture, and Environment in the US and Beyond.* Cambridge, MA: Belknap Press of Harvard University Press.

Buell, L. 2005. *The Future of Environmental Criticism: Environmental Crisis and Literary Imagination.* Malden, MA: Blackwell Publishing.

Carpentier, A. 1956. *The Lost Steps.* Trans. H. de Onís. New York: Knopf.

Carvajal, G. de 1934. *The Discovery of the Amazon According to the Account of Friar Gaspar de Carvajal and Other Documents.* Trans. E. L. Bertram, H.C. Heaton, ed. New York: American Geographical Society.

Chagnon, N. A. 1983. *Yanomamö: The Fierce People*, 3rd edn. New York: Holt, Rinehart, and Winston.

Clastres, H. 1975. *La terre sans mal: le prophetisme tupi-guarani.* Paris: Éditions du Seuil.

Coimbra, C. E. A. Jr., N. M. Flowers, F. M. Salzano, and R. V. Santos 2002. *The Xavánte in Transition: Health, Ecology, and Bioanthropology in Central Brazil.* Ann Arbor, MI: University of Michigan Press.

Conklin, B. A., and L. R. Graham. The shifting middle ground: Amazonian Indians and eco-politics. *American Anthropologist* 97(4): 695–710.

Coronil, F., A. Fix, P. Pels, *et al.* 2001. Current Anthropology forum on anthropology in public: perspectives on Tierney's Darkness in El Dorado. *Current Anthropology* 42(2): 265–276.

Cronon, W., ed. 1996. *Uncommon Ground: Rethinking the Human Place in Nature.* New York: W. W. Norton & Co.

Culler, J. D. 1997. *Literary Theory: A Very Short Introduction.* New York: Oxford University Press.

Culler, J. D, ed. 2003. *Deconstruction: Critical Concepts in Literary and Cultural Studies.* New York: Routledge.

da Cunha, E. 1986. *Um paraíso perdido*. Leandro Tocantins, ed., Rio de Janeiro: J. Olympia Editora.

Deleuze, G, and F. Guattari 1987. *A Thousand Plateaus: Capitalism and Schizophrenia*. Trans. and Foreword by B. Massumi. Minneapolis, MN: U. of Minnesota Press.

Diacon, T. A. 2004. *Stringing Together a Nation: Cândido Mariano da Silva Rondon and the Construction of a Modern Brazil, 1906-1930*. Durham, NC: Duke University Press.

Dryzek, J. S. 1997. *The Politics of the Earth: Environmental Discourses*. New York: Oxford University Press.

Eagleton, T. 2006. *Criticism and Ideology: A Study in Marxist Literary Theory*. New York: Verso.

Ellingson, T. J. 2001. *The Myth of the Noble Savage*. Berkeley, CA: University of California Press.

Elliott, A. 1994. *Psychoanalytic Theory: An Introduction*. Cambridge, MA: Blackwell.

Gandía, E. de 1929. *Historia crítica de los mitos de la conquista americana*. Madrid: Juan Roldán y Compañía.

Geertz, C. 1973. Thick description: toward an interpretive theory of culture. In *The Interpretation of Cultures: Selected Essays*. New York: Basic Books, pp. 3-30

Glotfelty, C. and H. Fromm, eds. 1996. *The Ecocriticism Reader: Landmarks in Literary Ecology*. Athens, GA: University of Georgia Press.

Greenblatt, S. 1992. *Marvelous Possessions: The Wonder of the New World*. Chicago, IL: University of Chicago Press.

Groden, M., M. Kreiswirth, and I. Szeman, eds. 2005. *The Johns Hopkins Guide to Literary Theory and Criticism*. Baltimore, MD: Johns Hopkins University Press.

Guha, R. 2000. *Environmentalism: A Global History*. New York: Longman.

Guha, R. and J. Martínez Alier, eds. 1998. *Varieties of Environmentalism: Essays North and South*. New York: Oxford University Press.

Handley, G. 2007. *New World Poetics: Nature and the Academic Imagination of Whitman, Neruda, and Walcott*. Athens, GA: University of Georgia Press.

Hawkes, T. 2003. *Structuralism and Semiotics*. New York: Routledge.

Heise, U. K. 2008. *Sense of Place and Sense of Planet: The Environmental Imagination of the Global*. New York: Oxford University Press.

Hemming, J. 2003. *Die If You Must: Brazilian Indians in the Twentieth Century*. London: Macmillan.

Hudson, W. H. 1904. *Green Mansions: A Romance of the Tropical Forest*. London: Duckworth and Company.

Jakobson, R. 1960. Closing statement. In T. A. Sebeok, ed., *Linguistics and Poetics in Style in Language*. Cambridge, MA: Technology Press of MIT and John Wiley and Sons, pp. 350-377.

Kosek, J. 2006. *Understories: The Political Life of Forests in New Mexico*. Durham, NC: Duke University Press.

Landy, J. and M. T. Saler 2009. *The Re-enchantment of the World: Secular Magic in a Rational Age*. J. Landy and M. Saler, eds. Stanford, CA: Stanford University Press.

Latour, B. 2004. *Politics of Nature: How to Bring the Sciences into Democracy*. Trans. C. Porter. Cambridge, MA: Harvard University Press.

Levin, J. 2002. Beyond nature? Recent work in ecocriticism. *Contemporary Literature* **43**(1): 171-186.

Lévi-Strauss, C. 1973 [1955]. *Tristes tropiques*. Trans. D. Weightman and J. Weightman. New York: Modern Library.

Lutz, C. A. and J. L. Collins 1993. *Reading National Geographic*. Chicago, IL: University of Chicago Press.

Mazel, D. 2000. *American Literary Environmentalism*. Athens, GA: University of Georgia Press.

McBeth, M. K., E. A. Shanahan, R. J. Arnell, and P. L. Hathaway 2007. The intersection of narrative policy analysis and policy change theory. *The Policy Studies Journal* **35**(1): 87–108.

Moi, T. 1985. *Sexual/Textual Politics: Feminist Literary Theory*. New York: Methuen.

Montaigne, M. de 1948. *On Cannibals. Essays*. Trans F. Carmody. Hillsborough, CA: L-D Allen Press.

Outka, P. 2008. *Race and Nature From Transcendentalism to the Harlem Renaissance*. New York: Palgrave-Macmillan.

Ralegh, W. 1997. *The Discoverie of the Large, Rich, and Bewtiful Empyre of Guiana*. Trans. N. Whitehead, ed. Norman, OK: University of Oklahoma Press.

Said, E. W. 1978. *Orientalism*. New York: Pantheon Books.

Selden, R., P. Widdowson, and P. Brooker 1997. *A Reader's Guide to Contemporary Literary Theory*. London and New York: Prentice Hall/Harvester Wheatsheaf.

Slater, C. 1996. Amazonia as Edenic narrative. In W. Cronon, ed., *Uncommon Ground: Rethinking the Human Place in Nature*. New York: W. W. Norton and Company, pp. 114–131.

Slater, C. 2002. *Entangled Edens: Visions of the Amazon*. Berkeley, CA: University of California Press.

Stepan, N. L. 2001. *Picturing Tropical Nature*. Ithaca, NY: Cornell University Press.

Strunk, Jr., W. and E. B. White 2007. *The Elements of Style*. New York: Penguin Press.

Tierney, P. 2000. *Darkness in El Dorado: How Scientists and Journalists Devastated the Amazon*. New York: W. W. Norton & Co.

Waugh, P., ed. 2006. *Literary Theory and Criticism: an Oxford Guide*. New York: Oxford University Press.

Wellek, R. and A. Warren 1949. *Theory of Literature*. New York: Harvest Books.

9

Water decision-makers in a desert city: text analysis and environmental social science

AMBER WUTICH AND CLARENCE C. GRAVLEE

INTRODUCTION

Text analysis encompasses a broad range of methods. For many researchers, the phrase "text analysis" likely connotes the close reading and interpretation of data that come in the form of words rather than numbers. Yet in this chapter, we argue for an inclusive approach to text analysis – one that recognizes the advantages of moving iteratively between words and numbers in analyzing texts. Our view is that both qualitative and quantitative methods belong in a complete methodological toolkit for analyzing texts. Instead of envisioning text analysis as occupying one side of a qualitative–quantitative continuum, we see text analysis as a suite of methods that can be used to investigate the full range of research questions, from exploratory to confirmatory.

Exploratory research questions are used to understand new phenomena – uncovering how they work and developing new models to describe them. Examples of exploratory research in environmental social science, which we discuss in greater detail below, include Paolisso and Maloney's (2000) exploration of environmental knowledge of the Chesapeake Bay, and Apostolopoulou and Pantis' (2009) investigation of failures in Greek conservation policy. Confirmatory research questions are used to test how well existing theories, hypotheses, or models describe a phenomenon of interest. Examples of confirmatory

Environmental Social Sciences: Methods and Research Design, ed. I. Vaccaro, E. A. Smith and S. Aswani. Published by Cambridge University Press. © Cambridge University Press 2010.

research, also discussed below, include Drieschova, Giordano, and Fischhendler (2008) study of flow variability regulations in international water treaties and Laurian's (2005) research on the efficacy of citizen input mechanisms in the toxic remediation process.

As Gravlee (2010) points out, the exploratory–confirmatory continuum of research questions runs roughly parallel to a methodological continuum, ranging from unstructured to structured research methods. Exploratory questions tend to be investigated using unstructured methods, such as participant-observation and focus groups. Confirmatory questions are generally investigated using structured data collection techniques, such as surveys and time allocation studies. Yet the distinction between unstructured and structured methods does not map neatly onto the usual distinction between qualitative and quantitative approaches. Semantic network analysis, for example, is a quantitative method but also unstructured in the sense that researchers do not impose a prior analytic framework. It is, therefore, appropriate for answering exploratory research questions using text.

Bernard and Ryan (2010) provide a helpful typology for understanding the data collection techniques and types of data frequently used in text analysis. Text analysis is commonly performed on data collected using archives, behavior trace studies, direct observations, self-reported data, or mixed method approaches. Archives may be used to gather data from laws and policies, newspaper articles, or home movie reels. Behavior trace methods examine physical evidence (e.g., traffic patterns or archaeological artifacts) or textual data (e.g., websites and correspondence). Direct observations may be collected using continuous monitoring, spot sampling, or time-allocation studies. Self-reported approaches to data collection may employ methods such as surveys, interviews, focus groups, and diaries. Mixed method approaches may include case studies, participant-observation, or combinations of any of the aforementioned methods.

Text analysis is typically used to analyze written words; however, these techniques can also be used to examine still images, video, sounds, and physical objects. Some examples of still image data are photographs, paintings, and drawings. Videos include data such as focus group recordings, films of ritual events, and Hollywood movies. Sound data may be audio-recorded conversations, music and songs, or historic radio addresses. Physical objects might include pottery, plant specimens, or industrial waste containers. In this chapter, we will present data from a case study of Arizona water decision-makers, collected using a self-administered, open-ended interview that yielded typewritten texts. But the analytic methods can be applied to a wide range of qualitative data.

CASE STUDY: WATER SCARCITY, CLIMATE MODELS, AND DECISION-MAKING IN A DESERT CITY

The case study is set in metropolitan Phoenix, an urban center in Arizona's Sonoran Desert with 4.2 million residents. Recent climate predictions indicate that this region will become warmer and drier, making it increasingly difficult to sustain current water provision levels (Ellis *et al.* 2008). The tension between climate uncertainty, economic growth, and water conservation is a major challenge for Phoenix's water decision-makers (Gober 2006). So far, uncertainty about the magnitude and economic impacts of future climate change has thwarted progress on water conservation policies in Phoenix.

To assist in decision-making under uncertainty, researchers at Arizona State University (ASU) created WaterSim, an interactive simulation model of water supply and demand. Simulation models such as WaterSim have become a common way for scientists to package and display climate information for policy-makers, planners, and other decision-makers. Some scholars, however, have suggested that policy-makers may not use simulation models because they perceive the models as lacking scientific validity, not meeting their needs and goals, and biased toward certain policy outcomes (Cash *et al.* 2003). The WaterSim study was designed to examine policymaker discourse around climate models to determine (1) if such critiques were common among Arizona water decision-makers and (2) whether these concerns could be alleviated through iterative, collaborative model-building (White, Wutich, and Lant 2010). The study is based at ASU's Decision Center for a Desert City (DCDC), a center funded by the National Science Foundation's Decision Making Under Uncertainty program.

A team of DCDC researchers conducted Phase I of the WaterSim study in 2006. We selected 62 decision-makers to participate, drawing from a list of 308 attendees of University of Arizona's Water Resources Research Center Annual Conference. We divided participants into groups, based on their self identification as scientists, policy-makers/planners, or lawyers/consultants, and invited them to a presentation of WaterSim. We conducted the WaterSim presentations and data collection in Arizona State University's Decision Theater, a decision-making laboratory set in a 360-degree immersive environment.

The decision-makers participated in an interactive presentation of WaterSim that explored how scenarios of climate change, population growth, urbanization, and policy changes would impact water availability in central Arizona. Immediately following the presentation, a facilitator asked participants to answer open-ended questions regarding (1) the relevance of the model to decision-makers' needs; (2) the quality of the technical evidence; and (3) whether the information presented was fair, unbiased, and respectful of stakeholder values. Participants entered their responses into a self-administered computer format, which enabled them to provide anonymous responses in a format that was appropriate for this computer-literate professional population.

The resulting dataset has been used to test a range of hypotheses. Wutich *et al.* (2010) used content analysis to assess decision-makers' willingness to discuss sensitive policy-related topics. White *et al.* (2010) also used content analysis to determine whether decision-makers perceived the WaterSim model to be salient, credible, and legitimate. In the analyses below, we use the dataset to demonstrate how a range of analytic methods can be used to ask both exploratory and confirmatory research questions about the same set of texts.

THE BASICS: INVESTIGATING TEXTS USING WORDS AND CODES

We distinguish between two broad classes of systematic methods for analyzing texts. The first focuses on the analysis of words in the raw texts. The second focuses on the analysis of codes that researchers assign to text segments to summarize the meaning of the text. In this section, we describe the building blocks for both types of analysis.

Building blocks of word-based text analysis

Cleaning and preparing texts

Word-based methods of analysis distill texts into their basic component – words – to detect patterns in usage or meaning. This focus on words makes it especially important to begin with clean, accurate texts to avoid miscounts and misleading results. If the texts are archival materials, the key is to produce an accurate digital copy that can be processed by text management software. If the texts are transcriptions of interviews or focus groups, it may be necessary to revisit the original recordings to verify that the transcripts accurately represent respondents' words. If the texts were collected using a self-administered questionnaire, you will have to assess whether making changes to respondents' statements are more likely to misconstrue their original meaning or to represent that meaning more faithfully.

In the Arizona water decision-makers' texts, for example, one respondent mentioned growth "moratoiums." This was clearly a typo, which we corrected to ensure an accurate count of how often people mentioned moratoriums. By contrast, we chose not to correct "maf," which our spellchecker flagged as incorrect but we recognized as a meaningful reference to million acre feet, a measure of water volume used in water management.

Building matrices for word counts and key words in context

The key idea behind word-based analysis – behind all analysis, really – is the data matrix. The most familiar type is the profile matrix. Typically, the rows of a profile matrix contain cases (corresponding to the unit of analysis), and the columns contain attributes (variables) of the cases. If you've ever used a spreadsheet in software like Excel®, you've used a profile matrix. The other type of data matrix is a similarity matrix (a.k.a. proximity matrix). In a similarity matrix, the rows and columns refer to the same type of things, and the cells contain a measure of the relationships among items to one another.

Although researchers are used to thinking about data matrices in relation to quantitative data, the concept applies to qualitative data as well. Figure 9.1 shows how words are converted to matrices in word-based analyses. We begin with a small sample of responses from the Arizona water decision-makers' texts (A). The frequency of words within texts can then be represented in a word-by-respondent profile matrix (B) in which the cells indicate the number of times each word appeared in each text. This matrix can be dichotomized (C) to indicate presence or absence of each word within the texts. Two different similarity matrices can be derived from the dichotomized profile matrix. The first (D) measures how often respondents used the same words. The second (E) measures how often each pair of words appeared in the same text. Converting free-flowing text into these data matrices opens a new realm of possibilities for analysis.

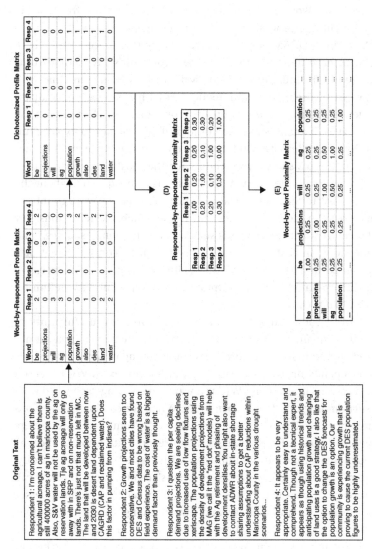

Figure 9.1   Transforming texts into profile and proximity matrices.

Exploring word-based datasets

With the matrices prepared, you can choose from different word-based approaches, such as word counts and key-words-in-context. Word counts are the simplest approach. Here you simply count the number of times each word occurs across all texts. A variety of software packages – including general-purpose text management packages such as MAXQDAplus, QDAMiner, and NVivo – make this process easy. These packages have functions to eliminate "stop words": recurring words that are not meaningful to the analysis, such as "the," "an," and "to". Software can also report word frequencies within each text or compare frequencies between groups of texts. Word counts can be useful in the early stages of analysis as a way of identifying themes to explore further (Ryan and Bernard 2003) or as an end in itself (Ryan and Weisner 1996). Figure 9.2 shows word counts for the most common words in the Arizona water decision-makers' responses to a question about the quality of WaterSim's technical evidence. We used the word count primarily to help identify themes and refine codebook definitions. For instance, frequent use of words such as "information," "sources," and "projections" indicated to us that decision-makers considered datasets to be important for assessing the quality of technical evidence. We then incorporated these descriptors into our preliminary definition for the "data" code.

Word count analysis assumes that words are useful units of meaning, but an obvious limitation is that the meaning of text cannot be reduced to individual words and the meaning of individual words often depends on context. The key-word-in-context (KWIC) method addresses this limitation. KWIC is a way of displaying each word with its surrounding text (see Weber 1990). When we conducted the word count shown in Figure 9.2, we noticed that "assumptions" were mentioned 23 times. A KWIC analysis then drew our attention to the way respondents discussed assumptions with regard to model validity. Respondents used the word "assumptions" to talk about the way calculations and parameters were used to construct the model; guesses about future water availability and climate change; and presumptions about how people behave when water is scarce – among other uses. As we discuss in the section on grounded theory, concerns about whether the model's assumptions are reasonable and whether they are sufficiently transparent played an important role in respondents' perceptions of bias in the model.

World	Frequency
water	60
model	52
not	41
would	33
data	28
information	26
have	24
assumptions	23
sources	19
used	19
there	19
use	18
population	18
know	16
may	16
was	15
will	15
river	15
projections	14
has	14
county	14
colorado	14
should	13
can	13
drought	13
demand	13
years	13
maricopa	12
growth	12
see	12
were	11
technical	11
question	11
very	11
been	11
based	11
recharge	10
scientific	10
available	9
per	9
supplies	9
presented	9
land	9
groundwater	9
flow	9

Figure 9.2   Word count results for narratives from Arizona water decision-makers.

Building blocks of code-based text analysis

Code-based methods, unlike word-based approaches, start from researchers' judgments about what the texts mean. There are a variety of approaches to code-based analysis, but all of them share a common set of building blocks. Two of the most important building blocks include (1) identifying themes and (2) building and applying codebooks.

Identifying themes

One of the first steps in code-based analysis is identifying themes. We define a theme as an underlying (dimension of) meaning that cuts across a variety of expressions. Themes can be identified deductively, based on theory, or inductively, based on occurrence of patterns in the data. In practice, most researchers use both inductive and deductive approaches to identifying themes. In the Arizona water decision-makers' study, for example, we identified two themes deductively, based on the literature: supply-side and demand-side water policies. We also identified some unanticipated themes inductively, based on a close reading of the texts. Below, we discuss in greater detail how we developed both types of themes as part of our analysis.

Many researchers identify themes intuitively and may be hard pressed to explain their process. Ryan and Bernard (2003), however, list 12 techniques for identifying themes and argue that making these techniques explicit improves the transparency and validity of text analysis (Figure 9.3). Some techniques require physically or electronically processing texts (e.g., word counts, cut and sort), but most focus on things that researchers can look for in text (e.g., metaphors, repetition, indigenous categories).

We used several techniques to identify themes in the Arizona water decision-makers study. As noted above, our word frequency and KWIC analyses drew attention to the word "assumptions," which led us to recognize "model construction" as an important theme in our analysis. We identified another important theme based on the indigenous concept of "paper water": water allocations that exist in law but may not coincide with the amount of surface and groundwater that is actually available. We also looked for co-occurrences that highlighted similarities or differences between concepts. We noticed, for example, that water decision-makers often contrasted "paper water" with "wet water" that actually exists underground and in waterways. This

Observational Techniques
Repetitions – repeated use of certain words or phrases may indicate their importance
Indigenous categories – unique terms that have special significance for a cultural group
Metaphors and analogies – use of symbolism that may convey an underlying meaning
Transitions – a topic switch can signify when one theme begins and another ends
Similarities and differences – finding these can help group and subdivide themes
Linguistic connectors – can point to underlying schemas, such as causality and time order
Missing data – things left unsaid can signal stigma or well-established cultural knowledge
Theory-related material – prior theoretical knowledge often suggests important themes

Manipulative Techniques
Cutting and sorting – pile sorting text fragments may suggest meta-themes and sub-themes
Word lists and KWIC – assists in using the repetition and similarity/difference techniques
Word co-occurrence – helps identify more complex themes involving multiple keywords
Metacoding – grouping themes or sub-themes is a way to identify broad meta-themes

Figure 9.3   Ryan and Bernard's (2003) twelve techniques for identifying themes.

contrast suggested several possible themes about hydrological uncertainty, environmental risks, and failed water policy. The cut-and-sort method also worked well in our study. We physically cut up the texts, and five team members – the WaterSim developer, the session facilitator, an anthropologist, and two student assistants – sorted them into groups that we labeled as themes such as "doomsday perspectives" and "alternative futures." This process was an excellent opportunity for us to brainstorm ideas for new themes as a team.

Developing a codebook

Once themes have been identified, the next major step is to develop a codebook. The codebook provides a conceptual and operational definition of each theme to indicate what it means and when it should be applied to segments of text. We suggest a format for developing codebook definitions that includes a definition, inclusion criteria, exclusion criteria, and exemplars (MacQueen *et al.* 1998). Figure 9.4 shows an example of this format from our codebook for the water decisionmakers study. The full codebook also specifies what units of analysis will be coded (e.g., words, sentences, or paragraphs), whether codes can overlap or not, and whether to code for presence (e.g., present/absent) or degree (e.g., high/medium/low).

Codebook development is an iterative process. Early definitions may reflect theory or initial hunches about what a theme means. These definitions are then refined through repeated engagement with the texts. To establish the validity and reliability of the codebook, multiple

Code 1: Supply-side Approaches to Water Development

Variable name Supply-side (supsi)

Theory area Development approaches —MACRO LEVEL (policy)

Detailed description Expression of the idea that *we need to make more water* (that is, make more water available, buy more water, create more water, etc.); the need to find *future water supplies* (**must mention water**)

Inclusion criteria Discussion of the need for more water or the ability to acquire water or ARE in the process of acquiring more water

Exclusion criteria Discussion of the need for or the ability to change water use or consumption

Typical exemplars Desalination, buying water, getting water rights for the Colorado River

Atypical exemplars Groundwater recharge, cloud seeding, reclamation

Close but no Xeriscaping, talk about growth that does not mention water

Code 2: Demand-side Approaches to Water Development

Variable name Demand-side (demsi)

Theory area Development approaches —REFERS TO MACRO LEVEL (policy)

Detailed description Expression of the idea that we need to *make the water we have last* (that is, we need to conserve water); the need to preserve *present water supplies*; expression of the idea that *growth causes over-consumption* (**must mention water**)

Inclusion criteria Discussion of the need to control human behavior to make water last

Exclusion criteria Discussion of the need for or ability to make more water

Typical exemplars Pricing structures, new laws, education about water use, discussion of the need to change values

Atypical exemplars None

Close but no None

Figure 9.4 Codebook definitions for two codes used in the Arizona water decision-makers study.

coders should independently code the text (Ryan 1999). A measure of such as kappa or Cronbach's alpha can then be used to evaluate inter-rater reliability. If inter-rater agreement is low, you should identify what makes the definition for a theme confusing or unclear, refine the codebook definition, and retest it as often as needed. In some cases, a theme cannot be operationalized in a valid and reliable way. In the Arizona water decision-maker study, we could not reach an acceptable level of inter-rater agreement for "robustness" even after ten itera-tions of code revision. As a result, we excluded this theme from our codebook and analysis.

Guidelines vary about how many themes should be included in a codebook, but a good rule of thumb is to include no more than three levels of sub-themes and no more than 50 codes total (Miles and Huberman 1994). It is often tempting to include many more themes, but a longer codebook increases coder fatigue and coding errors. The most successful codebooks are focused on achievable, theory-driven research goals.

TEXT ANALYSIS: THREE APPROACHES

We present three distinct approaches to text analysis in this chapter. The first is semantic network analysis, a predominately exploratory approach. The second is grounded theory, which can be used to con-duct both exploratory and explanatory research. The third is content analysis, which is used to conduct primarily confirmatory research.

Semantic networks

Semantic network analysis originated in linguistics and is used to describe the semantic relationships among concepts. These analyses are similar to factor analysis in that they are designed to identify under-lying dimensions of meaning that cut across categories. All analyses begin with a matrix that summarizes the relationships among words or codes, as shown in Figure 9.1. These relationships may be captured using categorical (e.g., presence/absence), ordinal (e.g., none/some/many), or continuous data (e.g., word counts). The results tend to be more illuminating when datasets contain many categories or variables, allowing for the analysis to capture more complexities of underlying meaning. Like factor analysis, these analyses can be performed in stat-istical software packages like SAS or SPSS. Additionally, researchers may use software designed specifically to conduct semantic network analyses, such as ANTHROPAC for cultural domain analysis (Borgatti 1992) or UCINET for social network analysis (Borgatti, Everett, and Freeman 2004). Semantic networks are generally used during the exploratory stage of analysis, and focus on semantic relationships that are not yet well understood or grounded in empirical findings. The output yields visualizations that can be particularly helpful for hypothesizing relationships and identifying models, which can later be tested using confirmatory methods. We discuss three approaches for creating semantic networks: correspondence analysis, multidimensional scaling, and hierarchical clustering.

Correspondence analysis is used to analyze a profile matrix, such as a respondent-by-word matrix or a respondent-by-code matrix. For instance, the dataset might contain information regarding the types of respondents and their use of words or codes. The correspondence analysis then computes the relationships between the rows and columns of the matrix. The analysis yields a correspondence map, in which items that are more similar are grouped more closely together, as well as quantitative output summarizing the results. Typically, researchers interpret this map by looking for dimensions (axes) and clusters of meaning.

Paolisso and Maloney (2000) demonstrate how correspondence analysis can be integrated with analysis of texts. They used informal ethnographic interviews, free listing, and triad tests to elicit farmers' and environmentalists' knowledge of nutrient runoff and *Pfiesteria* pollution on the Chesapeake Bay. Then, using a correspondence analysis, the authors found that (1) farmers and environmentalists had very similar knowledge of nutrient runoff and *Pfiesteria*, but (2) farmers and environmentalists viewed *each other* as very dissimilar. The correspondence analysis provided visual confirmation of trends the authors identified in their texts.

Multidimensional scaling (MDS) is used to analyze a similarity matrix, such as a word-by-word matrix or code-by-code matrix. For instance, the dataset might contain information regarding the number of times that words or codes co-occur across a set of narratives. MDS can also be used to analyze dissimilarities, such as the number of words, sentences, or paragraphs that separate distinct words or codes. MDS can handle ordinal data for non-metric analyses or continuous data for metric analyses. The MDS analysis computes statistically the distances among various items and maps a solution that best represents the distances among these items. Like correspondence analysis,

MDS yields a map as well as quantitative output summarizing the results. Again, the map can be interpreted based on dimensions and clusters of meaning.

Chhetri, Arrowsmith, and Jackson (2004) provide an example of how MDS can enhance the analysis of text. The researchers collected open-ended and closed-ended data from hikers in Australia regarding their experiences in nature-oriented tourism. An MDS of feelings evoked by natural landscapes revealed dimensions of positive–negative emotions with intrinsic–extrinsic properties. These results, along with other findings, were then used to develop a model of experiential landscapes for nature tourism.

Hierarchical clustering, like MDS, is used to analyze similarity matrices using similarities or dissimilarities. This method iteratively creates clusters, assigns items to new clusters, and collapses small clusters into larger ones. In contrast to MDS, hierarchical clustering offers the researcher more control in determining how items are clustered. The collapsing of clusters can be performed according to the single-link method (based on the distance between two clusters' closest members), the complete-link method (based on the distance between two clusters' furthest members), or the average of the two. Hierarchical clustering yields a dendrogram visualization and a quantitative output summarizing the results. The dendrogram can be interpreted by identifying clusters, the similarity of items within clusters, and the degree of division between clusters.

Tikkanen *et al.* (2006) used hierarchical clustering in a study of forest owners in Finland. Forest owners provided data on forest use objectives collected via conceptual mapping, free listing, and open-ended questions. The hierarchical cluster analysis yielded three clusters of objectives: income, future investment, and leisure activities. The authors argued that the analysis produced novel findings that complemented the results of previous research.

For the Arizona water decision-makers' dataset, we performed an exploratory analysis of words to identify themes and possible hypotheses. We began with the texts elicited in response to the following question: "How relevant is the model to your needs as a decision-maker (or the needs of decision-makers in your workplace)?" We first cleaned the text responses for word-based analysis, as described above. We then decided to analyze only words mentioned ten or more times, and created a word-by-word matrix containing correlations of word co-occurrence. Finally, we used the UCINET routine for hierarchical

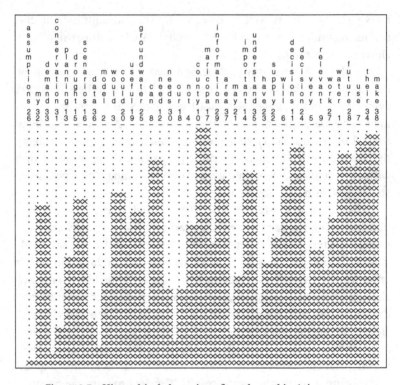

Figure 9.5   Hierarchical clustering of words used in Arizona water decision-makers' texts.

clustering on similarities with the average-link method. The results are displayed in Figure 9.5. Our analysis identified 37 clusters, but we focus on just one here to demonstrate the utility of this analysis. We began by identifying the two most similar words in the dendrogram: "Maricopa" and "county." It makes sense that these words would co-occur frequently because the WaterSim model simulates water scenarios for Arizona's Maricopa County. In this cluster, the next most closely linked word is "not." Following that, "information" and "area" are linked together. Finally, "our" is more distantly linked with this cluster. Based on the co-occurrence these words together, we hypothesized that WaterSim's scale of analysis – and particularly the focus on Maricopa County – would be perceived as less relevant for the informational needs of respondents' geographic areas. This was later confirmed in White, Wutich, and Lant's (2010) content analysis of the coded data.

Grounded theory

Grounded theory is a method designed to generate an explanatory theory of some problem, process, or outcome. Increasingly, grounded theory is also used as a phenomenological method to describe lived experiences (cf. Bernard and Ryan, 2010). In practice, the approach is used to examine questions that fall at different points along the exploratory–confirmatory research continuum. Grounded theory originated in Glaser and Strauss's (1967) classic *The Discovery of Grounded Theory*. Since then, the method has splintered into more inductive (Glaser 1992), deductive (Strauss and Corbin 1990), and constructivist (Charmaz 2000) versions. While grounded theory continues to grow and change, some core principles are shared across all of these approaches.

A grounded theory analysis begins with the identification of a topic of interest. Rather than drawing a probability sample, researchers use a theoretical sample of informants (or other data sources) selected to provide diverse perspectives on the topic of interest. Once a corpus of texts is assembled, open coding begins. Researchers code the text line by line, either naming concepts or using in vivo codes based on the informants' own words. Throughout this process, researchers also write memos that document their evolving understanding of the texts.

In the next stage, selective coding, researchers collapse the open codes into larger categories. Researchers may also conduct axial coding by looking for relationships among these categories. Throughout, researchers seek out additional informants who can add new or oppositional perspectives to the existing corpus of data. This iterative process of theoretical sampling, selective coding, and axial coding continues until no new perspectives are introduced. The point at which additional data collection yields no new information is referred to as theoretical saturation. In the final stage, the researcher draws together all of the information with a core category that summarizes the phenomena being theorized.

Apostolopoulou and Pantis' (2009) study of the Greek conservation policy failures provides an excellent example of grounded theory. The researchers conducted interviews with a theoretical sample of 91 people involved in Greek conservation policy via government, nongovernmental organizations, local agencies, and scientific research. After transcribing the interviews, they coded line by line, identified relationships among codes, and identified a core category. They concluded that the core category (absence of a Greek conservation strategy) could be explained by the lack of a history of Greek conservation policy, lack of state capacity to implement conservation policy, lack of public participation, and lack of involvement by conservation biologists. Other grounded theories of environment include Oreszczyn's (2000) research on the values assigned to English hedgerows and Farmar-Bowers and Lane's (2009) study of the conservation of native biodiversity on Australian farmland.

In the Arizona water decision-makers study, we were interested in understanding the perceived legitimacy of the WaterSim model. According to Cash *et al.* (2003), environmental models must be perceived as legitimate (that is, not inappropriately serving the interests of any constituency or group) to be accepted by decision-makers. We began with the aforementioned sample of water decision-makers working in science, policy/planning, and law/consulting. We believed this diverse group would be able to provide a range of perspectives on model legitimacy. We then asked them to tell us about the aspects of the model that contributed or detracted from its legitimacy.

We began our analysis with open coding – reading the text line by line to identify potentially important concepts. We named some of the themes we identified using respondents' own words ("in-vivo coding" in the language of grounded theory) to capture meaningful ways of expressing the concepts. Examples of such themes include "plug-ins," "what-if scenarios," and "garbage in, garbage out." We created memos to document our evolving understanding of the texts. One such memo noted that many decision-makers envisioned the ideal model as untainted by stakeholder influences or biased information. Such a model was described as "factual," "scientific," or "purely data driven." This was a revelation to us because it was at odds with our understanding of model construction, in which modelers create a stylized depiction of reality that necessarily excludes some pieces of information and thus cannot be purely data driven.

Our next step was to aggregate the initial concepts we identified through open coding into larger, more abstract categories. This process, known as selective coding, yielded 15 categories. Then, we focused on trying to understand and describe the relationships among the 15 categories – a process grounded theorists call axial coding. As this process continued, groups of categories began to emerge. We discovered that there were three main categories in which all of the subcodes were interconnected. We named these categories "the fit between data and reality," "the quality of the science," and "interactions with stakeholders and audiences." Based on our evolving understanding of the phenomenon, we determined that all of these codes and categories were part of a core category "the incorporation of appropriate information in the model."

We found that, in order to create an unbiased water simulation model, Arizona water decision-makers felt that the appropriate information must be incorporated in the model. First, this means ensuring the best possible fit between the data and reality by using the established data sources, the right variables, allowing users to manipulate these variables, and focusing on the appropriate scale of analysis. Second, the model should use rigorous scientific methods, including transparent and justifiable assumptions, historic trend modeling, correct calculations, and checks on scientific validity. Finally, the model should involve stakeholders and audiences appropriately – soliciting feedback from stakeholders, including the needs of underrepresented groups in the model, using the model for non-political purposes and audiences, and being careful not to stack the deck against particular outcomes. While our grounded theory was similar to Cash *et al.*'s (2003) findings, our analysis indicated that that modeling method was much more closely linked to perceived legitimacy among Arizona water decision-makers than previous research would predict.

Content analysis

Content analysis has its foundations in the political science and communications research of the early 1900s (Diefenbach 2001). Today the method is used across disciplines to test hypotheses about environmental themes. Such hypotheses deal with (1) the presence or prevalence of codes or words in a text, (2) the relationship between types of texts or respondents and codes or words, or (3) the relationship among different words or codes. Because it is used to test existing theories and hypotheses, this method falls squarely on the confirmatory end of the exploratory–confirmatory research continuum.

The focus on hypothesis testing means that classic content analysis generally favors deductive reasoning and relies on systematic methods of coding and analysis. Codebook development can take different forms in content analysis. In some cases, the approach may be entirely deductive. Themes are selected based on theory or prior empirical research, and codebook definitions are developed a priori. But themes can also be identified inductively using the techniques we described above. In this case, the ideal is to develop the codebook using one set of data and test hypotheses on another dataset. When researchers have only one dataset available, they generally split the original sample into two parts for code development and hypothesis testing.

Other sampling considerations in content analysis include the types of texts to be sampled, sample size, and generalizability. Researchers must also designate a unit of analysis – an entire text, a question response, a paragraph, or a word – for which the hypothesis will be tested. In content analysis, codes are generally exclusive and non-overlapping. Conventionally, the coding of texts is performed by human coders. Another option is the use of content dictionaries, in which a computer assigns codes according to algorithms established by the researcher. The coded texts then yield a respondent-by-code or respondent-by-word matrix; text analysis packages such as MAXQDA and QDAMiner will automatically generate a matrix from coded text. These matrices can be exported to standard statistical software, such as SAS or SPSS, to conduct statistical tests of association.

Content analysis has been used to test a variety of hypotheses in the environmental literature. Here we present a few recent examples to illustrate different approaches to research design. One common approach examines press coverage to test hypotheses related to public discourses around environmental issues. Consider Liu, Vedlitz, and Alston's (2008) longitudinal analysis of climate change in the *Houston Chronicle* newspaper (1992–2005). They identified newspaper articles that dealt with climate change, global warming, or greenhouse gases. They then coded the articles to determine the salience of climate change, how it was discussed (e.g., threat level), and the actors involved. The results indicated that climate change was increasingly salient, regarded as harmful, and seen as an international issue. Other recent applications of content analysis to media discourse about the environment include Johnston, Biro, and MacKendrick's (2009) study of language use in corporate websites for organic products and Cheng and Palacio's (2009) 45-year longitudinal study of water issues in Spain's national newspapers.

Content analysis has also been used to test hypotheses regarding environmental institutions by examining the texts of laws, regulations, or treaties. Drieschova, Giordano, and Fischhendler's (2008) study of international water treaties examined how flow variability is regulated. The researchers analyzed 50 water treaties that focused on water scarcity issues, were signed in the period 1980–2002, and met other exclusion criteria. They then coded the texts for regulations that establish allocation mechanisms, adaptation mechanisms, formalized communication, and cooperation related to flow variability. The results demonstrated the tension between flexibility and enforcement in water treaties. Other examples of institutional approaches to content analysis include Koski's (2007) research on regulations limiting environmental pollution by large-scale livestock operations in the United States and Paloneimi and Tikka's (2008) study of conservation policies that affect forest owners in Finland.

Content analysis is also appropriate for analyzing narratives recorded in interviews, focus groups, meetings, and other conversational settings to test hypotheses about respondents' beliefs and behaviors. An example is Laurian's (2005) evaluation of Community Advisory Boards (CABs) in Tucson, Arizona that were designed to facilitate citizen input to toxic remediation. Laurian used content analysis to examine minutes from 81 CAB meetings and interviews with 27 CAB members. She concluded that CABs are ineffective providing feedback to relevant agencies and in engaging the wider community, although they do accomplish the more modest goals of informing and collecting the feedback of CAB members. Other examples include Kaplowitz's (2001) study of community members' perceptions of mangrove products and services in Teacapan-Agua Brava Lagoon, Mexico and Shandas, Graybill, and Ryan's (2008) study of how urban planners incorporate the principles of ecosystem management into environmental policies in western Washington.

For the Arizona water decision-makers' dataset, we performed a content analysis to test for differences in respondent groups' tendency to discuss supply-side and demand-side approaches to developing water in Arizona. Supply-side approaches to developing water are focused on finding or acquiring new sources of water. In contrast, demand-side approaches to developing water are focused on conserving current water supplies by reducing consumption. Historically, Arizona's water decision-makers have focused on supply-side approaches to water development; demand-side approaches have been considered politically risky, a threat to economic development in the state, and likely to have a negative impact on the local economy. More recently, academics and environmental activists have pushed for recognition that conservation policies should be implemented to ensure that there is enough water for Arizona's growing population. We hypothesized, then, that policy-makers would be most likely to discuss supply-side approaches and least likely to discuss demand-side approaches. In contrast, we anticipated that scientists would be the most likely to discuss demand-side approaches and least likely to discuss supply-side approaches. We expected lawyers and consultants to be intermediate in both cases.

To begin, we developed and tested codes for supply-side and demand-side approaches to development, as shown in Figure 9.4. We determined that both reached an acceptable level of inter-coder agreement (supply-side kappa = 1.00; demand-side kappa = 0.67). Once the data were coded, we created variables for the number of times each respondent made a statement with the corresponding code. We then used ANOVA to compare how often policy-makers, lawyers/consultants, and scientists discussed supply-side and demand-side approaches to water development. The results indicate that there was no statistically significant difference in the discussion of supply-side approaches across the three groups (sci = 0.93; pol/pla = 0.57; con/law = 0.53; $F(2, 57) = 0.826$; $p = 0.44$). However, we did find that scientists were significantly more likely to discuss demand-side approaches, followed by consultants/lawyers, and finally policymakers/planners (sci = 0.80; pol/pla = 0.18; con/law = 0.24; $F(2, 57) = 4.553$; $p = 0.15$). We concluded that, although all three groups discussed supply-side approaches, scientists were more likely to discuss demand-side approaches than the other two groups. This finding has important implications for those seeking to change water policy in Arizona.

CONCLUSION

In this chapter, we introduced a variety of methods that can be used to analyze text. Beginning with the basics, we explained the preliminary steps used to prepare words and codes for analysis. We then discussed in-depth how to conduct three kinds of text analysis: semantic network analysis, grounded theory, and content analysis. Finally, using the case of Arizona water decision-makers, we demonstrated how each method works.

As a suite of methods, text analyses have three primary strengths (Ryan 2005). First, text analysis helps ground researchers in the words and experiences of the people being studied. This proximity to the data can help researchers develop an intimate understanding of and rich insight into the phenomena of interest. Second, many approaches to text analysis are particularly well suited to exploration and discovery. For this reason, text analysis is often used to develop new theories, models, and hypotheses. Third, text analysis is apt for capturing complicated, contested, or mutable phenomena. Because text analysis is so flexible, it allows researchers to track complex processes and to capture multiple perspectives and marginal voices.

Despite the advantages of text analysis, one chief disadvantage is the amount of time required to do it well. Transcription alone – often the first and simplest step of a text analysis project – takes about six hours for every hour of recorded talk. Beyond this, certain phases of text analysis projects, such as codebook development and line-by-line coding, have no clear end point and could go on indefinitely. The best way of avoiding this pitfall is to identify and execute clear research goals, even in exploratory projects. By focusing on a finite set of phenomena, themes, or relationships, researchers can ensure that their projects involve finite and feasible workloads.

The flexibility of text analysis helps explain why it is so often used in multi-method research. Text analysis can be combined with a range of approaches, as the research reviewed in this chapter demonstrates. For instance, Tikkanen and colleagues' (2006) study of Finnish forest owners and Chhetri, Arrowsmith, and Jackson's (2004) study of hikers in Austalia showed how text analysis can be integrated with findings from conceptual mapping, free listing, and surveys. We believe that qualitative and quantitative approaches are particularly powerful when combined in mixed-method research. We have observed that scholars from the biological and physical sciences are increasingly incorporating textual data in their analyses, as they become more interested in understanding human dimensions of environmental change. In coming years, we expect that the audience for mixed-method research, in which text analysis plays a prominent role, will grow significantly.

We suggested at the outset that different methods of text analysis can be used to answer questions along the exploratory–confirmatory continuum. To date, however, few studies in the environmental social sciences have used text analysis to derive new theories and then test those theories in confirmatory research. Bridging this gap remains a major challenge for the further development of text analysis in the environmental social sciences. Apostolopoulou and Pantis' (2009) study can be used to illustrate how this might work. The authors used grounded theory to derive a framework that explained failures in Greek conservation policy. Their exploratory analysis yielded a new theory of conservation failures but stopped short of testing whether the theory applied to other cases. Apostolopouou and Pantis' work raises important confirmatory questions about the extent to which their theory could help explain the failure of conservation policies in other national contexts. We look forward to a new generation of multi-method text analyses that advance important exploratory and confirmatory research in environmental social science.

REFERENCES

Apostolopoulou, E. and J. D. Pantis 2009. Conceptual gaps in the national strategy for the implementation of the European Natura 2000 conservation policy in Greece. *Biological Conservation* **142**: 221–237.
Bernard, H. R. and G. W. Ryan 2010. *Analyzing Qualitative Data: Systematic Approaches.* Los Angeles: Sage Publications.
Borgatti, S. 1992. *Anthropac 4.8.* Colombia, SC: Analytic Technologies.
Borgatti, S., M. G. Everett, and L. C. Freeman 2004. *UCINET 6.69.* Harvard, MA: Analytic Technologies.
Cash, D. W., W. C. Clark, and F. Alcock, *et al.* 2003. Knowledge systems for sustainable development. *Proceedings of the National Academy of Sciences* **100**(14): 8086–8091.
Charmaz, K. 2000. Grounded theory: Objectivist and constructivist methods. In N. K. Denzin and Y. Lincoln, eds., *The Handbook of Qualitative Research.* pp. 507–535. Thousand Oaks, CA: Sage Publications.
Cheng, L. and E. Palacio 2009. ¿El ciclo hidrológico o el ciclo de atención mediática? Estudio empírico de los encuadres noticiosos del AGUA en la prensa española. *Comunicación y Sociedad* **22**(2):197–221.
Chhetria, P., C. Arrowsmith, and M. Jackson 2004. Determining hiking experiences in nature-based tourist destinations. *Tourism Management* **25**: 31–43.
Diefenbach, D. L. 2001. Historical foundations of computer-assisted content analysis. ed., M. D. West. New directions in computer content analysis: theory, method, and practice. New York: Ablex Publishing.
Drieschova, A., M. Giordano, and I. Fischhendler 2008. Governance mechanisms to address flow variability in water treaties. *Global Environmental Change* **18**: 285–295.
Ellis, A. W., T. W. Hawkins, R. C. Balling, and P. Gober 2008. Estimating future runoff levels for a semi-arid fluvial system in central Arizona. *Climate Research* **35**(3): 227–239.
Farmar-Bowers, Q. and R. Lane 2009. Understanding farmers' strategic decision-making processes and the implications for biodiversity conservation policy. *Journal of Environmental Management* **90**: 1135–1144.
Glaser, B. 1992. *Basics of Grounded Theory.* Mill Valley, CA: Sociology Press.
Glaser, B. G. and A. Strauss 1967. *The Discovery of Grounded Theory: Strategies for Qualitative Research.* Chicago: Aldine.
Gober, P. 2006. *Metropolitan Phoenix: Place Making and Community Building in the Desert.* Philadelphia: University of Pennsylvania Press.
Gravlee, C. C. (2010). Research Design and Methods in Medical Anthropology. In M. Singer and P. Erickson, eds., *A Companion to Medical Anthropology.* Malden, MA: Blackwell Publishing.
Johnston, J., A. Biro, and N. MacKendrick 2009. Lost in the supermarket: the corporate-organic foodscape and the struggle for food democracy. *Antipode* **41**(3): 509–532.
Kaplowitz, M. D. 2001. Assessing mangrove products and services at the local level: the use of focus groups and individual interviews. *Landscape & Urban Planning* **56**: 53–60.
Koski, C. 2007. Examining state environmental regulatory policy design. *Journal of Environmental Planning and Management* **50**(4): 483–502.

Laurian, L. 2005. Public input in toxic site cleanup decisions: the strengths and limitations of Community Advisory Boards. *Environment and Planning B: Planning and Design* **32**: 445–467.

Liu, X., A. Vedlitz, and L. Alston 2008. Regional news portrayals of global warming and climate change. *Environmental Science & Policy* **11**: 379–393.

MacQueen, K. M., E. McLellan, K. Kay, and B. Milstein 1998. Codebook development for team-based qualitative analysis. *Cultural Anthropology Methods* **10**(2): 31–36.

Miles, M. B. and A. M. Huberman 1994. *Qualitative Data Analysis: An Expanded Sourcebook*. Thousand Oaks, CA: Sage Publications.

Oreszczyn, S. 2000. A systems approach to the research of people's relationships with English hedgerows. *Landscape and Urban Planning* **50**: 107–117.

Paloniemi, R. and P. M. Tikka 2008. Ecological and social aspects of biodiversity conservation on private lands. *Environmental Science & Policy* **11**: 336–346.

Paolisso, M. and R. S. Maloney 2000. Recognizing farmer environmentalism: nutrient runoff and toxic dinoflagellate blooms in the Chesapeake Bay region. *Human Organization* **59**(2): 209–221.

Ryan, G. W. 1999. Measuring the typicality of text: using multiple coders for more than just reliability and validity checks. *Human Organization* **58**: 313–322.

Ryan, G. W. 2005. *Qualitative Data Analysis*. Beaufort, NC: National Science Foundation Short Courses in Research Methods.

Ryan, G. W. and H. R. Bernard 2003. Techniques to identify themes. *Field Methods* **15**: 85–109.

Ryan, G. W. and T. Weisner 1996. Analyzing words in brief descriptions: fathers and mothers describe their children. *Cultural Anthropology Methods Journal* **8**: 13–16.

Shandas, V., J. K. Graybill, and C. M. Ryan 2001. Incorporating ecosystem-based management into urban environmental policy: a case study from western Washington. *Journal of Environmental Planning and Management* **51**(5): 647–662.

Strauss, A. and J. Corbin 1990. *Basics of Qualitative Research: Grounded Theory Procedures and Techniques*. Newbury Park, CA: Sage Publications, Inc.

Tikkanen, J., T. Isokaanta, J. Pykalainen, and P. Leskinen 2006. Applying cognitive mapping approach to explore the objective–structure of forest owners in a Northern Finnish case area. *Forest Policy and Economics* **9**: 139–152.

Weber, R. P. 1990. *Basic Content Analysis*, 2nd edn. Newbury Park, CA: Sage.

White, D., A. Wutich, T. Lant, *et al.* (2010) Credibility, salience, and legitimacy of boundary objects for environmental decision making: water managers' assessment of WaterSim: a dynamic simulation model in an immersive decision theater. *Science and Public Policy* **37**(3): 219–232.

Wutich, A., T. Lant, D. White, K. Larson, and M. Gartin 2010. Comparing focus group and individual responses on sensitive topics: a study of water decision-makers in a desert city. *Field Methods* **22**(1): 88–110.

10

Linking human and natural systems: social networks, environment, and ecology

JEFFREY C. JOHNSON AND DAVID C. GRIFFITH

INTRODUCTION

This chapter examines the methods employed in research exploring the relationships between systems of human relations, or social
networks, and people's interactions with various elements of natural
ecosystems. Social networks are fundamental to understanding cultural systems of resource sharing; cooperation in hunting, fishing, and
agricultural production; the diffusion of technological innovations;
the sharing and distribution of ecological and environmental knowledge; and in human adaptive responses to changes at various scales
from acute ecological disruptions, such as hurricanes, to major environmental shifts, such as global climate change. In addition, human
behavioral and ecological networks are interconnected in ways that
can foster change through direct and indirect network effects and
through system cascades. Thus, factors contributing to changes in ecosystem structure and function at one level (e.g., climate change) can
influence the structure of human behavioral systems and, conversely,
factors affecting changes in the structure of human behavioral systems (e.g., shifts in fishing effort due to prices or regulation) can ultimately impact elements of ecosystem function (e.g., top-down trophic
cascades).

Several interesting social network theoretical principles
may be at play in the linking of human and natural systems and in

Environmental Social Sciences: Methods and Research Design, ed. I. Vaccaro, E. A. Smith and
S. Aswani. Published by Cambridge University Press. © Cambridge University Press 2010.

understanding and modeling human environmental and ecological behavior. These include such things as homophily (e.g., "birds of a feather flock together"), preferential attachment (e.g., "the rich get richer"), and various topological motifs or features of both ecological and social networks (e.g., small worlds, clustering, transitivity, cohesion). In addition, social capital, a recent social scientific interest, is usually conceptualized in social network terms (Burt 1992; Lin 2002).

The chapter will briefly examine several case studies in terms of the relationships between social networks and the distribution of cultural knowledge, the role of social resources in coping with natural disasters, and links between human social networks and elements of ecological systems. Our discussion will include the nature of sampling in network studies and the particular methodological challenges unique to collecting and analyzing social network data. The examples will also reflect the range of different types of network approaches, including whole or complete social networks (sociocentric) involving both one- (people by people) and two-mode (people by events) networks, and ego or personal network analysis (egocentric). The chapter will emphasize the importance of a network perspective for producing a better understanding of systems structure and function, and for gaining a more holistic understanding of how human and natural systems interact.

SOCIAL NETWORK ANALYSIS

The basic building block of a social network is the dyad or link between two entities. These entities can be people, organizations, countries, etc. and the links can involve flows, communications, affective relations, emotions, interactions, etc. Links can be either present or absent, as in individuals knowing one another or not, or can take on a value, as in the degree to which people give and receive advice. The collection of dyads bounded in some way (e.g., all children in a classroom) is what constitutes a whole or complete social network, while the set of dyads for a single individual is what constitutes an ego network (e.g., the ties for a single child to others [termed alters] in a class and possibly the links among alters).

There are numerous books and articles on social network methods and applications that will aid anyone interested in social networks (Johnson 1994; Scott 1991; Wasserman and Faust 1994). This chapter, however, does not go into the specifics of social networks methods and measures, but rather provides examples of how social network analysis can be applied in the course of a social research involving aspects of ecology and the environment. What we hope to illustrate is how social networks help explain some phenomena of interest (e.g., the diffusion of agricultural innovations), as well as how non-network factors help explain the emergence of network structures (e.g., the evolution of cooperative networks in villages). In both cases, the social connections among social entities is critical for understanding a whole range of social phenomena of interest, such as norm formation, the development of social capital, the diffusion of knowledge and innovations, variation in cultural knowledge, and attitude formation, to name a few.

Example I: ego networks and natural disasters

The widespread destruction of property due to the floodwaters from a natural disaster such as Hurricane Katrina or Floyd is clearly evident. However, the psychosocial impact of an environmental disaster is usually less well understood. Earlier disaster studies have clearly observed a link between destruction, disruption, displacement, and psychological stress and trauma, including, for example, increases in suicide (Fullilove 1996; Peacock Morrow and Gladwin 1997; Provenzo and Fradd 1995). In addition, work on the sociology of disasters has found that the economic, social, and psychological problems faced by disaster victims, both during and after an event, varies by ethnicity, class, and gender (Dash, Peacock, and Morrow 1997; Gladwin and Peacock 1997; Peacock and Ragsdale 1997).

Less well understood are some of the social factors that help mitigate and lessen psychological stresses stemming from a disaster. Individuals vary on the amount of personal (e.g., personal savings), social (e.g., kin and friends), and institutional (e.g., insurance) resources available to them (Morrow 1997). Occasionally considered forms of social capital (Lin 2002), these resources in turn help in reducing the social, psychological, and economic uncertainties and impacts presented by loss and disruption (Fullilove 1996). For example, many victims have access to kin or friends who provide temporary shelter, clean-up help, or possibly financial assistance while yet others have limited social support because they recently moved to the region or lack linguistic skills. For this example, we ask one important and related question; what forms of social and other resources aid in lessening the social and psychological impacts of natural disasters? In some sense, this example examines how social resources, as manifested in social networks, influence an individual's ability to cope with and adapt to environmental disruptions. This example will provide an in-depth investigation of how these various forms of resources, as reflected in individual's ego network composition, help in mitigating social and psychological stress. In addition, it is the purpose of this example to illustrate the usefulness of the ego or personal network approach.

Data collection and study design

The data presented here derived from a pilot study examining longer-term impacts of Hurricane Floyd. The sample consisted of victims still without housing up to a year following the disaster, randomly sampled from residents in Federal Emergency Management Agency (FEMA) trailer parks still up and running in Eastern North Carolina a year after the event (2000 to 2001). Thus, it should be noted that most of the respondents in the study experienced catastrophic loss of property. The survey instrument used in this portion of the study consisted of an ego-centered network inventory to help in understanding the extent and quality of access to social resources (e.g., help in evacuating belongings, help in finding shelter, etc.) (Mueller, Wellman, and Marin 1999) and institutional resources (e.g., Red Cross, FEMA, etc.). Psychological well-being was determined with the use of the Profile of Mood States instrument (POMS) that reliably measures depression, anxiety, and vigor (Palinkas, Johnson, and Boster 2004).

Network background

It is important to make a distinction between strong and weak ties in social networks, particularly for the purposes of this example. Strong ties involve social relations between a focal individual (ego) and close friends and/or kin (alters). These relations tend to be dense and enduring involving high degrees of interaction. There is a high likelihood that ego's close ties involve people who also know one another leading to higher levels of network redundancy. Weak ties, on the other hand, are social relations between an ego and more passing acquaintances formed, for example, in the course of work, recreation, or interactions at other informal settings. These ties are often diverse involving people who may not know one another (i.e., non-redundant). Such ties are more instrumental than emotional but are extremely important for accessing novel information or resources (Grannovettor 1973). Generally, actors have many more weak ties than strong ties.

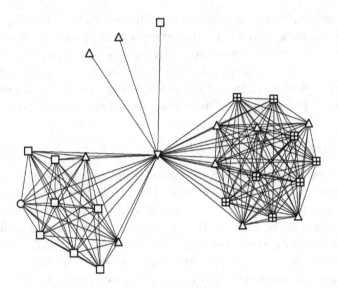

Figure 10.1   An example of an ego network where ego (in the center) has connections to two separate clusters of alters involving immediate kin (circles), extended family (squares), friends (triangle) and coworkers (box). The left cluster is primarily extended family and friends while the right cluster is primarily coworkers and friends.

Figure 10.1 provides an example of an ego network in which ego (in the center) is connected to two clear clusters of alters who are themselves not connected to one another. The composition of the network shows elements of network homophily in alter characteristics. Most of the cluster to the left of ego includes strong ties with immediate kin (i.e., mother, father, daughter) and some friends, while the cluster to the right includes mostly friendship and coworker ties. Thus composition based on various kinds of relations can be readily calculated for each ego.

The variables

The variables used in the analysis (Table 10.1) reflect both aspects of an individual's social networks and other factors hypothesized to affect the dependent variables. Most of the network-oriented variables are compositional in nature: that is, they reflect the extent to which an ego's network is composed of alters with characteristics or attributes of hypothesized interest. Since the main focus here is access to social and institutional resources, we are interested in the extent to which

Table 10.1. *List of independent and dependent variables.*

Dependent (from POMS)
Tension–anxiety, depression, anger, fatigue, and confusion.

Independent (demo and social and geographic proximity)
Education, age, household size, number helping, median days of help from alters, *log percent of alters that are immediate family, log percent of alters that are extended family, log percent of alters that are friends, log percent of alters that are neighbors,* log percent of alters that are local, log percent of alters from outside the immediate area (regional), log percent of alters from outside the state, and *number of organizations helping*
(Note: variables in italics were used in the multiple regression models)

---

an ego's network is composed of alters with various degrees of social (weak, strong ties) and geographic (in-state, out-of-state) proximities. Whereas this example is interested in access to social and institutional resources, other ego network studies may be interested in social capital, contagion, or the diffusion of behaviors (e.g., smoking), to name a few (see, for example, Lin 2002; McCarty 2002). Depending on the focus of the ego network, studying different compositional and classic network measures (e.g., centrality, density) may be of greater interest.

The models looked at several factors that might explain variation in an individual's psychological state. These include: social proximity – the type of social resources; geographic proximity – geographic distance from social resources; network size – amount of social resources; and institutional resources – support from formal institutions. What we are particularly interested in is the effect of network-oriented variables on mood states controlling for a number of standard demographic variables. The models involve standard OLS (ordinary least-squares) regressions, with some of the variables being log transformed to improve normality.

Table 10.2 shows the bivariate correlations among the variables from Table 10.1. As is evident, in the bivariate case the significant relationships between psychological states and network or other variable concern mostly the extent to which an ego's network is dominated by immediate kin or very strong ties. More moderate to weak ties (e.g., neighbors) are associated with more positive psychological states.

Table 10.3 shows the results for a series of multiple regressions looking at the effects of the various compositional ego network

Table 10.2. *Bivariate correlations between the various independent and psychologically oriented dependent variables (probabilities in parentheses are two-tail).*

	Tension/ anxiety	Depression	Anger	Vigor	Fatigue	Confusion
Immediate	0.339**	0.350**	0.358**	−0.237*	0.457***	0.415***
family	(0.023)	(0.027)	(0.016)	(0.116)	(0.002)	(0.005)
Extended family	−0.205	−0.012	−0.276*	−0.021	−0.122	−0.181
	(0.177)	(0.942)	(0.067)	(0.892)	(0.431)	(0.240)
Friends	0.040	−0.147	0.102	0.171	−0.154	−0.043
acquaintances	(0.796)	(0.366)	(0.505)	(0.260)	(0.319)	(0.780)
Coworkers	−0.204	−0.146	−0.035	0.011	−0.143	−0.219
	(0.179)	(0.370)	(0.822)	(0.942)	(0.355)	(0.153)
Neighbors	−0.109	−0.327**	−0.174	0.252*	−0.249*	−0.322**
	(0.476)	(0.039)	(0.253)	(0.096)	(0.103)	(0.033)
Local	0.003	−0.004	−0.033	−0.067	0.145	0.054
	(0.966)	(0.980)	(0.827)	(0.633)	(0.349)	(0.726)
Outside area	0.248*	0.293*	0.206	−0.181	0.264*	0.391***
	(0.100)	(0.067)	(0.175)	(0.234)	(0.084)	(0.009)
Outside state	−0.278*	−0.083	−0.043	0.060	−0.289*	−0.255*
	(0.064)	(0.611)	(0.777)	(0.694)	(0.057)	(0.095)
# Alters helping	−0.094	−0.118	−0.062	0.266	−0.119	0.013
	(0.528)	(0.458)	(0.679)	(0.071)	(0.430)	(0.931)
Organizations	−0.076	−0.038	−0.148	0.166	−0.119	−0.120
	(0.614)	(0.813)	(0.327)	(0.269)	(0.437)	(0.431)

$p < 0.1^*$, $p < 0.05^{**}$, $p < 0.01^{***}$.

variables on depression while controlling for a smaller set of demographic variables. The models use this smaller set of hypothesized independent variables due to potential problems with statistical power given the small sample size. Four models were run for the dependent variable in order to see the independent effect of each of the compositional ego network variables and also to avoid possible problems with multicolinearity. The results of the various models are in line with those from the bivariate regressions above in that an over-reliance on strong ties and an absence of more moderate to weak ties has an impact of an individual's mood state under these difficult circumstances. In the case of depression more moderate ties, in the form of neighbors, appear to mitigate, although weakly, the impacts of depression but less so with fatigue (results not shown). It should be noted that a similar series of models were run for geographic proximity of alters included with no real appreciable effects of the geographic proximity variables on mood states (percent of alters from outside the state, inside the state, and local).

Table 10.3. *Regression models comparing the effects of the various composition network variables on the dependent variable depression while controlling for demographic variables (included are standardized coefficients with t-values in parentheses).*

Effect	Model 1	Model 2	Model 3	Model 4
Education	−0.284*	−0.299*	−0.235	−0.224
	(−1.86)	(−1.64)	(−1.25)	(−1.41)
Organizations	−0.037	−0.120	−0.089	−0.094
	(−0.24)	(−0.71)	(−0.52)	(−0.60)
Age	0.042	−0.030	−0.014	0.056
	(0.24)	(−0.18)	(−0.09)	(0.35)
Immediate	0.412***	−	−	−
	(2.66)			
Extended	−	−0.131	−	−
		(−0.71)		
Friends	−	−	−0.019	−
			(−0.10)	
Neighbors	−	−	−	−0.320*
				(−2.00)
Constant	0.000	0.000	0.000	0.000
	(2.58)	(2.74)	(2.67)	(2.75)
Squared multiple R	0.226	0.079	0.066	0.163

$p < 0.1^*, p < 0.05^{**}, p < 0.01^{***}$.

There are bivariate relationships between over-dependence on strong family ties (lack of weak ties) and a range of psychological problems during extended recovery. There are bivariate relationships between the number of alters outside the area and a range of psychological problems during extended recovery. The relationship between lack of weak ties and psychological well-being holds when controlling for a number of demographic variables while the relationship with geographical proximity disappears.

Example discussion and summary

In this case it is not the strength of weak ties, but rather the lack of weak ties that has the biggest impact on extended recovery from a natural disaster. It is not simply the size of someone's ego network but more the composition of such networks that seems to matter, with a combination of strong and weak ties aiding in mitigating the negative psychological states following natural disaster. Understanding both the formal and informal social resources and mechanisms used by hurricane victims, or victims of any natural disruption, that helped reduce social and psychological trauma and disruption will aid in gaining a better understanding of social and other factors that lead to resilience in the light of disaster. First, knowing the types of formal resources (e.g., FEMA grants) most helpful to victims will further aid in better evaluating the extent to which formal services are effective. Second, the recognition and understanding of the form and kind of important informal social resources will help in better understanding resilience at the individual level (e.g., getting information out to important informal sources of information in communities such as local churches), particularly with respect to issues related to long term recovery and adaptation. Finally, an understanding of access to and use of these various resources will help those most affected by potential disasters, the people themselves, by providing information that will help them better prepare for the inevitable disruptions afforded by nature.

What this example shows is the importance of social network factors in individual and group adaptations to environmental and ecological changes at a variety of levels. Call this social capital or social resources, but access to people and institutions is important for understanding an individual actor's ability to adapt to changing environmental, ecological, economic, and social conditions. The ego network approach highlighted in this example has some distinct advantages. Ego network data can be easily incorporated into any standard survey. This alleviates the need to talk to everyone in the network (e.g., all actors in a given town), as in the whole or complete network case. Boundary specification issues occur at the ego level in terms of eliciting a fixed or unlimited set of alters from ego during the interview. However, the advantages and disadvantages of any elicitation approach are beyond the scope of this chapter. For a good review of these issues see McCarty (2002).

Example II: social networks and intracultural variation

We are often interested in knowledge people have, whether cultural, technological, environmental, biological, etc., and how it varies as a function of a variety of social and cultural factors (e.g., gender, class). There has been a long history of the study of intracultural variation, particularly among cognitive anthropologists studying various ethnobiological problems (e.g., people's knowledge of plants, birds, animals, fish, etc.) or environmental issues (Boster and Johnson 1989; Johnson and Griffith 1985; Kempton, Boster, and Hartley 1994). Stefflre (1985) in much of his work was attempting to pull together a diverse number of areas in the explanation of cognition. Thus, any variation in what he termed "heads" (cognition) is linked to material conditions (what he called technology and resources) and social structure and organization (e.g., social networks). Decision-making and ultimately behavior took place within this framework. These ideas have important implications in that they link cognition and its variation to aspects of culture at various levels (individual vs. cultural). Spheres of interaction that influence cognition, for example, are themselves linked more broadly to concepts of social organization, such as stratification and social class, while these are further linked to material and environmental conditions.

In this example we examine the relationship between social network position and variation in individual perceptions concerning different kinds of meats and how they are processed. Although the cultural domain examined here is food oriented, such an approach could be used to study any environmental or ecological cultural domain, including causes of environmental problems or ethnobiological knowledge (Johnson and Griffith 1996; Boster and Johnson 1989). So we ask two fundamental questions. Does the social network in which we interact influence individual cognition? If so, what is it about the content of these spheres of interaction that lead to fundamentally different ways of viewing the world?

The data from this example were taken from a larger study of seafood consumption in the United States (Griffith *et al.* 1988). One aspect of the study was concerned with seafood consumption in the landlocked Midwest. Data on perceptions of seafood relative to other sources of protein, such as beef, poultry, and pork and how they are presented and processed, were collected among informants selected according to a snowball sample of upper and lower middle class residents of a small Midwestern town. The data collected in this manner allowed for an examination of variations in perception as it relates to an individual's sphere of interactions within a given social class. Two hypotheses will be examined here, to illustrate the approach:

H1: Perceptions (approach to the cognitive task) will differ on the basis of network position (e.g., subgroup membership)

H2: There will be differences (distinctions) in the importance of food in the daily social affairs between network subgroups that will be reflected in the criteria used for categorization.

Setting and data collection

The setting for the study was a town in central Missouri, USA, with a population of approximately 13 000 people at the time of the research. The town, although in a rural area, had a mix of small industries, some employing as many as 1700 workers. Approximately 8500 jobs (81 percent of total employment) involved nonagricultural employment, reflecting a more industrial presence that is important for understanding the character of social class in this community. A series of preliminary in-depth interviews with city officials and real estate agents identified neighborhoods within the city that were predominately lower middle and upper middle class. One neighborhood of each type was chosen for the original seed for the two network subsamples. A block was chosen at random in each neighborhood and one house from each of the two blocks was chosen at random to initiate the snowball sample (see Johnson 1990). Each of the household heads was asked to name three other household heads with whom they discuss issues surrounding food. Each of the three household heads named would then be approached and so on until 15 households from each seed were interviewed for a total of 30 households. Interestingly enough, the two separate seeds led to a joining of the two subsamples at wave number three yielding a network that forms a single component in which each actor in the network can reach every other actor by some path no matter how long.

Interviews in the household were conducted with what was called the "key kitchen person" or the person who is most responsible for both the purchase of groceries and cooking of food. Two primary sources of data were collected. First, a series of network and demographic questions were asked obtaining information on the three households mentioned, such as the last time any one from the focal household ate a meal with any member from the three other households elicited. Finally, each informant was asked to complete an unconstrained pile sort task (also referred to here as a cognitive task) in which they were asked to place the stimuli, in this case photographs of different types of meats (i.e., beef, poultry, pork, seafood) processed in various ways (e.g., fresh, frozen, canned), into piles according to how similar they perceive each of the types of meat to be to one another.

The stimuli were created from a series of in-depth interviews with key kitchen persons concerning product brand familiarity. A listing of all meat products (e.g., Oscar Mayer® Wieners, Starkist® Tuna) found in grocery stores was compiled. This list was presented to the key kitchen informants and each was asked to check the items with which they were familiar. The most frequently checked items were then purchased at the store and photographed. The photographs of meats were then given an identification number on the back and laminated in plastic, for a total of 30 stimuli cards.

Results

In order to test the hypothesis (H1) that the subgroups are employing two fundamentally different models in their approach to the cognitive task, the cultural consensus model was used (Romney, Weller, and Batchelder 1986). The model views agreement as an indication of shared cultural knowledge, where agreement is determined by the extent to which there is a single factor solution in a minimum residual factor analysis. The pile sort data for the 30 informants was converted into a matrix where columns are informants and rows are the presence or absence of a judged similarity between any two items (e.g., between Starkist® Chunk Light Tuna and Oscar Mayer® Wieners). Columns were then intercorrelated, producing a correlation matrix representing inter-informant agreement. This matrix was then subjected to minimum residual factor analysis as a test of consensus, and multidimensional scaling as a means for visualizing the agreement among informants.

The factor analysis including both subsamples revealed a violation of one expectation of the cultural consensus model (the ratio of the first to second eigenvalue should be greater than 3), in that the ratio of the first to second eigenvalue is only 2.1. This suggests the presence of two or more subcultures, involving the existence of possible competing cognitive models.

Consensus by group

Separate analyses were performed on the two network subsamples. Again correlation matrices for each group were produced and subjected to minimum residual factor analysis. In each case there is a better fit to the model. This provides further support for the presence of at least two competing models.

Although the analysis to this point seems to point to alternative models being employed depending on subgroup membership, the exact nature of these models that ultimately influence the approach to the cognitive task are unknown. However, during the course of interviews informants were asked to explain their sorting behavior in terms of reasoning for shared membership of items in a given pile. Transcripts of these interviews revealed two primary criteria for sorting. The most evident of these was based on simple meat groupings such as beef, poultry, pork, and fish. A less clear set of criteria concerned aspects of processing including such things as fresh, frozen, canned, and so on. Based on the explanations provided by informants two hypothesized "models" were constructed for comparison across informants. These theoretical models consisted of a free pile sort based on grouping by type of meat, henceforth referred to as the meat standard or model, and by type of processing, henceforth termed the processing standard or model.

The theoretical models

Two theoretical pile sort models were constructed by categorizing on the basis of type of meat and processed state (e.g., frozen, canned). These purposely constructed pile sorts represented theoretical models reflecting aspects of the stimuli. Each theoretical model was entered into the analysis as if they were additional informants. Thus, the theoretical models themselves can be examined in the consensus analysis or a comparison can be made in terms of the mean differences between groups with respect to average distance (mean correlations) to each model and visualized using multidimensional scaling.

Figure 10.2 shows the results of a multidimensional scaling of the inter-informant agreement matrix including both theoretical models. As is evident, the upper middle class group is to the right of the configuration near the process model, while the bulk of the lower middle class group is to the left near the meat model. Figure 10.3 is a network visualization of the network relations among the informants with the size of the nodes proportional to the size of correlations to the meat theoretical model. This corroborates the results above in that there is a clear tendency for the lower middle class informants to use aspects of the meat model in their approach to the cognitive task. In a non-parametric statistical test of the differences between the groups with respect to the correlation to the meat model there is a clear and statistically significant difference in the expected direction

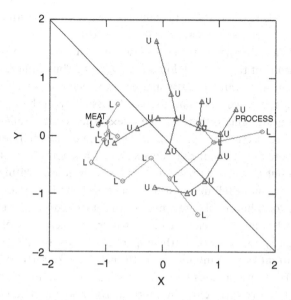

Figure 10.2 Multidimensional scaling of the inter-informant agreement matrix among the actors from the two seed samples (U for upper middle and L for lower middle) including the two theoretical models and spanning trees connecting members of each subgroup.

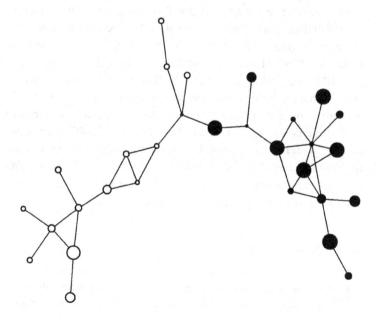

Figure 10.3 Network of informants in study with lower middle (solid black) and upper middle (white) groups. Node size is proportional to the size of each actor's correlation to the meat model (see text).

(Mann-Whitney U test statistic = 164.000, Monte Carlo exact estimate of p for 99.00% level of confidence = (0.0157, 0.0161)).

There is a difference between the two subsamples in terms of their perceptions of the cultural domain of interest. Thus, spheres of interaction appear to influence the manner in which individuals see the world. Although we have not discussed possible underlying reasons for these differences, they may be due to the possible salience of food to the respective groups (H2). In the course of the interviews, informants were asked about the households with whom they interacted, and about aspects of their interactions with household members. One of the more telling questions concerned the last time any one from the focal household ate a meal with someone from the elicited households, and the social setting in which the meal took place (e.g., dinner party, restaurant). For the upper middle class sample, food was an important part of interaction with members from the other households. Thus, interactions frequently took place at dinner parties or lunches at the country club. In contrast, the lower middle class members of the network from different households rarely if ever ate meals together. The primary place for interaction was at church meetings and weekly bible studies. This may have led people to employ different cognitive models, due to differences in possible orientations toward food in terms of such possible things as utility versus form (Boster and Johnson 1989). A correlation between the number of days since last eating a meal with other households and the correlation to the meat model was moderately strong and significant ($r = 0.407$, $p < 0.03$), supporting the inference that people whose social interactions involve little to no food have a more utilitarian view of the domain. Food is an essential component of social interaction for the upper middle class group and a finer grained classification scheme, one based on how something is processed, can be important in accruing cultural capital (Bourdieu 1984). For the lower middle class group, food is mostly absent from their spheres of social interaction, so takes on a more instrumental form.

Example discussion and summary

Bourdieu sees variation in internalized cultural codes, such as different perceptions of meats, leading to unequal access to cultural capital, where such capital can gain one "profits of distinction" (Bourdieu 1984: 562). A particularly relevant discussion from a footnote in *Distinctions* illustrates his view:

> In fact, through the economic and social conditions which they presuppose, the different ways of relating to realities and fictions, of believing in fictions and the realities they simulate, with more or less distance and detachment, are very closely linked to the different possible positions in social space and, consequently, bound up with systems of dispositions (habitus) characteristic of the different classes and class factions. Taste classifies, and it classifies the classifier. Social subjects, classified by their classifications, distinguish themselves by the distinctions they make, between the beautiful and the ugly, the distinguished and the vulgar, in which their position in the objective classifications is expressed or betrayed. And statistical analysis does indeed show that oppositions similar in structure to those found in cultural practices also appear in eating habits. The antithesis between quality and quantity, substance and form, corresponds to the opposition – linked to different distances from necessity – between the taste of necessity, which favors the most "filling" and most economical foods, and the taste of liberty – or luxury – which shifts the emphasis to the manner (of presenting, serving, eating, etc.) and tends to use stylized forms to deny function. (Bourdieu 1984: 6)

Thus, the social networks in which we are embedded reflect elements of class and ultimately such things as taste. These in turn influence our world views in terms of how we classify the world around us.

The important thing about this example is that by including actual dyadic ties among actors, that is their social networks, we can study the influences of both ties and other social attributes (e.g., social class) on the dependent variable of interest. This stands in contrast to standard survey methods involving random samples in that although we may have found similar social class influences on cognition using such standard approaches we would have been unable to understand network contextual effects on the outcome of interest giving us a more holistic understanding. Thus, we can understand not only how various traditional attributes (e.g., age, education) influence outcomes, but we can also determine the influence of actual social relations on such outcomes.

Example III: two mode behavioral networks and ecosystem links

Although there has been much recent interest in models that involve integration of natural and human systems (as in, for example, ecosystem-based management), there are relatively few empirical examples of such integration. Much of the emphasis in ecosystem-based management has been on the biology side, focusing on species population models or possible food web models. However, the behavior of resource extractors (e.g., fishermen) can also be considered in network terms. In fact, establishing these behavioral networks can take place concurrently with establishing ecological networks or other ecosystem models in order to best understand the full dynamics of the system. Thus, Johnson and Orbach (1996) show that the interdependencies of species/gear combinations employed by fishers (i.e., fishing behaviors) form a network revealing a number of important aspects of a given fisheries complex (i.e., a set of interconnected species and gears). Like any system, these behavioral networks form structures with various properties. Thus, such behavioral networks vary in terms of robustness, stability, sustainability, and vulnerability, just as with traditional food webs in ecology. As in food webs, understanding the nature of a behavioral network structure (e.g., connectance or graph density, degree distribution, keystone gears) can aid in understanding the potential direct and indirect impacts of both environmental change (e.g., global climate change) and changes due to fisheries regulations on the behavioral network structure and, hence, on the economic livelihoods and social lives of fishers and their communities.

Another benefit of viewing human fishing activities as a network is that it facilitates the direct linking of human behaviors with ecosystem properties, such as food webs, and has the potential to further our understanding of the complex interdependencies between the two. Changes in ecological networks (e.g., reductions in a food web compartment's biomass) can have direct impacts on behavioral networks as fishers adapt their fishing behaviors to meet new ecological realities. In both Mid-Atlantic and Northeast fisheries, Griffith (1999) and Griffith and Dyer (1996) documented that fishers generally respond to changes, whether ecological or regulatory, by switching behaviors or increasing effort along already existing network behavioral pathways. These behavioral adaptations will in turn have an impact on the ecological network given a reallocation of fishing effort within the food web system.

Constructing behavioral networks

Human behavioral networks can be constructed in a variety of ways from a variety of sources of both a primary and secondary data (e.g., interviews, government records). Figure 10.4 shows an example of a human behavioral network constructed for Pamlico Sound, North

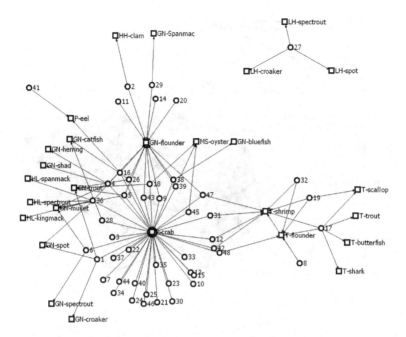

Figure 10.4 Pamlico Sound Commercial Human Behavioral 2-mode
Network (HL, hand line; P, pots; GN, gill nets; HH, hand harvest;
T, trawl; LH, long haul; MS, mechanical dredge) based on links between
fishers and the gear/species they incorporate in their operations
(squares are gear/species types and circles are fishers).

Carolina, USA, from interviews with fishers (Johnson and Orbach 1996).
The network was constructed from fisher's reports of gear and species
combinations used throughout a given year, often called an annual
round. A two-mode matrix was constructed where rows are individual
fishing units (e.g., captains) and columns are types of gears used and
species targeted during the time period of interest. The figure shows
a two-mode network of fishing gear types by individual fishers and
provides for a better understanding of the interrelationships among
gears and species and the fishers that employ them. These behavioral
networks can be looked at in terms of the relationships among either
gear/species combinations or the fishers themselves. The two-mode
network of gear/species combinations by individual fishing units can
be converted into an affiliation network of the relations among fishers
vis-à-vis the gear/species combinations they employ or the relations
among gear/species combinations vis-à-vis the fishing units employing
them. This allows for the identification of such things as clusters of

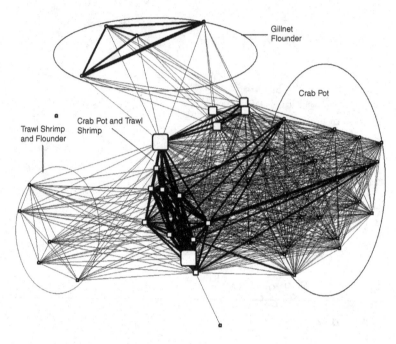

Figure 10.5   Pamlico Sound Commercial Human Behavioral Network based on affiliation among fishers vis-à-vis gear types. Clusters of fisher behaviors are circled and labeled.

fishing strategies, similarities among fishers based on annual round behaviors, interdependencies among gear and/species combinations, and the importance of a gear/species combination in maintaining the integrity of the behavioral network. In addition, an understanding of the interdependencies among gear/species combinations can be important for understanding the impacts of regulations, prices, and ecological changes on the overall behavioral network of fishing activities.

Figure 10.5 is an affiliation network showing the relations among fishers vis-à-vis the type of fishing in which they engage in a given year. This network helps in understanding how fishers themselves cluster on the basis of their fishing behaviors. So, for example, there are clusters of individual fishers who engage exclusively in crab potting, others crab pot in combination with either gill netting or shrimp/flounder trawling and a single unit engages in all of these.

Figure 10.6 shows network affiliations based on gear type, adding information on the species varieties most often targeted with

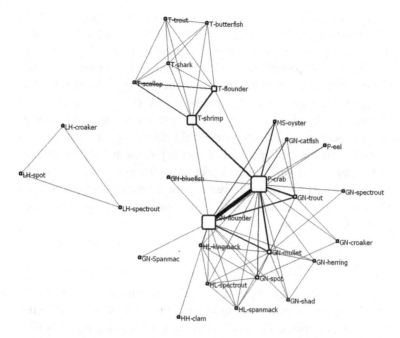

Figure 10.6   Pamlico Sound Commercial Human Behavioral Network
(HL, hand line; P, pots; GN, gill nets; HH, hand harvest; T, trawl;
LH, long haul; MS, mechanical dredge) based on affiliation among
gear types vis-à-vis fishers. Nodal size is a proportional to a gear type's
betweenness centrality and line thickness is proportional to the
number of fishers two gear types have in common.

each gear and thereby linking human and natural systems vis-à-
vis gear, fish, and fisher networks. The figure reveals the interdependencies among the various types of fishing in which fishers engage.
The thickness of the lines in the network graph is a function of the
number of fishers jointly engaged in a given gear and species combination. So, for example, fishers who crab pot also have a tendency to
gill net for flounder and to some extent trout. The size of the nodes is
a function of the betweenness centrality (the extent to which a node
is on the shortest path between all other nodes in the network) of the
gear/species combinations. This can be thought of as index of broker-
age and importance in social networks and reflects gear/species combinations that link other types of combinations that are not directly
linked to each other (Freeman 1977). These interdependencies form
a fishing behavioral network that can be important for identifying
keystone gears and species in a given fisheries complex. The network

can also be analyzed to understand the direct and indirect effects of fish reductions on behavior as in, for example, the impact of the keystone gear/species combination on other components of the network, in this case crab potting. Reduction in or the outright removal of crab potting would have a huge impact on the structural integrity of the behavioral network. This is not unlike the direct and indirect impacts of removing species from a food web, particularly keystone species (i.e., a species critical to the structural integrity of the food web). In Pamlico Sound, the disappearance of crab potting due to ecological or regulatory factors would have a proportionally greater impact on the behavioral network than the removal of a component such as long hauling (LH) that already forms a separate and disconnected component of the network.

Application example

To illustrate the usefulness of this idea we provide a comparative example from a study by Johnson and Orbach (1996) that characterized and documented commercial fishing efforts in North Carolina for the purposes of producing a comprehensive management plan for the state. The study broke the state into five different areas based on ecosystem type and fishing activities. Data on fisher's annual rounds were collected in each of the areas, and two-mode matrices were constructed. These were then converted to affiliation matrices such as illustrated in Figure 10.5, reflecting the relations between the various gear/species combinations found in the respective areas. Behavioral networks of this form can be analyzed in a number of ways, such as system robustness or resilience (e.g., the impact of node removal on the structure of the overall network). We will look briefly at two methods for the purposes of this example.

The first measure is network density, meaning simply the number of ties observed in the network divided by the total number of possible ties. Network density can range from zero to 1.0; a density of 1.0 would mean every node in the network is connected to every other node in the network, whereas a zero measure would indicate the network is completely disconnected. We would expect a network with high density to be impacted less by the removal of a single node, and thus to be more robust in the face of change, given the high degree of tie redundancy in the network. The second measure, network fragmentation, is a dynamic index of the effect of node removal on the structure of a network in terms of the number of separate components

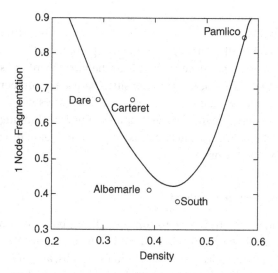

Figure 10.7   Relationship between network fragmentation based on key gear/species removal and behavioral network density, where fragmentation concerns the number of network components produced by removal of a keystone behavior (i.e., species/gear combination).

produced by the removal of one or more nodes. A network component is a network in which each node in the network component can reach every other node in the component by some path no matter how long. This is an index of the extent to which the removal of a node (e.g., a gear/species combination) disconnects the network into separate components. In Figure 10.6, for example, there are two network components. There is the main component including crab potting and a much smaller component involving long hauling (LH).

Figure 10.7 is a scatter plot showing the relationship between density and network fragmentation for the five areas. The programs Keyplayer and UCINET (Borgatti 2003; Borgatti, Everet, and Freeman 2002) were used to calculate network fragmentation and density when a single key gear/species combination was removed from the network that would maximize the fragmentation index. As you can see from the figure, there is initially a trend downward in fragmentation as density increases reflecting the possible mediating effects of density on system robustness. However, the area with the highest density also is the area with the highest fragmentation with the removal of a single node. This is interesting in that, although it is generally true that the higher the density the potentially more robust the system, there are cases in which a single node connects dense areas of the network that are themselves not connected to one another. This is the case with the Pamlico Sound and it illustrates nicely how important crab potting (e.g., due to high betweenness centrality) is to the integrity of the system despite the high levels of network density. There are a number of other cohesion measures that can be used in such an assessment, but this example illustrates the insights that can be gained by thinking of these productive behaviors as a network as opposed to a set of disconnected productive endeavors.

Example discussion and summary

There are a number of advantages to conceptualizing behavioral networks in the manner described above. These behavioral networks can be linked directly to ecological networks, as in food webs, and this connection can help identify important causal dynamic pathways from the ecosystem side up and from the human behavioral side down. Each of those gear/species combinations can be thought of as predators in a food web. But more importantly, they play the role as predators at the interface between the ecological and behavioral elements of the overall system. Thus, models can be conceptualized and developed that look at the direct and indirect effects of human behavior on the food web and conversely how changes in the food web directly and indirectly impact the human behavioral network. Further, supply chains and webs (seafood dealers, processors, wholesalers, retailers, consumers) can also be added to understand how changes in consumer preferences, for example, can have cascade effects through both the human behavioral and ecological networks. Modeling networks in this manner has real potential to help produce a more comprehensive ecosystem management framework.

OVERALL CHAPTER SUMMARY AND DISCUSSION

We opened this chapter with the promise of using social network research methods to enhance our understanding of interactions between human and natural systems. To this end, we discussed three illustrative case studies. In our Hurricane Floyd example, we demonstrated the importance of weak network ties, combined with strong ties, in reducing problems associated with recovering from a natural disaster, pointing to the critical role of networks in a person's ability to access social resources and institutional support as well as other forms of aid. In our example from Missouri on meat classification, it was clear that networks (as well as class affiliations, which manifest themselves in networks) influenced perceptions of a cultural element shared by all humans but which enjoys wide variation: food. Collecting network data from two social classes further elucidated the relationships among food events, class background, and perceptions of food. Finally, the study of North Carolina fishing networks demonstrated how network-based linkages between natural and human systems can be constructed from interview data regarding fishing behaviors (e.g., gear varieties, annual rounds, species targeted). This work demonstrated that direct and indirect impacts on fish stocks and other dimensions of marine environments could be dynamically linked to network structure and the network affiliations of fishers, increasing our understanding of how regulatory measures such as mandated gear modifications are likely to influence fishing behaviors and, in turn, marine environments.

These examples demonstrate that a variety of methods are available for constructing and representing social networks, and that these can be applied to various issues of theoretical importance in the social sciences. In this chapter, we have focused on how social and natural systems interact with one another and result in very real social problems and solutions, understanding those linkages with reference to social networks. Combined with more traditional lines of research (e.g., more classical survey and linear approaches), social network methods and theories can lead to a more valid and comprehensive understanding of the link between human and natural systems.

REFERENCES

Borgatti, S. 2003. *KeyPlayer*. Boston: Analytic Technologies.
Borgatti, S., M. G. Everett, and L. C. Freeman 2002. *UCINET for Windows: Software for Social Network Analysis*. Harvard, MA: Analytic Technologies.
Boster, J. S. and J. C. Johnson 1989. Form or function: a comparison of expert and novice judgment of similarity among fish, *American Anthropologist* **91**: 866–889.
Boster, J. S. and J. C. Johnson 1994. South Pole III. Paper presented at the annual *Sunbelt Social Network Conference*, New Orleans, LA.
Bourdieu, P. 1984. *Distinction: A Social Critique of the Judgment of Taste*. Trans. R. Nice. Cambridge, MA: Harvard University Press.
Burt, R. S. 1992. *Structural Holes: The Social Structure of Competition*. Cambridge, MA: Harvard University Press.
Dash, N., W. G. Peacock, and B. H. Morrow 1997. And the poor get poorer: a neglected black community. In W. G. Peacock, B. H. Morrow, and J. Gladwin, eds., *Hurricane Andrew: Ethnicity, Gender and the Sociology of Disasters*. New York: Routledge, pp. 206–225.

Freeman, L. C. 1977. A set of measures of centrality based on betweenness. *Sociometry* **40**: 35–41.

Fullilove, M. T. 1996. Psychiatric implications of displacement: contributions from the psychology of place. *The American Journal of Psychiatry* **153**: 1516–1523.

Gladwin, H. and W. G. Peacock 1997. Warning and evacuation: a night for hard houses. In W. G. Peacock, B. H. Morrow, and J. Gladwin, eds., *Hurricane Andrew: Ethnicity, Gender and the Sociology of Disasters*. New York: Routledge, pp. 52–74.

Granovetter, M. 1973. The strength of weak ties. *American Journal of Sociology* **78**(6): 1360–1380.

Griffith, D. 1999. *The Estuary's Gift: A Mid-Atlantic Cultural Biography*. University Park, PA: Penn State University Press.

Griffith, D. and C. Dyer 1996. *Appraisal of the Social and Cultural Aspects of the Multispecies Groundfish Fishery in the Mid-Atlantic and Northeast Regions*. Washington, DC: NOAA, July. (Available on the Wood Hole Oceanographic Institute website.)

Griffith, D. C., J. C. Johnson, J. D. Murray, and S. Kemp 1988. Social and cultural dimensions of consumer knowledge among seafood and seafood analog consumers in the southeast: implications for consumer education. Technical Report to the Gulf and South Atlantic Fisheries Development Foundation.

Johnson, J. C. 1990. *Selecting Ethnographic Informants*. Newbury Park, CA: Sage.

Johnson, J. C. 1994. Anthropological contributions to the study of social networks: a review. In S. Wasserman and J. Galaskiowicz, eds., *Advances in Social Network Analysis: Research in the Social and Behavioral Sciences*. Sage: Newbury Park, pp. 113–151.

Johnson, J. C. and D. C. Griffith 1985. *Perceptions and preferences for marine fish: a study of recreational fishermen in the Southeast region*. UNC-SG-85-01, 104 pages, University of North Carolina Sea Grant: Raleigh.

Johnson, J. C. and D. C. Griffith 1996. Pollution, food safety, and the distribution of knowledge. *Human Ecology* **24**(1): 87–108.

Johnson, J. C. and M. K. Orbach 1996. *Effort management in North Carolina fisheries: a total systems approach*. UNC-SG-96-08, 258 pages, University of North Carolina Sea Grant: Raleigh.

Kempton, W., J. S. Boster, and J. Hartley 1994. *Environmental Values in American Culture*. Cambridge, MA.: MIT Press.

Lin, N. 2002. *Social Capital: A Theory of Social Structure and Action*. Cambridge: Cambridge University Press.

McCarty, C. 2002. Measuring structure in personal networks. *Journal of Social Structure* **3**: 1.

Morrow, B. H. 1997. Disaster in the first person. In W. G. Peacock, B. H. Morrow, and J. Gladwin, eds., *Hurricane Andrew: Ethnicity, Gender and the Sociology of Disasters*. New York: Routledge, pp. 1–19.

Müller, C., B. Wellman, and A. Marin 1999. How to use SPSS to study ego-centered networks. *Bulletin de Methode Sociologique* **69**: 83–100.

Palinkas, L. A., J. C. Johnson, and J. S. Boster 2004. Social support and depressed mood in isolated and confined environments. *Acta Astronautica* **54**: 639–647.

Peacock, W. G., B. H. Morrow, and H. Gladwin 1997. *Hurricane Andrew: Ethnicity, Gender, and the Sociology of Disasters*. New York: Routledge.

Peacock, W. G., and A. K. Ragsdale 1997. Social systems, ecological networks and disasters. In W. G. Peacock, B. H. Morrow, and J. Gladwin, eds., *Hurricane*

Andrew: Ethnicity, Gender and the Sociology of Disasters. New York: Routledge, pp. 20–35.

Provenzo, Jr., E. F. and S. H. Fradd 1995. *Hurricane Andrew, the Public Schools and the Rebuilding of Community.* Albany, NY: State University of New York Press.

Romney, A. K., S. Weller and W. H. Batchelder 1986. Culture as a consensus: a theory of culture and informant accuracy. *American Anthropologist* **88**: 313–338.

Scott, J. 1991. *Social Network Analysis: A Handbook.* Newbury Park: Sage.

Stefflre, V. 1985. *Developing and Implementing Marketing Strategies.* Santa Barbara, CA: Praeger Publishers.

Wasserman, S. and K. Faust. 1994. *Social Network Analysis: Methods and Applications.* Cambridge, MA: Cambridge University Press.

11

Khat commodity chains in Madagascar: multi-sited ethnography at multiple scales

LISA L. GEZON

INTRODUCTION

This chapter addresses theoretical and methodological concerns of multi-sited research with reference to a study of khat in Madagascar. The bushy khat plant, whose leaves are chewed fresh for a mild amphetamine effect, grows well in the cool temperatures of the Mt. d'Ambre region in northern Madagascar. Khat first arrived in Madagascar with Yemeni dock workers, hired under a French colonial regime, in the early to mid twentieth century. Its growing local popularity has meant a significant increase in revenues for farmers over the last 10–15 years. Today khat is primarily chewed in Yemen, in parts of the Horn of Africa, Somalia, Kenya, Ethiopia, and in immigrant communities from those regions abroad (Carrier and Gezon 2009).

By localizing Malagasy khat production within a broader context, this chapter investigates links between the economic processes of production, distribution, and consumption – often referred to as a commodity chain. These interconnected dynamics occur in multiple geographically dispersed locations, involving many different actors. Understanding the effects of khat requires research in multiple locations to determine how geographically dispersed variables affect each other. The draw toward a multi-sited approach emerged from a general interest in explaining forest degradation, with the question: What are the major pressures on the Mt. d'Ambre forests? Upon learning that khat production had increased tremendously on the north and east

Environmental Social Sciences: Methods and Research Design, ed. I. Vaccaro, E. A. Smith and S. Aswani. Published by Cambridge University Press. © Cambridge University Press 2010.

sides of the Mt. d'Ambre, a more focused question emerged: What is the relationship between the expansion of khat production and deforestation? *We hypothesized that people are cutting down forests in order to grow khat.* A multi-sited approach, focusing on the commodity chain, made sense for understanding how demand outside of the immediate region of production influenced local decision-making and land use patterns.

Preliminary research (in 2003), which included interviews with local people, revealed another concern with khat. Many educated people, including policy-makers, were concerned that khat was being cultivated to the detriment of food crops. What had once been a region rich with rice and a major supplier of vegetables seemed to have become dominated by khat production while the cultivation of food crops declined. People worried about food security. So the focus expanded to inquire into the ways that land cover change informs broader discussions of food systems. *The working hypothesis, which mirrored local concerns, was that khat expansion had displaced food production and was therefore responsible for weakening the food security of the north by making them reliant on imports from other parts of the country.* This concern broadened the geographic perspective to include extra-local suppliers of food staples. Because of the large scope of this research, it was conducted over several field trips between 2003 and 2007.

While the first hypothesis was weakly supported, the second was not. The reasons for the decline in local food production are complex and not directly related to khat in most cases. On the contrary, khat provided a way of coping with the declining viability of previous subsistence strategies. This study revealed that analysis of commodity chains at multiple scales and in multiple locations is important for understanding local land use patterns. Concerns about protected area management in particular benefit from moving beyond local and contemporary levels of analysis. Interrogating larger issues of consumer demand as well as the political, economic, and historical contexts of production, trade, and consumption permits a nuanced and multi-faceted understanding of why and how land cover is changing, at the same time revealing how people in particular locales survive on the margins of globalization.

MULTI-SITED RESEARCH IN PERSPECTIVE

Theoretical underpinnings

Multi-sited research, with its interest in analyzing systematic connections between dynamics in geographically distant locales, can be theoretically grounded in world system theory, globalization, and political ecology, with particular interest in issues of scale. It also emerges from the Manchester School of British social anthropology, under Max Gluckman. An interest in globalization in anthropology coincides with the first global oil crisis and has underpinnings in the world system theories of Immanuel Wallerstein (1974), Andre Gunder Frank (1967), Samir Amin (1977), and Francis Moore Lappé (Lappé and Collins 1977). The crux of these theories is that the world is interconnected, and that dynamics occurring in one location cannot be explained without reference to those in other locations. This was particularly used for understanding poverty and relationships of global domination. These theorists developed what became known as dependency theory, identifying the poverty of former colonized nations and the wealth of colonizers as being the result of the political and economic manipulations of colonial power. These theories laid forth universal/macro theories of the results of global processes on local people. These are based in the increasing disparities of wealth that stem from resource extraction, practices that excluded people in peripheral countries from competing with those from the economic core, and forced subordination through such practices as taxation and manual labor. This entrenched hierarchy has rendered the peripheral nations dependent for survival on the wealthy nations.

Theorists of globalization have looked to such factors as transnational capital flows, the transformation of local economies in service of the global economy, the related weakening of the nation-state, technological advances hastening pace and shortening distance (Harvey 1989), horizontal integration via the networks such as the internet (Castells 1996), and the relationship of capitalism to uneven economic development (Smith 1984) as keys to understanding processes of globalization (T. L. Friedman 2000).

In anthropology, theorists such as Tsing, Hannerz, and Appadurai have responded to an assumption of globally homogeneous processes and top-down dictation of local lifeways. Throughout her work, Tsing points out that what we refer to as global is not a top-down project, but that it is co-produced across scales (1993, 2000, 2005). Her concept of "friction" captures this sense: "As a metaphorical image, friction reminds us that heterogeneous and unequal encounters can lead to new arrangements of culture and power" (2005: 5). Hannerz (1996) and Appadurai (1996) analyze the cultural dimensions of globalization addressing the popular alarm that globalization will lead to homogenization. Hannerz traces transnational influences back and forth between the core and periphery, while Appadurai introduces concepts such as ethnoscapes, mediascapes, and financescapes for understanding the fluidity and irregularity of global flows.

Environmental anthropologists look to early work by Julian Steward (1955) and his students, including Sidney Mintz and Eric Wolf, as inspiration for a multi-sited approach that considers connections between the processes of industrialization and its effects on urban expansion and agricultural change. Mintz originally worked on Steward's larger project focusing on understanding the ecological base of complex contemporary societies in Puerto Rico. In his study of sugar cane plantations, Mintz's influential book, *Sweetness and Power* (1985) identifies the implications of increasing consumption and production of sugar. He connects the consumption of sugar to an intraclass struggle for profit, the growing hegemony of industrial capitalism, and the control of slave and industrial wage labor.

Eric Wolf (1982) wrote a broader global history, identifying the connections among nations in their quest for wealth and power. He called for rigorous attempts at formulating theory capable of taking connections into account and noted the shortcomings of a theoretical and empirical focus on a single geographic location. Political ecology emerged within anthropology with an explicit interest in understanding how extralocal dynamics affect local environmental processes. Wolf is credited with making the first written mention of a manner of inquiry that he called "political ecology" (1972), when he argued that local ecological and social practices must be understood in the context of non-local interests.[1] In later political ecology, scholars have used the concept of scale to refer to relationships between geographical spaces of progressively wider span, considering how local, regional, national, and international levels of analysis inform each other. Zimmerer and Bassett (2003) point out that scale involves social and biophysical dimensions, and that the process of identifying scalar units is highly political. Scale refers not only to geographical space, but also to levels of political inclusiveness. Place is not static and bounded, but is rather a historically situated and culturally constructed space, deeply connected to flows of power and

---

[1] Important references in the study of political ecology include Bassett (1988), Biersack and Greenberg (2006), Blaikie and Brookfield (1987), Escobar (2008), Hecht and Cockburn (1990), Martinez-Alier (2002), Moore (2005), Paulson and Gezon (2006), Peet and Watts (1993) and the entire special issue of the *Annals of the Association of American Geographers* 1993, Volume 8, Issue 2, Peet and Watts (2004), Robbins (2004), and Schmink and Wood (1987).

control (Chalfin 2004; Massey 1994). Identification of relevant levels of scale and the relationships between them are to be contextualized in each instance.

The commodity chain has been useful in conceptualizing the on-the-ground economic processes of globalization. Commodity chain analysis moves away from conceptualizing progressively inclusive levels of scale in favor of identifying links between places and processes. Early analyses of commodity chains by Hopkins and Wallerstein (1986) and Gereffi and Korzeniewicz (1994) represent an offshoot of dependency theory, focusing on the labor and productive aspects of commodity formation (Kenney and Florida 1994). A later approach built on these earlier formulations but identified itself with the term *filière* (commodity chain), which emphasizes "the series of relations through which an item passes, from extraction through conversion, exchange, transport, distribution and final use" (Ribot 1998: 307). It differs from the early approach in that it does not privilege production, per se, and includes greater focus on distribution and consumption. Jesse Ribot and others developed this framework to emphasize empirical investigation of market relationships, moving away from formal neoclassical models (Bernstein 1996; Ribot 1998), which ignore the embeddedness of markets in broader historically situated political and social systems, including production and consumption. In all, the *filières* approach builds on earlier commodity chain conceptualizations, but is more closely aligned with an anthropological emphasis on ethnography and holism. In his early edited volume, *The Social Life of Things*, Appadurai (1986) similarly called attention to studies of commodities from cultural as well as political, economic, and social perspectives. He proposed that relations and contests of power connect the processes of production, distribution, and consumption. This perspective has influenced many current commodity chain and multi-sited perspectives in anthropology.

The challenge of the multi-sited approach is to identify systematic connections between scales and zones of influence, identifying how political, economic, and cultural processes, in Eric Wolf's words "transcend separable cases, moving through and beyond them and transforming them as they proceed" (1982: 17). Part of this challenge is remembering that multi-sited research can never be divorced from theory. As Jonathan Friedman points out, "[g]lobal systemic relations are not visible as such." Rather, they are about "analytical or theoretical properties of processes that are posited by the researcher" (J. Friedman 2000: 639).

Methodological approaches

This theoretical interest in transnational processes and global connections requires new methodological approaches. In his influential
review, George Marcus notes that the world system does not structure
local contexts, but rather that "cultural logics ... are at least partially
constituted within sites of the so-called system" (Marcus 1995: 97).
Understanding the local remains critical to globalization studies, and
macro-theory does not obviate the need for ethnography. He identifies
a strategy that requires "quite literally following connections, associations and putative relationships" (1995: 97). It involves fieldwork in
multiple geographic sites, with sensitivity to tracing the connections
between them.

This approach recalls important scholarship coming out of the
Rhodes-Livingstone Institute in Northern Rhodesia (now Zambia)
and the Manchester School under Max Gluckman (Burawoy 1991;
Gluckman 1958; Van Velsen 1979). They embraced the extended case
method for identifying connections in time, space, and topic. Epstein
wrote that "cases have their sources in the ceaseless flow of social life
and, in turn, contribute to that flow" (1979: 230). Kottak and Colson
(1994) took inspiration from the Manchester School, as well as from
Mintz (1985), Wallerstein (1974), and Wolf (1982), in formulating their
linkages methodology. This approach combines many facets, including
"a network approach (to trace the far flung sets of relationships associated with geographical mobility and external interventions)" (Kottak
and Colson 1994), ethnography combined with survey techniques, longitudinal research, and the collection of records through archives or
government reports. This kind of research often takes time and a team
approach, including experts from the country being studied.

Scholars writing about a multi-sited approach underscore the
need for multiple methods and extensive knowledge of the phenomena of interest. A thread that runs through all is the need for a flexible
research strategy that is ultimately based in sensitivity to discovering
processes and connections.

Marcus and others point out some of the challenges of multi-sited
fieldwork. For one, because of the fluidity and complexity inherent
in these relationships, the object of study is never entirely knowable
ahead of time (Marcus 1995: 102). Susan Friedberg (2001), who studied green bean commodity chains between Africa and Europe, noted
several additional constraints including the inability to speak multiple languages fluently and time constraints that make it hard to do

in-depth ethnographic work in every relevant locale. She also noted the difficulty of gaining access to privileged spaces (such as corporate boardrooms), people, and information, since "studying up" (referring to Laura Nader's [1972] call to study those at all levels of power hierarchies) is critical when trying to understand high-level decision-making processes. Karen Hansen identifies a similar difficulty in her study of secondhand clothing in Zambia (2000: 18). Marcus notes that "multi-sited ethnographies inevitably are the product of knowledge bases of varying intensities and qualities" 1995: 100). A single ethnographer cannot hope to have equal knowledge at all points in a multi-sited research project, because of both time constraints and the exclusivity of political and economic information.

A further challenge is presented when the "field" does not emerge as a specific location in the Malinowskian tradition of a homogeneous village community – the traditional standard-bearer of ethnographic fieldwork. Passaro (1997), for example, a contributor to Gupta and Ferguson's (1997) volume on fieldwork, found this as she designed and carried out her research on homelessness in Manhattan. She resisted suggestions that she narrow her study to an ethnography of a homeless shelter, recognizing that this would be inadequate for understanding the wide range of places that homeless people occupy. Studies that involve transient or dispersed populations require flexible strategies of investigation into multiple levels of knowledge and experience.

The case study below presents a unique situation, where the principle multiple sites are primarily in the same region of the same country. The majority of the nation's khat is produced within 50 miles of the northern city of Diego Suarez, and the main consuming population is within that city. Khat is not exported outside of Madagascar on a large scale, but urban populations in other parts of the country increasingly consume it.

STUDY SITE

Background on Madagascar

Madagascar has been a hotspot in global conservation since the 1980s. Natural and social scientists have flocked to this island nation, drawn by the uniqueness of its flora and fauna – 85 percent of which is endemic to the island (Goodman and Benstead 2005). Concurrent with the biodiversity are threats to it from human activities, which have often been unfortunately blamed almost exclusively on local people's subsistence practices. International donor institutions such as the World Bank and USAID also took an interest in funding conservation and development activities, especially after receiving strong criticism for sponsoring environmentally insensitive projects elsewhere in the world. USAID opened its Madagascar office in 1983 and had a strong environmental program. By the late 1980s, the World Bank became the leading donor institution and coordinated the activities and policies of an association of donors (Gezon 1999; Kull 1996; Marcus and Kull 1999).

In 1984, the Malagasy government drafted the National Strategy for Conservation and Development, which is recognized as being one of the first national environmental plans established in Africa. The Government of Madagascar organized the International Conference of Conservation for Sustainable Development in 1985. In 1987–88, the government, in collaboration with donor institutions, developed the National Environmental Action Plan (NEAP), to be executed in three 5-year phases, beginning in 1991 (Gezon 1999). During that time, the national park service (ANGAP) was established to manage and eventually fund basic conservation efforts.

My research in Madagascar began in 1989. My first project focused on the politics of managing what was then the Ankarana Special Reserve protected area (it has since been reclassified as a National Park), which lies just south of the Mt. d'Ambre. That study revealed that local political processes intersect with regional ethnic, state, and NGO politics in the context of claims to the legally protected forest (Gezon, 1997, 1999, 2000, 2006). It was focused primarily on sites on the western side of the reserve.

In a more recent study, I sought to move away from an approach common in conservation studies that is grounded in the activities immediately surrounding a protected area. I took the actual ecological pressures on forests as my point of departure, recognizing that this would lead me to explore commodity chains and require a multi-sited research design. I focused on a different protected area – Mt. d'Ambre in northern Madagascar, which is located about 30 km from the regional capital city of Diego Suarez, and where non-staple food and cash-crops predominate. Mt. d'Ambre has been a protected area since the colonial era, and the majority of it is currently managed as a National Park (Gezon 1997, 2000, 2003; Gezon and Freed 1999). Cash cropping of fruit and vegetables to serve the French population of the city dates to the early colonial era in the early twentieth century.

Because of the relationship between production and external markets, it became apparent that studying production alone would not reveal the complexities of contemporary forest degradation, local livelihoods, or conservation efforts. I thus developed a research design based on an interdisciplinary commodity chain approach.

After doing preliminary research in the early 2000s, it became apparent that the most significant dynamic was the expansion of khat production in the vicinity and on the edges of the Mt. d'Ambre National Park. I nevertheless continued to inquire into the significance of vegetable production. As the case study will reveal, the khat and vegetable commodity chains became interlinked in ways I could not have anticipated.

Background on khat

Khat is an internationally controlled substance that is illegal throughout most of Europe and in the United States and Canada, but it is legal in Madagascar and many other Indian Ocean countries where it has traditionally been grown and consumed (Carrier and Gezon 2009). The World Health Organization has placed khat into two different categories, or Schedules. When it is fresh, it contains cathinone, which is in the category of substances that are the most highly potent and subject to abuse (Schedule I also includes narcotics, cocaine, and methamphetamine). After 24 to 48 hours, cathinone breaks down into cathine, which is a Schedule IV drug, defined as having low abuse potential, currently accepted medical use, with some risk of low-level dependence.

Wherever khat is grown throughout the world (mainly Yemen, Ethiopia, and Kenya), it tends to be cultivated by small holders (with most farming under 2 ha) and distributed through small-scale traders (Carrier 2005; Gebissa 2004; Kennedy 1987). This is also the case in Madagascar. A well-maintained khat field must be weeded about once a year, but other than that the labor input is minimal (it is somewhat higher for those farmers who irrigate), and so it is a good investment for just about any household that has available land.

Consumers of khat in Madagascar were traditionally those of Yemeni descent, known locally as "Arabou." During the French colonial era, Yemeni dock workers brought khat with them to the city of Diego Suarez, or Antsiranana, in the far north of Madagascar and planted it on a small scale in kitchen gardens. The first to grow it commercially, according to interviews, were the Creoles – white farmers of French descent who came over from Ile de la Reunion around the turn of the century – who established small plantations on Mt. d'Ambre, about 20 miles inland. When the French were forced to leave the country in the mid 1970s amidst a socialist revolution, they either sold or abandoned the khat farms. One of the oldest and most productive establishments on Mt. d'Ambre today is owned by a family that bought their land from a Creole family and who identify as a mix of Yemeni, Malagasy, and Creole descent.

Since the 1980s, more and more Malagasy of non-Yemeni descent have begun chewing it. Many concur that taxi drivers were among the first to chew it, in order to stay awake while they worked at night. Khat has also become popular as a recreational drug, most visibly among urban youth and men. The pulse of the street economy of the northern city of Diego Suarez is fueled by khat, with sellers and chewers, and people stopping to shop and chat along well-traveled streets. When trucks with khat arrive, people flock around the most popular street merchants to buy their share. Khat has become the lifeblood of the informal economy of the north, providing significant income to small-scale farmers and producers.

Methods[2]

In designing this study, many of the challenges of multi-sited research noted above presented themselves: namely that while my research question into commodity chains was clear, I did not know exactly where my leads would take me. My subjects were also dispersed over the landscape and not assembled into one neat community, as in Passaro's (1997) study of homelessness. I would not be able to have an in-depth experience at every point of interest, as I could have while conducting dissertation research, living primarily in a single village site for 16 months. In attempting to place khat within the context of legality and regulation, I also realized the strong possibility of encountering silence and gaps in trying to reach policy-makers and community leaders. Finally, I faced the challenge of identifying political, economic, and cultural processes that connect and mutually define the various locales.

The three processes in the commodity chain each led me to a different set of methods and locations. The overall method was a

[2] This research was supported by funding from the US Department of Education (Fulbright-Hays Faculty Research Abroad Fellowship), the National Science Foundation (Award Number BCS-0318640), and the National Geographic Society (Grant Number 7413.03).

purposive, or judgment, sampling, which, according to Bernard (2000) is when "you decide the purpose you want informants (or communities) to serve, and you go out to find some" (Bernard 2000: 176). More specifically, for each part of the study of human dynamics, I adopted a network sampling, or a chain referral approach. This is commonly used for populations that are hard to find (Bernard 2005). Snowball sampling, a particular kind of chain referral, involves beginning with one or two primary informants who then share the names of others who also share characteristics desired by the researcher. Each person interviewed, then, is asked to share other names. Note that this method differs from random, or probability, sampling, where each member of the target population would have an equal chance of being selected. Random sampling was not possible at any point along the chain, either because of the nature of the question, which explicitly involved tracing leads, because of the goal of gathering data about cultural systems and not generalizing individual experience, or because of logistical constraints in gaining access to people (Bernard 2000: 175).

Studying production and its effects on forest cover required a multidisciplinary study of land cover change. For this, I assembled a team of researchers in 2004 to examine these dynamics through satellite images and ground-truthing. The goal of that segment of research was to investigate the original hypothesis that people are cutting down forests in order to grow khat. The study of production on the ground around the Mt. d'Ambre has so far lasted from 2003 to 2007 and will surely continue over time. It has involved participant observation, open-ended interviews, and a structured interview schedule.

Studying distribution was less clearly definable as I set up my research design, since I knew very little about it. I proposed to trace out distribution networks with both farmers and retail sellers in the city as points of departure. Studying consumption involved two main methods: one involving network sampling, where chewers were identified and their milieu studied. The second was a structured interview schedule administered at the end of the study, in 2007, in an attempt to collect broader and more generalizable data about khat chewing in the general population of Diego Suarez.

The links along the commodity chain flow easily from one to the other, with overlaps, as with fibers in a rope. The variable of khat takes on different forms, or values, along the chain, as it goes from being a cash crop for farmers, a tradable commodity for distributors, and a recreational stimulant for consumers. Rural and urban areas link through the intermediary of distributors, who, as research revealed, are sometimes also producers. In the khat commodity chain, the various geographic nodes mutually define each other's conditions. The thread of supply from producers affects the type and amount of work available for distributors and the amount and quality of product for consumers. Consumer demand, in turn, lays the framework for producer decisions and opens or closes opportunities for distributors. Government policy affects each of the three areas, through practices of agricultural extension and conservation; regulation and taxation of commodity trade; and legality and public health concerns with khat as a drug.

Taken together, these processes make up what can be referred to as the khat commodity chain, a general set of processes where supply and demand come together to set price, but where the unique practices and unexpected additional variables at each of the nodes define the conditions to which all others must respond. Tracing those unique practices and local contingencies is the task of a multi-sited ethnography that, as Marcus (1995) and other advise, flexibly follows the connections – anticipated or not – that arise in the course of study. The dynamics of khat will be presented in the case below in a focus on issues raised in the study of production, considering studies of remote sensing and the effects of khat production on vegetable production.

EXTENT AND HISTORY OF PRODUCTION: VIEWS FROM SPACE

Methods

Answering questions about khat's effects on forests is a first step in understanding the overall environmental and food system sustainability of khat production. A systematic inquiry into regional land cover change required an interdisciplinary team. For this, I collaborated with Glen Green and Sean Sweeney, remote sensing scientists from the Center for the Study of Institutions, Population, and Environmental Change (CIPEC), Bloomington, Indiana. In this, the earliest phase of the study, we acquired and analyzed satellite images in a university computer laboratory. With funding from the National Geographic Society, we acquired nine Landsat images from between 1972 and 2000. Sweeney and Green digitally processed the images at CIPEC (Gezon et al. 2005) and generated two-date multi-temporal composites.

The three investigators (Gezon, Green, and Sweeney) then met in May 2004 in Bloomington to study the images and identify locations that had either undergone significant change or that remained basically the same throughout the north of Madagascar. We located 27 sites for further investigation on the ground, including two in the heaviest khat-growing areas of Madagascar – one in vicinity of Joffreville on the northeast side of the Mt. d'Ambre protected area, and one in the vicinity of Antsalaka on the eastern side. We briefly described these based on what we expected to find, drawing on evidence of change in the digital information and our familiarity with the environment based on previous research in Madagascar (Kottak and Colson 1994). For the khat growing area from the northeast to the southeast of Mt. d'Ambre, we noted that there was little change digitally evident between 1972 and 2000. The most dramatic change occurred in one area close to the protected area to the south of Antsalaka on the east side.

During June–August, 2004, we visited each of the sites directly relevant to khat production with the intention of ground-truthing what we observed in the satellite data. To learn about the social context of environmental change or stability, I gathered socioeconomic and ethnographic data by interviewing people using purposive sampling as we walked along the road, and in more structured, often recorded, interviews in villages at the investigation sites, often with community leaders. These interviews focused on questions of migrations and residential patterns, social differentiation, infrastructure access, political and social organization, production and distribution, and histories of resource use. I supplemented this fieldwork with both interviews of professionals in Diego Suarez and studies of grey literature reports, especially the Plans Communals de Developpement (PCD) – community development plans mandated by the donor community, which provided a socioeconomic overview of the areas they cover (for the full report, see Gezon *et al.* 2005).

Results

The results suggested that in the Joffreville site there had been some forest degradation due to underplanting and clearing for bananas, but little to no damage due to the expansion of other crops. Cultivation of most other commodities occurs on permanent fields, most of which are irrigated, thus reducing the need to expand production through swidden. We learned that in the greater Joffreville area, while there is some primary forest clearing for khat production, it is not the most important means of expanding production. Much khat is irrigated, growing on former rice fields. Most other fields are rain-fed, planted on grassy hillsides. In Antsalaka (to the southeast), we gathered that cyclone damage accounted for the change we had seen, and that people had indeed gone in and planted khat in the aftermath. There was some, though minimal, evidence of people cutting down forests in or near the protected area to grow khat. Although the images revealed little change through 2000, we surmised from observation that there had been more forest removal for khat in more recent times. During his research in 2009, primatologist Ben Freed reported that he found some evidence of khat cultivation having spread to the northwestern side of Mt. d'Ambre. There, a well-established farmer planted fields that butted up to the protected area. Freed felt, however, that this did not pose a threat to the forest, but rather a physical and economic buffer against encroachment (Ben Freed, personal communication, September 2009).

Significance: khat production and environmental change

These findings provide an historical and a regional perspective on the effects of khat production on land cover change, based on empirical observation from above, using satellite images, and on the ground. This knowledge is critical when questioning the overall sustainability of khat production in this region. The relationship of khat production to forest and species integrity has political, economic, and ecological consequences. In terms of the larger question of food security to be explored below, knowing khat's effect on forests is critical for evaluating whether it is even a sound possibility for regional livelihood sustainability, given parallel concerns for forest conservation.

KHAT AND VEGETABLES: METHODS FOR LINKING
BETWEEN PROCESSES

That some khat production does threaten forests suggests that formal attention be paid to this phenomenon by agronomists and conservation personnel. That most production does not threaten forests opens it up for further consideration as a possible source of sustainable livelihood for the north. The question of food security still remains. If khat provides cash to producers and traders but undermines regional food security, its production is not sustainable in a larger sense. Understanding this requires a multi-sited examination of the production, distribution and consumption of khat and food crops in order to understand opportunities and constraints in each domain.

In terms of methods, the challenge was in studying processes – of following khat and vegetable crops from production, through distribution, to consumption in order to understand the extent to which khat production was displacing food production. Focusing on the movement of material items required methodological and geographic flexibility. In this case, the sites were relatively localized, with the core area spanning the city of Diego Suarez and agricultural areas within 100 km of it.

In collecting data on each of the processes studied, basic methods of traditional ethnography were used, including participant observation, open-ended ethnographic interviewing, elicited reporting to a structured set of questions, interviews with officials, and consultation of written reports – contemporary and archival. For six months in 2004, extensive ethnographic research involved general ethnographic observation and interviews, including systematic inquiry into urban consumption of vegetables through targeted interviews and food diaries. In 2005, a one-month trip to Madagascar allowed a follow-up on the study of urban vegetable and khat consumption, and a one-month stay in France yielded research into archival documents in Paris and the colonial archives in Aix-en-Provence. In 2007, a team that included Malagasy university students administered a set of structured interview schedules on production, distribution, and consumption of khat (Gezon and Totomarovario 2008).

Participant observation and the identification of study sites

Study of production took place primarily in the khat-producing regions of the Mt. d'Ambre. Study of consumption took place at all points, since even producers consume khat. Distribution took place in the zones of production as well as in the cities of Diego Suarez and Ambilobe to the south. The airport south of Diego Suarez was an additional point of distribution, as people sent khat to contacts in cities throughout Madagascar (but not abroad). Important in early observations, in order to learn about the basic paths of the commodity chain, were daily informal connections with anyone who knew about khat. For my research, several key informants lived in the city of Diego Suarez and had family in the rainforest edge town of Joffreville, where we would occasionally visit together. They revealed where consumers and sellers could be found in town, where traders go to sell or transport their khat from villages of production to the city, and how best to contact producers. Emic models for conceptualizing the role of khat in society also began to emerge.

Interviews with leaders

Consultation with local leaders took place throughout the entire period of observation. Among those interviewed were a judge, bureaucrats with the tax service, economists at the chamber of commerce, medical doctors, the mayors of the cities Diego Suarez, Joffreville, and Antsalaka, the regional governor, political leaders at the village level, local conservation NGOs, the National Park Service (ANGAP), Malagasy university professors, and religious leaders. Each of them provided valuable analyses of khat at different points along the commodity chain. Interviewing them not only provided critical information for understanding commodity chains, but it also helped make the study relevant to their own concerns. The research project evolved in an iterative process, as their insights and questions refocused the study somewhat. The question about food security, for example, emerged from interviews with high-level politicians who were genuinely concerned about what to do about khat.

Food diaries

The study of vegetables as well as khat formed an initial focus of research, since both are crops grown around the Mt. d'Ambre. Even though khat is a more important economic force, the study of the vegetable commodity chain remained important because of the tight relationship between vegetable and khat production. For the vegetable consumption survey, 14 people were identified in the city of Diego Suarez through a network sample and asked to keep a log of what they ate each day. In choosing participants, I used a purposive sampling technique. The individuals were selected in consultation with my primary research assistant, who had extensive ties to the population in which khat consumption was increasing rapidly – the *quartiers populaires* of the city or in recently colonized edges of the city. Notebooks were distributed to people in charge of meal preparation (mostly women), and we interviewed them once before they filled out the notebooks and again afterward. The first interviews inquired about general socioeconomic information, such as household composition and sources of income. To gain an understanding of gendered social networks, these interviews also inquired into conjugal or other important relationships that contribute to livelihood sustainability. In the post-notebook interviews, they were asked about their own generalizations about what they eat and their perceptions of various kinds of foods. This questionnaire was significant in helping understand the kind of market there is for vegetables among the common people in the city. Knowing the dietary basis of people in the city was critical for evaluating the role of khat production in displacing vegetables and the impact of lowered vegetable production on local food security.

Structured interview schedules: khat

In 2007, three separate structured interview schedules were developed with the help of Malagasy associates on the production, distribution, and consumption of khat. The goal of this set of structured interviews was twofold: first, they helped gauge the generalizability of the information received ethnographically from primary informants. Second, open-ended segments revealed new dynamics that had not yet been considered.

For each of the structured interviews, we asked for basic demographic information and general opinions about khat. We administered the structured production interviews in the two major production areas of khat. We took popular beliefs about the implications of khat production as hypotheses, namely: (1) People are abandoning the cultivation of vegetables as a cash crop (introduced in the colonial era) in favor of khat as a cash crop. People fear this because it means a decline in the availability of local vegetables for the regional market and a decline in local nutrition. (2) People are planting khat on former rice fields, thereby substituting this tree crop and cash crop for a subsistence-oriented food crop. According to these hypotheses, people are thereby farming less rice. In both of these cases, people suspect that the high price of khat, combined with lesser labor requirements, leads to the abandonment of other forms of cultivation.

More specifically, we asked general questions about agricultural production, without privileging questions about khat, per se. We asked what people grow, how long they had been growing it, how they acquired the land for it, their labor arrangements, whether or not they chew khat (making a connection to the study of consumption), and where and how they sell their crop (making a connection to the study of distribution). We also asked about the value of growing khat compared with other crops and about any opportunities and constraints they face.

In the questionnaire for distributors and traders, we asked about their history of selling khat, to whom they sell, the economic return, any other sources of income, economic partnerships they have with spouses, family in rural areas, or others; and general open-ended questions about the state of the khat market. This questionnaire explored whether and how khat traders felt effects from the increase in khat production and consumption. It gave a sense of the socioeconomic position of traders and the extent of stratification among them.

In the consumption questionnaire, we asked about personal habits of consumption as well as about common stereotypes that khat makes people lazy, inhibits economic growth, and leads to tension within households over how money is spent. General observation and ethnographic interviews had revealed that many educated people, who do not chew khat and do not sympathize with it, believe that khat is detrimental to individuals and society for these reasons. The questionnaire was designed to see how pervasive these beliefs are within the khat-chewing community.

Together, the questionnaires were meant to investigate the workings of each process of the commodity chain and the connections between them: how demand in cities affects incentives to produce and the livelihoods of traders; how growing conditions affect the type and quantity of khat available; how public opinion about khat consumption provides constraints or opportunities for producers and traders.

Thirteen students from the Université d'Antsiranana in Diego Suarez provided most the labor of actually administering the interview schedule face to face (Gezon and Totomarovario 2008). The questions were designed to elicit structured but open-ended answers that could later be coded for statistical analysis. There were 154 respondents to the consumer questionnaire; 83 to the producer questionnaire (for which we traveled to Joffreville and Antsalaka, the major zones of production); and 45 to the trader/merchant questionnaire (found in the centers of production, in Diego Suarez, and at the airport). The respondents were selected again through a snowball, or network, sample based on the contacts of the person doing the interview. Since students were from various parts of the city and had varying socioeconomic backgrounds, the sample covers a fairly broad range of people.

This collection of methods suggests how khat connects the various locations. Time spent among farmers yielded access to distributors, and time among distributers provided one means for accessing consuming populations. Time among consumers helped understand the nature of demand for khat. The information in each of these locals revealed connections among them and the ways that supply or demand, for example, in one locale affects opportunities and constraints in another. The food diaries provided critical data for assessing the market demand for vegetables by local urban people, which suggested the larger context within which farmers are making production decisions. Interviews with experts provided a broader political, economic, and cultural context for interpreting activities as observed in practice.

RESULTS

Issues of consumption: khat

General ethnographic research revealed that khat chewing has gradually caught on among Malagasy people who identify themselves as people from coastal Madagascar (les côtiers). Many also chew by themselves and not in a social group, contrary to khat chewing practices in other parts of the world, like Yemen and Somalia. People report little to no direct social pressure to chew, although many cited the reason they began chewing was because they wanted to join friends who chewed. The main categories of chewers are men with stable incomes and barbo, or shiftless youth in search of distraction. When permitted, many formal sector laborers chew during work hours. Even though most work places no longer allow chewing, that is where many men became attached to chewing khat and now only do so on the weekend.

The barbo are often involved in the informal economy in one way or another, often with the stated goal of making enough money to purchase more khat. Some are students and few have stable employment. Most are not practicing Muslims and drink beer after spitting out their wad of khat in order to "kill the effect" (mamono ny dosy) of the stimulant. This contrasts with the Yemeni chewers, who are generally practicing Muslims and drink cold water or milk while chewing. The barbo often chew khat in groups on the street – playing cards, sitting quietly, or conversing. Khat is indeed becoming a source of youth identity for the barbo, much as it is in Kenya (Carrier 2005).

We analyzed the portion of the questionnaire that investigates perceptions of khat. The results are as follows (see Table 11.1). For

Table 11.1 *Perceptions of khat.*

Perceptions of Khat	Yes	No	Depends	Don't Know
Does khat pose any problems with regards to money?	41%	52%	7%	–
Does khat lead to social problems, such as domestic tension or illegal behavior?	10%	85%	–	–
Does khat make people lazy?	7%	77%	8%	3%
Should khat be made illegal?	3%	73%	3%	5%

the question, "Does khat pose any problems with regards to money?", 52 percent ($N = 154$) responded in the negative, 41 percent in the affirmative, and 7 percent said that "it depends." The open-ended part of the question invited people to cite reasons why it is or is not a problem. One common stereotype is that people buy khat instead of food. Some cited this as a problem, but not as many as would be predicted by how often this is mentioned as a concern. Those who thought it does not pose a financial problem noted, for example, that others buy it for them, or that they earn enough money so that they don't have to worry about the cost, or that they do not buy it in the dry season when it is expensive.

Another question asked whether khat leads to social problems, such as domestic tension or illegal behavior. To this, 85 percent responded in the negative and 10 percent in the affirmative. Many of the 10 percent cited that the social problem was that many people do not accept khat chewing as legitimate. A minority cited that it led to domestic disputes. For the question, "Does khat make people lazy?", 77 percent responded in the negative, 7 percent responded in the affirmative, 8 percent said that "it depends," 3 respondents said that they "didn't know," and 7 did not answer.

Finally, for the question, "Should khat be made illegal?", 73 percent responded in the negative, 12 percent in the positive, 3 percent could see both sides of the issue, and 5 percent "didn't know." When asked for any additional open-ended comments, many strengthened their statement that khat should not be made illegal. Several reasons cited are that it is an important source of income locally, it is pleasurable, and people would have a hard time stopping because they have the habit of taking it.

Consumption is the end point of the commodity chain. Increasing consumption of khat provides a context for understanding the growth in production. Because of its illegality and stereotype as an obstruction to economic development, this consumer trend has stirred up some social anxiety, especially among the elite and professional classes. Its distribution practices (sold informally on the street, outside of the open-air market place) and its most visible consumption practices (by young men without formal sector jobs) contribute to this concern over the good of khat for the population. Perceptions of khat by consumers and others in the *quartiers populaires* suggest that fears about khat do not tend to be shared widely. This anxiety is critical, nevertheless, for understanding the political climate of legalization, and for putting practices of production, distribution, and consumption into a broader perspective.

What this implies for the general research question is that khat has become embedded within the urban cultural milieu, particularly among the working poor. Most people felt very strongly that khat should not be made illegal and conveyed the sense that they would contest any attempts at making it illegal. What this means for producers is that the local market for khat is not going away. While increased consumption confirms simple economic models that link growing production to increased demand, ethnographic research reveals dynamics that might or do affect production, such as the popularity of khat as fashionable among youth (see also Carrier 2005) and the social anxiety over whether it should be legal or not. These dynamics also affect distribution practices, whereby distribution outside of the region is increasing within Madagascar through the medium of air transport, and is minimal outside the country because of its status as illegal in many nearby locales (Reunion Island, in particular). The commodity chain comes to life as a process localized at multiple points through this analysis.

Khat and food security

The question of vegetable production became relevant to the study of khat because of the misunderstood relationship between the two. Multi-sited analysis focusing on the processes of globalization has a wide lens, being attuned to unexpected contingent variables that significantly inform core research questions. The study of vegetables began because they have been an important cash crop grown around the protected area. Their study may have become subordinated entirely to the study of khat if it were not for the suspicion that khat was responsible for their decline.

With regards to the decline in vegetable production, we determined that the reasons are complex and only minimally connected to the growing popularity of khat. Interviews with over 80 farmers on the east side of Mt. d'Ambre provided the data on which this assessment has been made. Many farmers expressed constraints regarding the marketing of vegetables. For one, the condition of the roads is so poor that in some areas, people find it difficult to get their vegetable crops out. Either the roads are not easily passable even by ox-drawn cart or they are so bumpy that the crop would be ruined. During the colonial era, when vegetable crops were introduced, the roads were sufficient to get crops out to the main road. Khat is by far the easiest to transport, leaving them little choice in what to produce. Relatedly, transportation from the field to the main road is too expensive for many who do not own their own ox-drawn cart. Seeds for vegetable crops are very expensive, and often not of good quality. In addition, the price of vegetables is low, and sometimes farmers claim that they actually farm at a loss with vegetables. Finally, there is not a large local market for many of the vegetables that farmers traditionally cultivated since their introduction in the colonial era (confirmed by the urban vegetable consumption logs I collected), and they have difficulty finding buyers for their produce. Other markets for vegetables, to supply ships and restaurants, for example, are cornered by large-scale operations out of the central highlands in the region of the nation's capital, Antananarivo.

With regards to the suspicion that farmers are converting rice fields into khat fields, we learned that while many did make this transformation, as most new khat fields were a result of expansion into formerly unfarmed areas – most often non-irrigated grassy fields or hillsides, where it would be difficult to grow rice. Those who did transform rice fields retained some fields for rice and other crops. Surprisingly, we learned that some people are increasing rice farming and even converting khat fields back into rice fields because of the high prices of rice in the last few years. Despite the profitability associated with khat, people highly value food crops in general.

One deterrent to khat production regards labor. Despite the stereotype that farmers prefer to grow khat because it takes less work to cultivate, many farmers pointed out that they did not find this to be the case. Khat needs weeding, water management (for the irrigated fields), surveillance, and harvesting, for example. While wealthier farmers could afford to hire help with weeding and picking, the poorer ones could not. In addition to farming-related tasks, theft is becoming an increasing risk and requires nearly constant surveillance. Especially for poorer farmers, khat did not provide a great relief from labor.

A multi-sited research strategy revealed the constraints on vegetable farming. Without the study of urban vegetable consumption through food diaries, for example, and interviews with vegetable market sellers, confirmation of the diminishing local market for vegetables would be merely anecdotal. Interviews in the offices of urban business and political leaders also provided insight into larger scale vegetable markets that local producers knew very little to nothing about.

DISCUSSION

This research revealed significant issues regarding the production of cash crops around the Mt. d'Ambre and their implications for conservation and food security. These results would not have been possible without a flexible multi-sited ethnographic approach that revealed far-flung relationships between people and commodities, tracing the flow of khat through multiple social and material contexts (see Table 11.2).

The 2004 study based on satellite image analysis suggested that most khat production does not pose a significant threat to forests. Furthermore, our findings only weakly supported the hypothesis that khat production is displacing food crops. The study suggests that the amount of rice that has been displaced is minimal and not a threat to food security. While khat displaced some rice production, farmers are also capable of responding to market demands for more rice when the prices for it increase. In terms of vegetable production, it appears that khat has not *caused* decrease in vegetable production, but rather has provided a security net for farmers who have no longer been able to grow vegetables successfully. This finding is corroborated by Minquoy, who wrote that while some farmers in the area once survived well growing vegetables, after the French departed, "ce marché s'écroule faute de clientele" (2006), many took to growing khat instead.

Multi-sited analysis of global processes is based on the premise that production, distribution, and consumption are interconnected, and that concern about issues of production – and, in this case,

Table 11.2 *Methods in time and space.*

	Scale	Time
Ethnographic interviewing	Local	Present
Open-ended interviews with local people	Regional	
Structured interviews/questionnaires	National	
Semi-structured interviews with local leaders	International	
Satellite image analysis		Past
Governmental reports (gray literature)		
Longitudinal research		
Archival research		

conservation – need take the entire market system into consideration. Pressures felt by farmers, and challenges felt by conservation
personnel, can only be understood in a context that includes urban
consumers and decision-makers. The market forces affecting khat in
Madagascar have to do with increasing consumer demand (as observed
in urban sites) and decreased demand for other crops, such as vegetables (as observed in discussions with farmers, in the homes of urban
consumers and in urban market places). These two variables will be
likely to shape khat in the future as demand for a variety of cash crops
fluctuates and as the climate for the consumption of khat evolves.
While this study focused on production-related dynamics of khat, it is
worth noting that this latter variable – the climate for consumption –
may become increasingly influenced by the global war on drugs and
on discourse condemning its consumption in powerful nations such
as the United States. The study of khat consumption must heed this
additional international site of research.

CONCLUSION

The limitations of this approach might also be its strength: it is not
really a tight method in and of itself, but rather requires the researcher
to carefully assemble methods that address specific questions. Because
of the holism and fluidity of this approach, it combines well with
many methods, such as with micro-level studies of cultural ecology
and economics (Chapter 5, for example), perception and narrative
analysis (Chapter 8), and statistical analysis. Staying on track with the
multi-sited approach involves developing a tight research question

and linking it with appropriate methods. It may not be possible to do in-depth research in each of the locales implicated in a research question. More important than the number of research sites, however, is attention paid to the connections between one locale and others and the ways that dynamics in one co-construct the others. Gaps in ethnographic focus can be informed by interviews and extant written sources, including popular media

Multi-sited research addresses critical questions of scale and the processes of globalization. It calls for a creative re-visiting of traditional ethnography, incorporating the strengths of this central anthropological method in new contexts. One of the most valuable tools of ethnography that has not been lost in multi-sited approaches is the openness to discovering new connections and challenging received understandings.

REFERENCES

Amin, S. 1977. *Unequal Development: An Essay on the Social Formations of Peripheral Capitalism*: Monthly Review Press.

Appadurai, A. 1986. *The Social Life of Things: Commodities in Cultural Perspective*. New York: Cambridge University Press.

Appadurai, A. 1996. *Modernity at Large: Cultural Dimensions of Globalization*. Minneapolis, MN: Univ. of Minnesota Press.

Bassett, T. J. 1988. The political ecology of peasant-herder conflicts in the Northern Ivory Coast. *Annals of the Association of American Geographers* **78**(3): 453–472.

Bermard, H. R. 2000. *Social Research Methods: Qualititative and Quantitative Methods*. Thousand Oaks, CA: Sage Publications, Inc.

Bernard, H. R. 2005. *Research Methods in Anthropology: Qualitative and Quantitative Methods*. Lanham, MD: AltaMira Press.

Bernstein, H. 1996. The political economy of the maize filiere. *Journal of Peasant Studies* **23**(2 and 3): 120–145.

Biersack, A. and J. B. Greenberg 2006. *Reimagining Political Ecology*. Durham, NC: Duke University Press.

Blaikie, P. and H. Brookfield 1987. Defining and debating the problem. In *Land Degradation and Society*. London: Methuen, pp. 1–7.

Burawoy, M., ed. 1991. The extended case method. In M. Burawoy, ed., *Ethnography Unbound: Power and Resistance in the Modern Metropolis*. Berkeley, CA: University of California Press, pp. 271–287.

Carrier, N. 2005. "Miraa is cool": the cultural importance of miraa (khat) for Tigania and Igembe youth in Kenya. *Journal of African Cultural Studies* **17**(2): 201–218.

Carrier, N. and L. Gezon 2009. Khat in the Western Indian Ocean: regional linkages and disjunctures. *Etudes Océan Indien* **42–43**: 271–297.

Castells, M. 1996. *The Rise of the Network Society, The Information Age: Economy, Society and Culture* Vol. 1. Cambridge, MA, and Oxford, UK: Blackwell.

Chalfin, B. 2004. *Shea Butter Republic: State Power, Global Markets, and the Making of an Indigenous Commodity*. New York: Routledge.

Epstein, A. L. 1979 (1967). The case study method in the field of law. In A. L. Epstein, ed., *The Craft of Social Anthropology*. Oxford, UK: Pergamon Press.

Escobar, A. 2008. *Territories of Difference: Place, Movements, Life, Redes*. Durham NC: Duke University Press

Frank, A. G. 1967. *Capitalism and Underdevelopment in Latin America*. New York: Monthly Review Press.

Freidberg, S. 2001. On the trail of the global green bean: methodological considerations in multi-site ethnography. *Global Networks* **1**(4): 353–368.

Friedman, J. 2000. Globalization, class and culture in global systems. *Journal of World-Systems Research* **6**(3): 636–656.

Friedman, T. L. 2000. *The Lexus and the Olive Tree: Understanding Globalization*. New York: Anchor.

Gebissa, E. 2004. *Leaf Of Allah: Khat and Agricultural Transformation* Athens, OH: Ohio University Press.

Gereffi, G. and M. Korzeniewicz 1994. *Commodity Chains and Global Capitalism*. Volume 149. Westport, CN: Greenwood Press.

Gezon, L. 1997. Institutional structure and the effectiveness of integrated conservation and development projects: case study from Madagascar. *Human Organization* **56**(4): 462–470.

Gezon, L. 1999. From adversary to son: political and ecological process in Northern Madagascar. *Journal of Anthropological Research* **55**: 71–97.

Gezon, L. 2000. The changing face of NGOs: structure and communitas in conservation and development in Madagascar. *Urban Anthropology and Studies of Cultural Systems and World Economic Development* **29**(2): 181–215.

Gezon, L. 2003. The regional approach in northern Madagascar: conservation after the integrated conservation and development project. In S. R. Brechin, P. R. Wilshusen, C. Fortwangler, and P. C. West, eds., *Contested Nature: Power, Protected Areas and the Dispossessed – Promoting International Conservation with Justice in the 21st Century*. Albany, NY: SUNY Press, pp. 183–194.

Gezon, L. and B. Z. Freed 1999. Agroforestry and conservation in Northern Madagascar: hopes and hinderances. *African Studies Quarterly* **3**(2).

Gezon, L. L. 2006. *Global Visions, Local Landscapes: A Political Ecology of Conservation, Conflict, and Control in Northern Madagascar*. Lanham, MD: AltaMira Press.

Gezon, L. L., S. Sweeny, G. Green, and B. Z. Freed 2005. Forest loss and commodity chains in Northern Madagascar. National Geographic Society.

Gezon, L. L., and A. Totomarovario 2008. Encountering the Unexpected: Appropriating the Roles of Researcher, Teacher, and Advocate in a Drug Study in Madagascar. *Practicing Anthropology* **30**(3): 42–45.

Gluckman, M. 1958. *Analysis of a Social Situation in Modern Zululand*. Manchester, UK: Manchester University Press.

Goodman, S. M., and J. P. Benstead 2005. Updated estimates of biotic diversity and endemism for Madagascar. *Oryx* **39**(1): 73–77.

Gupta, A. and J. Ferguson 1997. Chapter 1: culture, power, place: ethnography at the end of an era. In *Culture, Power, Place: Explorations in Critical Anthropology*. Durham, NC: Duke University Press, pp. 1–29.

Hannerz, U. 1996. *Transnational Connections: Culture, People, Places*. London: Routledge.

Hansen, K. T. 2000. *Salaula: The World of Secondhand Clothing and Zambia*. Chicago, IL: University of Chicago Press.

Harvey, D. 1989. *The Condition of Postmodernity: An Enquiry into the Origins of Cultural Change*. Malden, MA: Blackwell.

Hecht, S. and A. Cockburn 1990. *The Fate of the Forest: Developers, Destroyers and Defenders of the Amazon*. New York: HarperCollins Publishers.

Hopkins, T. K. and I. Wallerstein 1986. Commodity chains: construct and research. In G. Gereffi and M. Korzeniewicz, eds. *Commodity Chains and Global Capitalism.* Westport, CT: Greenwood Press, pp. 17–20.

Kennedy, J. G. 1987. *The Flower of Paradise: The Institutionalized Use of the Drug Qat in North Yemen* Norwell, MA: Kluwer Academic Publishers.

Kenney, M. and R. Florida 1994. Japanese maquiladoras: production organization and global commodity chains. *World Development* **22**(1): 27–44.

Kottak, C. and E. Colson 1994. Multilevel linkages: longitudinal and comparative studies. In R. Borofsky, ed., *Assessing Cultural Anthropology.* New York: McGraw-Hill, Inc., pp. 396–412.

Kull, C. A. 1996. The evolution of conservation efforts in Madagascar. *International Environmental Affairs* **8**(1): 50–86.

Lappe, F. M. and J. Collins 1979. *Food First: Beyond the Myth of Scarcity.* New York: Ballantine Books.

Marcus, G. 1995. Ethnography in/of the world system: the emergence of multi-sited ethnography. *Annual Review of Anthropology* **24**: 95–117.

Marcus, R. R. and C. Kull 1999. Setting the stage: the politics of Madagascar's environment efforts. *African Studies Quarterly* **3**(2): 1–7.

Martinez-Alier, J. 2002. *The Environmentalism of the Poor: A Study of Ecological Conflicts and Valuation.* Cheltenham, UK: Edward Elgar.

Massey, D. 1994. *Space, Place, and Gender.* Minneapolis, MN: University of Minnesota Press.

Minquoy, V. 2006. Quand la logique dépasse l'éthique : le khat à Madagascar. *Les Cahiers d'Outre-Mer* **233**: 133.

Mintz, S. 1985. *Sweetness and Power: The Place of Sugar in Modern History.* New York: Viking.

Moore, D. S. 2005. *Searching for Territory: Race, Place, and Power in Zimbabwe.* Durham, NC: Duke University Press.

Nader, L. 1972. Up the anthropologist: perspectives gained from studying up. In D. Hymes, ed., *Reinventing Anthropology.* New York: Random House.

Passaro, J. 1997. "You can't take the subway to the field!": "Village" epistemologies in the global village. In *Culture, Power, Place: Explorations in Critical Anthropology.* Durham, NC: Duke University Press, pp. 147–162.

Paulson, S. and L. L. Gezon, eds. 2006. *Political Ecology, Across Spaces, Scales and Social Groups.* New Jersey: Rutgers University Press.

Peet, R. and M. Watts 1993. Introduction: development theory and environment in an age of market triumphalism. *Economic Geography* **69**(3): 227–248.

Peet, R. and M. Watts 2004. *Liberation Ecologies: Environment, Development, Social Movements.* New York: Routledge.

Ribot, J. C. 1998. Theorizing access: forest profits along Senegal's charcoal commodity chain. *Development and Change* **29**: 307–341.

Robbins, P. 2004. *Political Ecology: Critical Introductions to Geography.* Oxford, UK: Blackwell Publishing.

Schmink, M. and C. H. Wood 1987. The political ecology of Amazonia. In P. D. Little, M. M. Horowitz, and E. A. Nyerges, eds. *Lands at Risk in the Third World: Local-Level Perspectives.* Boulder, CO: Westview Press, pp. 38–57.

Smith, N. 1984. *Uneven Development: Nature, Capital and the Production of Space.* Oxford, UK: Blackwell.

Steward, J. H. 1955. *Theory of Culture Change: The Methodology of Multilinear Evolution.* Urbana, IL: University of Illinois Press.

Tsing, A. L. 1993. *In the Realm of the Diamond Queen.* Princeton, NJ: Princeton University Press.

Tsing, A. 2000. Inside the economy of appearances. *Public Culture* **12**(1): 115–144.

Tsing, A. L. 2005. *Friction: An Ethnography of Global Connection*. Princeton, NJ: Princeton University Press.

Van Velsen, J. 1979. The extended-case method and situational analysis. In A. L. Epstein, ed., *In The Craft of Social Anthropology*. London: Pergamon Press, pp. 129–149.

Wallerstein, I. 1974. *The Modern World Systems*. New York: Academic Press.

Wolf, E. 1982. *Europe and the People Without History*. Berkeley, CA: University of California Press.

Zimmerer, K. S. and T. J. Bassett 2003. Future directions in political ecology: nature–society fusions and fusions of interaction In K. S. Zimmerer and T. J. Bassett, eds., *Political Ecology: An Integrative Approach to Geography and Environment-Development Studies. Political Ecology*. New York: The Guilford Press, pp. 274–296.

12

Spatiotemporal methodologies in environmental anthropology: geographic information systems, remote sensing, landscape changes, and local knowledge

EDUARDO S. BRONDÍZIO AND RINKU ROY CHOWDHURY

INTRODUCTION

Spatial tools such as remote sensing (RS) and geographic information systems (GIS) are increasingly used in a variety of research and public applications. The popularization of geospatial data and tools in the media and society has significantly changed the way we perceive, understand and manage our landscapes. A variety of social actors have become familiar with these technologies, whether they be an extractivist cooperative disputing borders in the Brazilian Amazon, a US resident checking his property on a cadastral map, or a school teacher in India, using a satellite image to teach regional geography. Today, geospatial technologies are recognized as valuable assets of civil society and essential tools to address social and environmental problems (NAS 2002). The proliferation of satellite and public-domain spatial data, Global Positioning Systems (GPS), affordable computer hardware and software, and data processing and analytical techniques continue to expand the use of these technologies in anthropology generally, and environmental anthropology in particular. Such spatial information is frequently used in visualization (e.g., displays of aerial photography or satellite imagery for a study region) using Google Earth or

Environmental Social Sciences: Methods and Research Design, ed. I. Vaccaro, E. A. Smith and S. Aswani. Published by Cambridge University Press. © Cambridge University Press 2010.

other public domain software that allow quick online data access/display without requiring specialized training. More in-depth research and analyses entail the use of designated RS/GIS software programs (e.g., ERDAS Imagine, ArcGIS, Idrisi, Multispec, among many others), and the actual acquisition of the relevant GIS datasets (as opposed to merely accessing them for online displays and/or simple queries).

This chapter reviews uses and issues in the application of RS and GIS in anthropological research. We briefly present fundamental geospatial concepts and provide a concise history of RS and GIS applications in anthropology. Next, we review the range of geospatial concerns in anthropological research design, highlighting research questions, units of analysis, data search and temporal sampling, and assessments of data processing needs and analysis. In order to illustrate these geospatial concerns, we focus in particular on land use/cover change research, and provide guidelines for data planning and research design. Finally, we present critical ethical and pragmatic issues in the (re)presentation of spatiotemporal data and maps, reflecting on the positive potential as well as perils of using these tools in anthropological research.

FUNDAMENTALS OF REMOTE SENSING AND GIS

RS, GIS, and GPS are complementary suites of geospatial technologies and methods, collectively implicated in GIScience (Goodchild and Janelle 2004; Jensen 1996). RS involves the collection of surface reflectance data from a distance, such as in analog/digital aerial photography or satellite imagery recording information about the earth surface in gridded (raster) products. These data constitute the most significant sources of quantitative information about land cover and land use changes in the tropics and elsewhere (Sader *et al.* 1994). GIS, on the other hand, involve hardware, software, database systems and methods for the storage, representation, processing, integration, and analysis of diverse spatial data and their attributes. Both spatial and non-spatial information may be recorded in raster data or vector features such as points, lines, and polygons, referenced to a common cartographic system of spatial location. GIS enable the collation and processing of RS products for further representational or analytical tasks, such as modeling deforestation by linking data on forest (change) patterns with ancillary, spatially explicit socioeconomic variables. The following sections briefly review key elements of RS and GIS.

Remote sensing technologies enable the mapping of the earth's surface and subsurface features based on their differential reflectance of incident electromagnetic energy. A fundamental distinction among remote sensing technologies is based on the source of that energy: passive sensors record reflectance of incident solar radiation (i.e., the energy source is independent of the measurement device, exemplified by optical systems such as Landsat), while active sensors record the return of wavelengths generated by the sensor system (e.g., microwave RADAR or LiDAR). Since the military surveillance systems of World War II, sensors have improved to capture reflectance in a wider range of optical wavelengths with greater resolution, for progressively more information content. The level of detail (resolution) in digital imagery can be related to at least three aspects: spatial, spectral, and radiometric. These resolutions trade off with each other, and with the overall areal extent covered by each image scene/snapshot. Spatial resolution refers to the size of individual pictoral elements (pixels), corresponding to rectangular portions of the earth surface being imaged. Higher spatial resolution systems such as IKONOS or Quickbird map earth surfaces in great detail, with sub-meter pixels. Spectral resolution refers to the precision with which sensors partition the electromagnetic spectrum (into "bands") to record reflectance. The human eye is sensitive to wavelengths in the visible range, or 300–750 nm (blue to red wavelengths). NASA's Landsat Thematic Mapper sensor system captures the visible range in three ranges or reflectance bands (blue, green, and red), and additionally records reflectance in four infrared bands (three mid/near infrared and one thermal), as opposed to up to 220 bands in hyperspectral remote sensing (NASA's EO-1 Hyperion sensor). Radiometric resolution refers to the levels of quantization (referred to as bit depth) with which the sensor captures spectral reflectance intensities in a pixel, typically ranging from 0 to 255 (8 bits). Additionally, temporal resolution refers to the revisit frequency of the sensor for a specific point on the earth. Landsat TM has a temporal resolution of 16 days, compared to the NOAA AVHRR satellite's twice-daily imaging frequency. Processing satellite imagery or digital aerial photographs of varying spatial, spectral and radiometric characteristics involves three essential steps: geometric correction (georeferencing), radiometric correction (noise removal) and various methods of information retrieval relevant to the chosen application or research question. Subsequent sections will discuss some of these image processing techniques utilized in anthropological research on landscape characterization and change detection. Most RS applications, however, involve the analysis of RS-derived data with GIS tools.

Geographic information systems center on linked spatial and attribute (non-spatial) data, structured within a chosen model to represent real-world spatial objects and relations. Typically, GIS data models are of two basic types: raster and vector. Raster data represent a space-filled, *field-based* view, in which the geographic world is made up of continuously varying data values in gridded layers covering a study region. Spatial and attribute data are embedded within the same data structure: the spatial grid is divided into square/rectangular units, typically of uniform dimensions, each cell recording qualitative or quantitative attributes of interest (e.g., land use codes, distance to nearest road network, degree of fire risk, etc.). Vector data, on the other hand, subscribe to a *feature-based* view of the world, recording precise boundaries and information about specific objects of interest, rather than all space within a study area. Three types of features typically used are points (e.g., houses), lines (e.g., roads) and polygons (e.g., land parcels). In a vector data model, spatial and attribute data are stored separately but linked through a common identifier, often within a relational database.

The development of modern GIS was application driven, and dates to the computerization of spatial data management tasks in the US Census and Canadian Land Inventory during the 1960s. GIS software offers tools for spatial and relational data entry and storage (including coordinate and attribute data capture or importation), representation (e.g., through various data models), transformation and management (e.g., projections, editing, reduction/summarization), and visualization (various output formats and symbolization, alternate/dynamic renderings of two- or three-dimensional products, often embedded with internet mapping). Most significantly, GIS techniques enable the integration of data from disparate sources, and the analysis of multiple spatial data layers. Analytical tools range from simple querying, distance and buffering tools, to map algebra and spatial statistics/interpolation, as well as complex network/topological/terrain analyses, multi-criteria evaluations, and environmental modeling. Several of these techniques entail the integration of research/methodological approaches as well as diverse data sources such as ethnographies and field-derived surveys, cadastral information, digital elevation models, satellite or station derived climate data, land cover information, or utilities and infrastructure networks. These characteristics explain the increasing use of GIS in research and planning, as well as environmental and spatial decision-making. GIS are embedded, however, within a broader theoretical framework of *GIScience*, drawing from geospatial technologies (RS, GIS, GPS) as well as informed by information theory, mathematics and statistics, cartographic and cognitive sciences as well as linguistics. Thus, anthropological research (e.g., on spatial social relations and environmental perception/cognition) may draw from and contribute to both GIS applications, and GIScience more broadly.

A BRIEF HISTORY OF RS-GIS APPLICATIONS IN ANTHROPOLOGY

In anthropology, as in other disciplines, the use of geospatial technologies has expanded greatly since the 1970s, commensurate with the broad proliferation of GIS and RS, and with a trend towards interdisciplinarity in anthropological paradigms and methods (Aldenderfer and Maschner 1992; Conant 1978, 1984, 1994). Today, GIS and RS frequently contribute to methodological training in environmental anthropology, archaeology, and social sciences in general, aiding in the study of local populations and sociocultural phenomena (Behrens 1994, 1992; Fox *et al.* 2003), the history of landscape (Guyer *et al.* 2007; Nyerges and Green 2000), understanding and quantifying socioenvironmental transformation (Brondízio 2008; Galvin *et al.* 2001), preparation of field research (D'Antona, Cak, and VanWey 2008; DeCastro *et al.* 2002), and practical applications relevant to local populations and policy (Cultural Survivor 1995; Smith, Pariona, and Tuesta 2002). Conversely, anthropological concerns with local scales and richly detailed human–environment processes have also contributed to refining spatial categories and methods of analysis (John 1990; Liverman *et al.* 1998; Moran 1998). For instance, researchers in anthropological and related fields have engaged in the development of participatory field techniques, image interpretation, validation of land cover classification products, discussion of ethical and confidentiality issues in spatial data use representation and use, and disseminating geospatial products to local communities and indigenous groups (Brondízio *et al.* 1994; D'Antona, Cak, and VanWey 2008).

During the 1970s, anthropologists began to utilize newly available Landsat (Morain 1998) and radar data in addition to longer-used aerial photography (Reining 1979), expanding their applications in archaeology (Fisher and Feinman 2005; Gibbons 1991; Heckenberger *et al.* 2003; Lyons and Avery 1977; Server and Wiseman 1984; Stone 1993). These data have helped locate and contextualize villages in remote areas, and provided a lens by which to understand subsistence activities, assess infrastructure and environmental resources, and track the mutual transformation of social groups and landscapes, assisting in planning fieldwork, testing hypotheses, and generalizing local findings. In some cases (e.g., Conklin 1980), geospatial methods allowed the presentation of long-term ethnographic data over regional landscapes. Interestingly, by offering new perspectives and modes of analysis, geospatial methods have driven a pluralization of anthropological questions, demands for more, not less fieldwork (Conant 1994), and interdisciplinary collaborations amidst the emerging research agenda on global environmental change (Aldenderfer and Maschner 1992; John 1990; Moran and Brondízio 2001). Likewise, it has provided important resources to grassroots social movements concerned with environmental degradation and land demarcation since the 1980s (see Cultural Survival 1995; special issue of Human Organization, Herlihy and Knapp 2003; Wilkie 1987, 1990).

GIS and RS methodologies to explicitly link distinct spatio-temporal scales have greatly benefited human–environment studies in anthropology, geography, and ecology. Across these disciplines, efforts to conceptualize boundaries and relations among human populations and their environment have focused on households, sociocultural/ethnic groups, communities, cultural areas, territories and territoriality, niches, ecosystems, landscapes, biomes, and states and nation-states, among other units. An illustration of historical approaches to conceptualize units of analysis anthropology include Brondízio (2005), Fairhead and Leach (1995), Geertz (1963), Kroeber (1939), Moran (1990), Steward (1955), Vayda and McCay (1975), Vayda and Rappaport (1968), and Walker and Peters (2007). Various traditions within environmental anthropology favor particular articulations of scales/units, such as individuals and cultural groups (symbolic ecology); localistic approaches (ethnobiology); sociodemographic units and their biophysical environment (ecological anthropology); local connections to national and global scales (political ecology); groups with shared/contrasting interests in common pool resources (institutional analysis), or local/regional landscapes or a nexus of these (historical ecology). This diverse legacy has been enriched by the spatial resolution and relational analyses offered by GIS/RS (Brondízio, Fiorini, and Adams n.d.).

ASSESSING GEOSPATIAL DATA NEEDS IN
ANTHROPOLOGICAL RESEARCH

The specification of research questions and analytical units are the most fundamental tasks in planning anthropological research.

Geospatial data and the articulation of spatial information with non-spatial attributes afford particular opportunities and challenges in research design. This section outlines key considerations in the integration of GIS and RS with research foci in environmental anthropology, focusing on units of analysis, the formulation of spatiotemporal research questions, and pragmatic aspects of referencing data availability to research design. Finally, these considerations are linked to implications for data manipulation and analysis by focusing on a particularly relevant environmental anthropological research application: the detection and analysis of landscape change.

Analytical questions and units

The selection of units of analysis lies at the heart of understanding processes of socioenvironmental change, including deforestation or urbanization, and the roles of different forces such as cultural diffusion, environmental constraints, and political economy. This analytical choice is also the single most important step in preventing scalar mismatch between agents and outcomes of change, and the "ecological fallacy" (ascribing relationships detected at one scale to a lower level of analysis). A common example of this problem is presuming correlations between population growth and deforestation in a given area, without considering population distribution patterns and the role of external agents. Along the same lines, the selection of units of analysis is important to avoid "adaptation fallacies," or assuming a perfect match between a given population and the local resources, perhaps ignoring alternative relationships, such as external subsidies or exported environmental costs.

Defining units of analysis requires negotiating boundaries which may be ephemeral, fuzzy, open, circumstantial, and/or seasonal, thus requiring a flexible and critical approach. With few pre-defined units in human–environment analysis, a central guiding principle is to consider the hierarchically nested scales relevant to research questions of interest. For a given region, these decisions should account for local forms of social organization, spatial distributions of environmental resources, human populations, infrastructure, and land use systems. Thus, the researcher may identify questions, involving distinct political (e.g., states, municipalities, districts), institutional (government, private, communal areas), biophysical (e.g., watersheds, edaphic zones), sociocultural (e.g., ethnic groups, clans), demographic (e.g., households, cohort groups), and contextual units (e.g., distinct

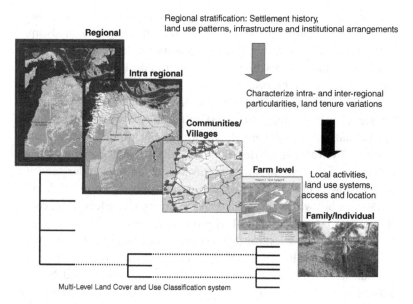

Figure 12.1   Regional stratification approach.

distance buffers relative to village centers/markets/rivers/roads). The diversity of environmental, historical and economic factors that mitigate against easy generalizations in a given region (Tucker 2005) necessitate the integration of local detail and knowledge into remote sensing and GIS data.

Intraregional analysis accommodates such complexity, recognizing environmental and social variations within a region (Brondízio 2005, 2006; Lambin 2003). In this context, hierarchically nested units can be defined according to one's research questions and regional structures, such as farm lots within a settlement, settlements within a community, rural communities within a municipality, or in relation to a conservation reserve, reserves within a region, and so forth. Biophysical units such as vegetation types or watersheds can also be nested in this context (Miller *et al.* 2009). Intraregional analysis thus entails regional stratification according to spatiotemporal patterns of social settlement or ecological change, a process that can be very useful during image classification (described in following sections). Figure 12.1 illustrates a regional stratification according to historical occupation and spatial scale (Brondízio 2006). While histories are not units of analysis per se, the institutions, social groups, and forms of resource use and ownership created through time can be. Thus, accounting for such variations may help to avoid unwarranted comparisons and to improve the level of detail in the analysis of landscape change, as well as offering image segmentation by social, historical, and environmental variation as opposed to classical remote sensing partitioning by pixel reflectance values.

Closely related to the selection of observational units in environmental anthropology is the task of defining a study region's precincts, and matching them to political, sociocultural, institutional, and biophysical boundaries that typically do not co-align. These overlaps (or mismatches) are important not only to understand if, where, how, and when a given population uses different parts of a landscape, but whether resource management at one level (e.g., community) is appropriate to deal with problems resulting from another level (e.g., watershed) (Brondízio, Ostrom, and Young 2009). An additional challenge lies in matching social and spatial/environmental boundaries with chosen units of observation (Boucek and Moran 2004; Fox *et al.* 2003; McCracken *et al.* 1999; Ostrom and Nagendra 2006). For instance, researchers investigating agricultural management in a given region need to consider whether prevailing relationships are one-to-one (e.g., each household in a study site cultivates a farm lot), one-to-many (e.g., each household farms several plots), or many-to-one (e.g., a given parcel managed by multiple households over time) (Evans and Moran 2002). RS derived data on land cover and/or change, when integrated with ancillary GIS data on agents of change and their connectivity to parts of the land, can reveal patterns and processes of management/social relations. GIS also aids in the creation/consideration of contextual (proxy) boundaries for areas lacking clear administrative/jurisdictional cartographies. For instance, if one wants to estimate land use change associated with a given village where no clear bounding coordinates are defined, researchers may generate buffer zones at different distances from a village center or utilize a common alternative, Thiessen polygons (Sirén 2007; Sirén and Brondízio 2009). Fundamentally important in such boundary definitions are considerations of their fluidity, contingency, and contestation, as well as of who is defining them (e.g., whether customary boundaries are more meaningful than formal ones), and how they change through time (including between seasons). Geospatial tools allow such manipulation of analytical units, thus rather than being constrained to given units, it allows comparison and testing of human–environmental relationships according to various spatial nexus and comparative frameworks.

Cross-referencing available data in preparing a research design

Preparing a research design integrating RS, GIS, and other methods from the toolkit of anthropologists require the definition of clear research questions, the searching of available data, estimation of field efforts, and understanding the limitations inherent to the resolution of different datasets (including not only spatial data, but surveys and ethnographic material). Figure 12.2 provides a practical guide to define, search, cross-reference, and evaluate the extent to which available RS and GIS data can be used to address one's needs. In preparing for this exercise one should identify: (1) the research question of interest; (2) the time frame of interest and/or the sequence of relevant events affecting an area; (3) the seasonality of the area: how climate or land cover/use may change through the year; (4) the spatial dimensions of important social and environmental features and/ or ideal data requirements. Once the above questions and data needs are outlined, potential sources of eligible RS/GIS data may be identified. Image scenes for specific regions may be quickly located using global referencing systems (e.g., the World Reference System[1] [WRS I or II] to identify Landsat images) and/or locational (e.g., Universal Transverse Mercator (UTM) or geographic) coordinates. Several search engines and public data archives (see Appendix Sites of interest) allow one to locate geographic coordinates in relation to image footprints.

As the scope of research frequently includes temporal trends/ processes, it is helpful to develop a temporal nesting of identified datasets by seasonal versus inter-annual/longer time intervals (Figure 12.2, 2–4). If seasonally referenced data are available, they enable discerning vegetative/land cover phenology and calendars of land-based/economic activities in a given area, and may suggest the need for proxy measurements/adjustments (e.g., considering bare soil in/as agricultural fields in an image captured outside the growing season). Longer-term datasets (e.g., image snapshots over years or decades), on the other hand, can reveal the impacts of historical events and period effects (e.g., major policy or economic changes, important conflicts, a major development project, changes

---

[1] The Landsat 1–3 WRS-1 notation assigns sequential path numbers from east to west to 251 nominal satellite orbital tracks, starting with number 001 for the first track. The Landsat 4 and 5 WRS-2 system notation assigns sequential path numbers from east to west to 233 paths numbered 001 to 233.

1. Define study area name and location
(e.g., use UTM coordinates X and Y):
Latitude: from _____ to _____
Longitude: from _____ to _____

1.2 Find, select, and bookmark area using Google Earth, with overlays of roads, rivers, administrative maps, and other relevant layers. Observe the regional topography and land cover, with particular attention to settlement patterns vis-à-vis land use and land cover.

1.3 Landsat WRS grid location:
WRS 1 (Landsat 1, 2, 3) Path _____/Row _____
WRS 2 (Landsat 4, 5)   Path _____/Row _____
Quadrant (if applicable): _____
Data quality (e.g., cloud cover)

1.4 Identify other data/sensors:
Sensor (airflight mission, satellite, and sensor)
Data type (analogic or digital)
Format (if applicable)

1.5 Carry out systematic search using image/maps data archive
(e.g., USGS Earth Explorer)

2. Define a time-line of relevant events

Temporal (yearly to decadal)

Spatial
┌─────────────────────────┐
│ Historical events   │
│ Socio-Economic change   │
│ Natural events   │
│ Others....   │
└─────────────────────────┘

3. Characterize seasonality and vegetation phenology

Spatial
┌──────────────┐
│ Climate   │
│ Land cover   │
│ Land use   │
└──────────────┘

Temporal

4. Graph or cross-tabulate 'IDEAL' sampling and IDENTIFIED available remote sensing data and maps in the context of each research question
Temporal resolution and data
(e.g., bi-yearly, Spring and Fall)
Spatial resolution and data
(e.g., Landsat TM, Path 20/Row 47)

5. Decide on data selection, refine/revise research questions according to available data (temporal sampling) and data resolution (spatial). Consider data temporal availability and spatial resolution to land use and cover spatial–temporal patterns, and define minimum mapping units and processing needs.

Figure 12.2   Steps in image/data search and research design.

276

in technology, or the occurrence of natural events such as droughts or floods, etc.).

Data quality concerns are important when selecting among alternate short- or long-term RS datasets that may match research needs. These include considerations of scene cloud cover, and patterns of geometric or radiometric corrections that are likely necessary. Quality and informational content is equally important in ancillary GIS data, and researchers need to assess the type and detail of thematic information about features of interest, as well as their cartographic aspects (e.g., projection system, scale and minimum mapping units, and metadata detailing types of corrections/transformations applied). These features will fundamentally influence data input as well as the quality of registration/overlay with other data layers. Plotting available data and information pertaining to an area over time as well as explicitly evaluating its quality helps the researcher adjudicate among available data or spatiotemporal sampling designs. It also helps to define the field-work strategies that might be needed to collect additional data or to validate and correct existing ones, and the costs associated with these choices: key issues in the progressive refinement of research questions and strategy. Figure 12.3 summarizes the major training activities and concepts in data organization and manipulations common to anthropological applications.

RESEARCH APPLICATION: DETECTING AND UNDERSTANDING
LAND CHANGE

A comprehensive discussion of data processing in RS and GIS, even within the field of anthropology, would be well outside the scope of a book chapter. In this section, we therefore highlight data processing and analytical considerations as exemplified in one common area of application of RS/GIS in environmental anthropology: the characterization of land cover and/or use, and depicting and understanding its change over time. Digital image processing in RS for land change analysis includes three main phases: preprocessing, land cover characterization with classification and/or continuous indices, and change detection, with field data collection at various phases throughout. GIS analysis may assist during the process of change detection, as well as enable a deeper investigation of the processes of historical change and/or future projections and scenarios.

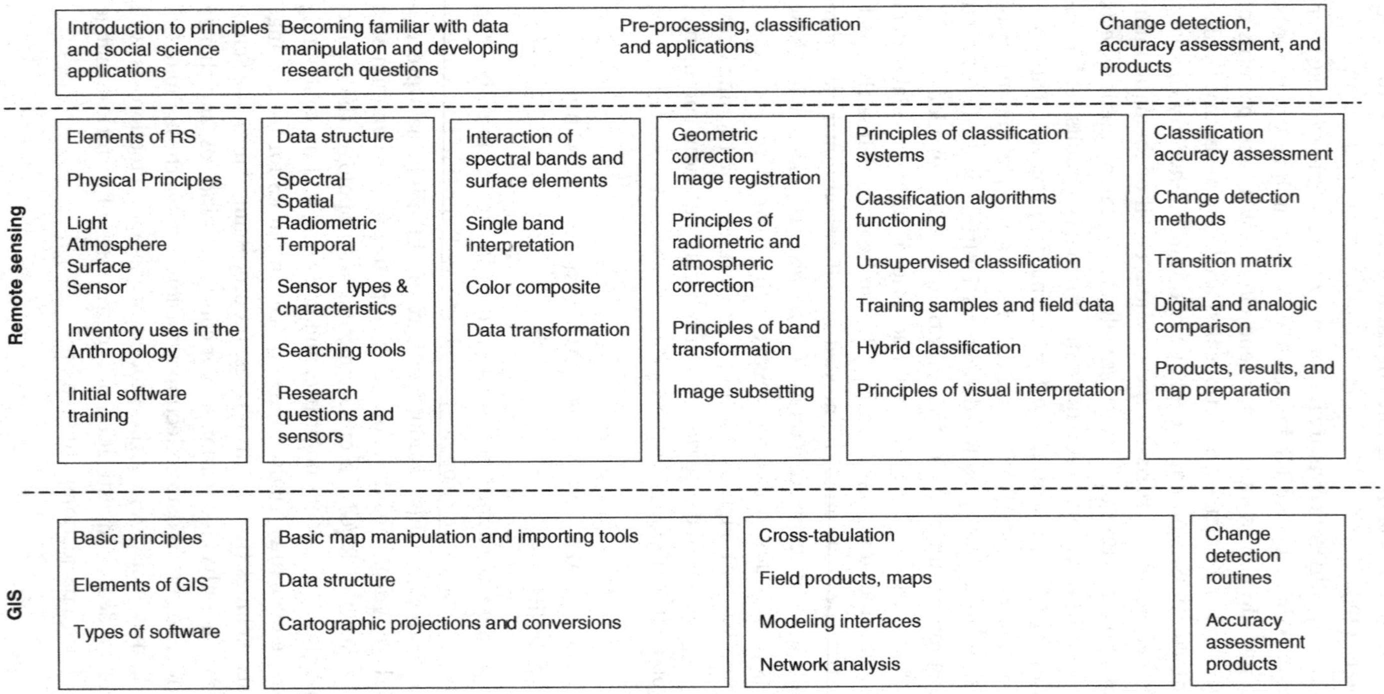

Introduction to principles and social science applications	Becoming familiar with data manipulation and developing research questions	Pre-processing, classification and applications	Change detection, accuracy assessment, and products

Remote sensing

Elements of RS
Physical Principles
Light
Atmosphere
Surface
Sensor
Inventory uses in the Anthropology
Initial software training

Data structure
Spectral
Spatial
Radiometric
Temporal
Sensor types & characteristics
Searching tools
Research questions and sensors

Interaction of spectral bands and surface elements
Single band interpretation
Color composite
Data transformation

Geometric correction
Image registration
Principles of radiometric and atmospheric correction
Principles of band transformation
Image subsetting

Principles of classification systems
Classification algorithms functioning
Unsupervised classification
Training samples and field data
Hybrid classification
Principles of visual interpretation

Classification accuracy assessment
Change detection methods
Transition matrix
Digital and analogic comparison
Products, results, and map preparation

GIS

Basic principles
Elements of GIS
Types of software

Basic map manipulation and importing tools
Data structure
Cartographic projections and conversions

Cross-tabulation
Field products, maps
Modeling interfaces
Network analysis

Change detection routines
Accuracy assessment products

Figure 12.3   A general training guide for social scientists developing expertise in RS and GIS.

Data preprocessing

Digital image processing usually begins with the importing/conversion, display and examination of each image layer (band) and statistics. Depending on the specific research objectives, data source, and study region, the researcher makes choices at this stage regarding image mosaicking or sub-setting (to cover a study area in adequate spatial extent and/or detail), the use of spectral bands (i.e., whether all bands are necessary, and whether transformed bands are needed), and radiometric/atmospheric correction algorithms to improve signal-to-noise ratios before further analysis (Green *et al.* 2005). In some cases, such corrections are necessary to correct for atmospheric problems in different parts of the same image (Sirén and Brondízio 2009). Advanced image processing software programs include pre-defined routines for radiometric enhancement, some of which are well-understood and commonly used to improve image quality (e.g., the Tasselled Cap transformation used to reduce atmospheric haze that especially affects lower wavelength bands), aiding in the preparation of clear image printouts for fieldwork, etc. Principal component analysis can dramatically reduce both random noise and systematic noise in imagery, and has been successfully applied to Landsat TM bands to enable high-resolution land classification in the tropics (Roy Chowdhury and Schneider 2004). As a rule of thumb, however, it is advisable not to undertake major radiometric transformations of the data if one is not experienced with their theoretical/empirical character (the nature of those changes and how they can affect the image).

One of the most important steps during preprocessing is geometric correction (used interchangeably with geocorrection and georeferencing). Geometric correction involves spatial transformations to map (or reassign) pixels to a geographic (latitude/longitude) coordinate system or a standard map projection, such as the Universal Transverse Mercator (UTM) (Jensen 1996; Wilkie 1996). While images can be ordered with vendor-applied georeferencing, performing the corrections "in-house" enables greater control of positional accuracy and error distribution. Geometric correction is a necessary step to most applications in environmental anthropology and to anyone interested on assembling a GIS and cross-referencing any kind of spatially explicit data. Similarly, it is necessary to prepare images for use during fieldwork, particularly if one wants to use a GPS in the field to locate a place on an image. The actual steps involved in geometric correction include the use of reference data (a pre-georeferenced map or image, in the absence of which field-derived GPS points may be substituted) alongside the target image to be transformed, and the selection of key locations/landmarks or Ground Control Points (GCPs) clearly visible in both reference and target images. The number (the greater, the better) and spatial distribution (widely and evenly distributed is better) of GCPs are important to minimize the magnitude of locational inaccuracy, captured as root mean square error (RMSE) after the coordinate transformation (Jensen 1996). A basic rule of thumb is to aim for a RMSE equal to or less than half the image pixel size, and use the lowest-order transformation function feasible (e.g., the nearest neighbor or affine transformation, for faster processing and least alteration of pixel attribute values). After georeferencing, the transformed image may be overlaid with the reference maps check for the quality of their spatial matching.

Preprocessing may further entail band transformations, and/or the integration of GIS techniques. For instance, a variety of algorithms allow the generation of indices of vegetation, soil, impervious surfaces and spatial texture. As mentioned earlier, principal component analysis can yield transformed bands that reduce image noise and data redundancy/dimensionality. Quantitative measures derived from transformations of red and infrared bands, such as the normalized difference of vegetation index (NDVI), are useful indices of relative biomass in many regions. NDVI as well as spatial texture measures have been found to enhance the ability to distinguish between land cover classes when overlaid with dehazed bands prior to image classification (e.g., Roy Chowdhury and Schneider 2004; Lu *et al* 2004b). Ancillary GIS data (e.g., digital elevation, soil, or vegetation layers) may also be used as prior probability images in image classification (described in the next section), to improve land cover discrimination and classification accuracy (Maselli *et al*. 1994; McIver and Friedl 2002; Pedroni 2003).

Characterizing land cover and land use: continuous and discrete approaches

Land cover can be described with continuous or categorical data. Continuous approaches derive indices of aspects of land cover features such as vegetation, bare soil, built-up or impervious surfaces and/or their moisture conditions can captured in image band transformations as described in the preceding section. Such measures include ratio or soil-line based indices, such as simple ratio (SR), NDVI, and numerous variants, including the enhanced vegetation index (EVI), soil adjusted vegetation index (SAVI), modified soil adjusted vegetation index (MSAVI), soil adjusted total vegetation index (SATVI), etc. (Jordan 1969; Lawrence and Ripple 1998; Rondeaux, Steven, and Baret 1996; Rouse *et al.* 1973). These indices represent the physical condition of the landscape through continuously varying values across space.

Land cover categorical classification, on the other hand, reduces continuously varying spectral reflectance (or vegetation index) values to fewer, discrete categories (nominal/qualitative data) that are meaningful to local social and/or ecological conditions. While it may seem desirable to always aim for the greatest number of detailed land cover classes, precision/accuracy trade-offs mean that numerous classes of finely detailed cover categories are typically classified with lower per class accuracy, while fewer and (spectrally) broader cover classes have greater classification accuracy/reliability. It is important to aim for similar accuracy among classes, and a minimum accuracy of 85 percent is widely accepted. In case of low accuracy, one should consider aggregating a class one level up where a more general definition may improve accuracy.

Optimizing detail and accuracy is thus a particular challenge in image classification. Other considerations include: that the system should be reproducible by another interpreter; that classes should apply over extensive areas; that aggregation of classes across levels should be possible; and, if necessary, that classes should recognize temporal and seasonal dynamics (Anderson *et al.* 1976; Di Gregorio and Jansen 2000). A further challenge lies in the distinction between land use and cover. While environmental anthropologists may be interested in locating particular forms of land use (e.g., pastures) in a regional landscape, those uses need to be translated to biophysical land cover characteristics (e.g., herbaceous/grassy cover) for the purpose of land classification. This is important since different land uses (e.g., crops and pastures) may actually produce very similar land covers which may be or not spectrally distinguishable (e.g., coffee agroforestry vs. secondary vegetation). The spectral signature of land cover features is defined by a combination of vegetation, moisture and soil conditions. The challenge we then face is to translate these conditions to land cover classes, and then relate them to relevant land use information.

Manual digitization (using digitizing tablets for analog products such as printed aerial photography, or on-screen digitization for digital photos/images) may be used to derive land cover maps without digital image classification. This method relies on the photo/satellite image interpreter's ability to discriminate features on a given image corresponding to distinct land cover classes. A number of spatial elements aid in the discrimination of land cover classes and/or features, including shape, size, pattern, and proximity/context of different features, as well as texture, tone, and shadows. Digital image classification, on the other hand, entails two main suites of techniques: supervised and unsupervised classification; hybrid classifications entail iterative combinations of the two.

Unsupervised classification allows the definition of classes without requiring knowledge of the image or study area, enabling the user to classify a large region into distinct categories of land cover in a time and cost-effective way at the beginning of research. The process identifies natural groupings of pixels in an image based on their location in multispectral feature space (their reflectance patterns in multiple bands). The number of clusters is defined by the user according to research questions. After classification, "the analyst then attempts a posteriori to assign these natural or *spectral* classes to the *information* classes of interest" (Jensen 1996: 231). Spectral classes may be difficult to interpret sometimes, with little resemblance to local reality. This assignment of unsupervised spectral classes to informational, "real world" classes entails ancillary knowledge of the area and GPS-assisted field visits. Nevertheless, many analysts prefer to use only unsupervised classification, often beginning with larger numbers of clusters, later aggregating similar spectral classes and using field-based information to identify the land cover categories they represent. Others prefer to use unsupervised classification only as the first step, then collecting field information to inform supervised or hybrid classification.

The first step in supervised classification is to develop a target classification scheme of land use/covers of regional interest. Such schemes are usually developed in an interactive process which involves the examination of land cover variability within an image, as well as thematic and field knowledge. Many researchers prefer to adopt hierarchically nested classification categories: the advantage of a hierarchical scheme is that detailed land cover classes may be aggregated to address questions about land use and cover change at different levels of analysis. For most studies, a classification scheme can be divided into three levels. The first level, suitable for regional analysis, divides the area into major land cover classes. A second level, more appropriate between the regional and local scales, divides the first level into more specific categories of land cover structure/composition and/or physiographic (e.g., topographic) characteristics of major landscape elements. The third and most detailed level aims at defining land cover classes for use in site-specific analysis, attentive to subtle differences in land cover classes relevant to ethnobotanical and land use questions. For instance, a general level I class of "successional forest" can be divided into two structural/seral stages of secondary forests at level II, and three or even four in level III.

Based on target classes, "the analyst uses 'training samples' to define areas with pixels of known identity (through a combination of fieldwork, aerial photos, ancillary data, etc.) and uses its 'statistics' to classify pixels of unknown identity" (Jensen 1996: 231). The user defines areas of interest (AOIs) representing training sites (TS) for each target class, which can then be used by the selected classification algorithm[2] to classify pixels of unknown identity, and also to support accuracy assessment.[3] TS need to be collected for as many as samples as possible for each of the proposed land use/cover classes, and be largely relative to image resolution (e.g., minimally 9 pixels or about 1 ha in the case of a Landsat TM image). Depending on field conditions, TS can be collected by observing areas along a roadside or river, during field visits with local farmers or informants, and many other creative ways. It can also be collected through aerial surveys and in some cases using high-resolution images available through Google Earch™. It is also important to ensure a wide spatial distribution of TS for land cover classes of interest, in order to avoid clustered samples biased towards only one part of the image/landscape. TS areas can be located with GPS in georeferenced image printouts or through real-time links to the digital imagery loaded on portable laptops, to allow for immediate adjustments/revisions.

A supervised classified image output is generated containing the classes represented by training samples. This procedure has a number of advantages: the user "trains" the classification algorithm based on their expert knowledge and desired targets; field (and other ancillary) data can be integrated into the classification process, and it is generally

---

[2] Common supervised algorithms can be parametric or non-parametric depending on the statistical assumption about the normality of data distribution. Non-parametric classifiers include spectral angle, Euclidian distance, parallelepiped, neural networks, among others, while parametric classifiers include maximum likelihood, ECHO (combines textural/spectral classifier and maximum likelihood), and tree classifiers.

[3] Accuracy assessment is based on "areas of reference" representing classes from your classification system; these areas are used to assess whether your classification performance is acceptable; a common reference to consider a thematic class as acceptable for most purposes is to present a classification accuracy above 85%. Kappa statistics (expressed in percentages), which represent a measure of omission and commission errors, are the most standard measure of accuracy for thematic classifications (Janssen and van der Wel 1994).

easier to test the overall classification accuracy. However, it also has several disadvantages: it requires high quality and broadly distributed field data, collected intensively and extensively to represent variability among landscape feature classes. It also assumes that a given training sample represents some level of homogeneity in order to serve as a reference to other pixels of that cover class in the image.[4] Several users prefer to use a combination of supervised and unsupervised methods. For instance, preliminary spectral clusters derived from unsupervised classification may be used as training sites in combination with field-derived data in a second-stage classification using supervised techniques. In either case (i.e., unsupervised, supervised or hybrid), one should use a combination of visual, spectral, and statistical tools to evaluate classes and improve class discrimination, making use of overlay techniques such as blending, swiping, and flickering layers, and charting spectral signatures and their separability statistics (e.g., using transformed divergence statistics).

Preparing and using images for fieldwork and interviews

Preparing data products for fieldwork is an important step for anthropologists using RS and GIS. Preparation of maps usually involves the use of GIS to represent an image (black and white or color composite) within a coordinate grid, juxtaposed with other layers of interest (e.g., municipal/community/reserve boundaries, roads, river systems), and, if applicable, legends (symbols representing different thematic features). Although basic cartographic information is always important, the degree of detail varies according to the goals of the map, but should at least include scale, north orientation, data source, and legend.

The selection of the area/subset to be used for preparing image printouts depends on the stage of research and sampling goals. In general, image printouts can be prepared at three scales which can be used from exploratory to advanced stages of research and fieldwork, as illustrated in Figure 12.1. These include a regional scale (i.e., relative to the whole area of the image and representing the larger landscape), a subregional scale (i.e., representing compartments/areas within an image that reflect social/environmental variability relevant

---

[4] These descriptions emphasize "hard" classification procedures, i.e., each pixel is assigned to only one class. Algorithms to account for fuzzy membership and probability assignment are available, but require advanced technical expertise.

to the research questions), and a local scale (i.e., representing the most disaggregated level of interest). While the definition of map/printout scale will depend on the size of the whole area of interest and the spatial resolution of the image, experience shows that the following scales for print-outs are useful to most applications of Landsat and SPOT data: Regional (~1:50 000), Subregional (~1:30 000 to 1:50 000), and local (~1:15 000 to 1:30 000). The subregional and local-scale maps may be defined in a systematic sampling of the whole image (e.g., subdivided into quadrants), or led by particular regions/strata of interest (e.g., topographic gradients, institutional regimes, or forest protection status). Likewise, preparing images to be used at the local level with land managers and key informants will depend on sampling goals, but in general these images should represent the landscape most immediate to those managers or residents (Figure 12.1).

Additional considerations in preparing these images for use in interviews include the selection of color composition, coordinate systems, and their production using materials durable in field conditions. The selection of spectral bands and colors to depict their combinations (composites) should aim to balance familiarity of human vision with detailed information about the environment. Using data from Landsat series 4, 5, or 7 as an example, the most common color composite used for image printouts (one which offers a good trade-off between appearance and spectral information) assigns spectral bands 5 (mid-infrared), 4 (near-infrared), and 3 (red) to the red, green and blue color guns respectively. This will produce an image which resembles somewhat our own perception of the environment, i.e., vegetation will be greenish, water will be bluish, and soil will be reddish.

Image printouts should also include a coordinate system (e.g., geographic latitude/longitude or UTM) which one can use, for instance, to locate a reference point collected with a GPS. Since one can measure distances more easily in planar coordinates (e.g., meters), a UTM coordinate system or equivalent is the most practical for field purposes. A GPS locational reading can then be easily located within the image's UTM grid. Although the interval for a coordinate grid will depend on the scale of the map, 1 km or 500 m grid spacings are very useful for subregional and local scales (e.g., printed at a scale of ~1:15 000–1:30 000). One should also consider whether an image printout can sustain field conditions, i.e., rain and humidity, constant manipulation, etc. If possible, it is always advisable to laminate image printouts/maps before going to the field and use permanent markers to make notations on top of it. Finally, one should always have extra copies of images to be donated during fieldwork to collaborators and/or institutions, such as to the interviewed farmer, to a community, or to a public agency that may benefit from it.

Using images in interviews during field research require a series of steps to avoid possible intimidation of interviewees, confusions during interpretation, and to maximize benefits to both parties. The use of images and maps should be preceded by a clear explanation of the project, confidentiality guarantees, and the interviewee's informed consent. One can start by explaining the origin of the image one is using, including its availability to the public (vis-à-vis privileged or exclusive data). One can donate/present an image to the interviewee at this stage or later depending on the situation. Depending on interview goals, the researcher may consider a three-step process for using images, addressing discussions from the regional to local scales (e.g., Figure 12.1). Following an explanation of the research project and imagery provenance, the regional-scale image may be used to contextualize the specific place where the conversation is occurring within the broader study area, utilizing major landmarks familiar to the interviewee. Concurrently, the researcher should explain to the interviewee the symbology and color composition utilized in the map products, enabling the interpretation of how colors map to landscape features and cover classes recognizable by local land managers/farmers (e.g., in the Landsat 543 composite described above, light-dark shades of green representing herbaceous-arboreal vegetation, blue as water, and reddish/yellowish as exposed soil or infrastructure). This preliminary orientation may then be followed by detailed images at larger cartographic scales (subregional or local) to discuss landscape features in environments progressively more immediate to the interviewee. Patterns of environmental variability, management practices, land tenure, land use systems and local environmental knowledge are appropriate themes at this level of detail. Depending on research interests, a more local-scale (e.g., farm-level) image can then be utilized in conjunction with interviews eliciting calendars of land use/economic activities, management practices, and land tenure, or ethnoecological research to distinguish landscape compartments and spatially explicit land use histories, further aided by local-scale sketch maps (e.g., D'Antona *et al.* 2008).

Detecting land change

As with land cover characterization, analysis of land transformation over time may refer to continuous or categorical changes using multi-temporal datasets. Techniques vary with research/application goals (e.g., urban expansion, agricultural intensification, deforestation, forest degradation, etc.). Continuous land cover change analyses can focus on shifts in reflectance (as captured in noise-corrected spectral bands), or on changes in computed land cover indices (e.g., vegetation/soil/impervious surface indices) across multiple image dates. Categorical change detection, on the other hand, proceeds with comparisons of classified images from multiple dates. The reliability of change analysis results is linked to the change detection technique employed, and depends fundamentally upon the quality of image georeferencing and registration (i.e., precision of alignment between dates), the quality of atmospheric and radiometric correction (especially when comparing spectral reflectance directly across dates), and the consistency and robustness of the classification system used for each date. A comprehensive review of change detection techniques is presented by Lu and colleagues (2004a).

Continuous change detection between two image dates includes techniques such as image differencing (calculating differences in per-pixel reflectance values, vegetation indices, etc.), image ratioing (performing a per-pixel ratio operation between the two images), or image regression (wherein the image from time 1 is treated as an independent variable and time 2 as dependent variable to estimate a regression coefficient for each pixel, which is used to create a "predicted" image for time 2 for comparison with the actual time 2 image). These techniques need to be used with care, since their applicability is affected by underlying data quality (e.g., atmospheric effects) as well as patterns of spatial autocorrelation (e.g., violating regression assumptions of independence of observational units), necessitating refinements (e.g., radiometric enhancement or modifying spatial sampling regimes). Once applied correctly, these techniques are typically followed by thresholding (Singh 1989) to determine whether calculated shifts are significant changes or part of "natural" variability. Again, research objectives (e.g., type of land cover change of interest) will influence the application of these techniques, e.g., the choice of specific bands to compare (Lillesand and Kiefer 1987: 650–655).

Continuous change analysis using multiple (more than two) image dates may entail multi-temporal composites for visualization or further processing, change vector analysis (CVA) or other time series analysis (TSA) techniques. Creating multi-temporal image composites (after geocorrection and image-to-image registration) is a powerful tool for depicting and detecting change over time. Subtle color differences produced by spectral change among dates may reflect changes in land cover that can be further assessed. For instance, a multi-temporal, unsupervised classification of composited bands from different dates can yield output classes representing different kinds of change. These forms of output may be validated or investigated (e.g., fieldwork, ancillary data, historical records) to characterize the kind of changes being detected.

CVA calculates (1) the Euclidean distance between a pixels position in n-band space in time 1, and its corresponding band-space location in time 2, and (2) the direction (angle) of the change vector as measured by its angle. The direction of change indicates the quality/type of change (e.g., vegetation loss or regrowth). Lambin and Strahler (1994), for instance, used CVA successfully to capture distinct processes of land cover change operating at distinct time scales, by using NOAA AVHRR imagery and applying the technique to three RS indices of land cover: vegetation, temperature, and landscape structure. Another powerful analytical approach to TSA involves principal component analysis (PCA). When PCA is applied to time series images, it can serve to array the sources of change in order of most to least significant. Eastman and Fulk (1993), for instance, applied PCA to examine vegetation changes over a 3-year period in Africa. They found that the first standardized principal component captured the typical NDVI signal over the time period for the region, while successive components described changes in the NDVI signal over the period (with components 2–4 summarizing seasonal changes, 5–6 capturing satellite orbital shifts, and 7–8 depicting rainfall anomalies related to the 1987 El Niño/Southern Oscillation).

Categorical change detection is appropriate if images are not atmospherically and radiometrically corrected, or if the primary research objective is to assess changes in locally relevant land use/cover categories rather than continuous cover indices. In this case, each image is geometrically corrected and subjected to unsupervised, supervised or hybrid classification (with comparable/identical target classes in each time), following which a post-classification comparison is performed using GIS overlays. The categorical change detection produces a third, transition image depicting spatial changes along with a transition matrix indicating the frequencies of transitions from classes in date 1 to those in date 2. For instance, a pixel classified as forest in date 1 and herbaceous cover in date 2 can be interpreted to reflect deforestation, while the reverse may indicate reforestation. Inconsistencies in transition matrices and images may appear because of differences in geocorrection (pixels in some parts of the image may not match exactly between dates), or classification error (similar pixels classified differently in each date, or impossible transitions, such as a pixel of bare soil transitioning to dense forest in 5 years). It is worth remembering that spatial errors compound multiplicatively with data integration: two land cover maps of 90 percent overall classification accuracy, when overlaid for change detection, will yield a transition image whose accuracy may not exceed 81 percent overall.

Understanding and analyzing land patterns/change

Research in environmental anthropology focuses on multiple spatio-temporal processes of human–environment interaction. RS and GIS tools have the potential to aid in the analysis of causal, contextual, and cognitive realms of these interactions. Many anthropologists, particularly archaeologists, are interested on the study of spatial patterns (e.g., the distribution of land cover and settlement classes across landscapes) and the processes structuring them. One may seek to understand factors affecting land use decision-making, and changes in population, environment, food supply, technology, and productivity relationships (Hunt 1995: 176–177). Land change studies are frequently concerned with the extent, direction, and rate of land use/cover change across multiple units/scales of analysis (e.g., buffer zones, farm lots, settlements, community areas, indigenous reserves, municipalities, etc.). Spatially explicit GIS models are frequently used to explore causal relationships (e.g., Evans and Moran 2002; Roy Chowdhury 2006), permitting the examination of space and time as variables in human–environment interaction. For instance, the distribution of cultural artifacts and/or land use patterns may be analyzed in relation to varying "bins" (classes) of spatial variables derived in GIS, such as concentric/nested zones of varying widths from a river, road or another feature of interest, distinct elevation classes, etc. Such secondary data are readily produced from primary spatial layers (e.g., elevation models, river networks) with basic GIS tools for distance and buffer generation and attribute data reclassification.

Historically, however, anthropologists have used RS and GIS to gain a comparative perspective of how these processes unfold in distinct social/environmental contexts (Reining 1979). This interest continues today, investigating complex questions regarding the location, association, and spatial-historical contexts within which human groups, settlements, biophysical resources, and infrastructure influence each other over time (Guyer *et al.* 2007; Hirsch and O'Hanlon

1995; Pinedo-Vasquez *et al* 2002). Within such contexts, geospatial technologies can offer ancillary help (e.g., locating a village within a large region, or considering rural–urban linkages). They also offer empirical datasets and analytical power (e.g., cross-referencing kinship alliances and the organization of territories, or assessing agricultural intensification/disintensification in the context of regional transformations).

Anthropologists concerned with environmental cognition are increasingly using geospatial tools to represent local environmental perceptions, local topology (designation of places/features and their interrelations), and symbolic meanings. Ethnoecological methods have long provided tools to relate etic and emic views of landscapes and land use systems, and understanding how social groups understand, materially and symbolically, their local and regional landscapes. These tools can range from ethnohistorical descriptions of landscapes, to ethnobotanical knowledge, and the construction of agricultural calendars and symbolic representations of territories. These methods, in conjunction with GIS and RS tools, can now aid in the development of classification systems, image interpretation, and resource mapping in general.

CONCLUDING REMARKS: ETHICAL ISSUES, REPRESENTATION, AND CHALLENGES IN SPATIAL-TEMPORAL ANALYSIS

The challenges of incorporating geospatial technologies in anthropological and social sciences have not been ordinary (Behrens 1994; Fox *et al.* 2003; Goodchild and Janelle 2004; Liverman *et al.* 1998; NAS 2007). While GIS/RS tools have enabled anthropologists to scale up their research from local to regional scales and engage with applied problems, they have simultaneously raised theoretical, methodological, and ethical issues. Rindfuss and Stern (1998) summarized some of these issues within the social sciences as related to (sub)disciplinary differences in favored perspectives and variables, such as how to bridge "why" questions about the underlying basis of human behavior with those examining the manifestations of that behavior ("where," "when" and "how much"). Another important challenge lies in reconciling alternative classifications of the environment emanating from distinct cognitive and cultural standpoints (Hirsh and O'Hanlon 1995).

Whether intentionally or not, RS and GIS convene different forms of representation of people and their landscapes, rendering some aspects visible and others invisible (Pickles 1995; Porro 2000; Turner and Taylor 2003). The nature of these problems can be related to the spatial, temporal, and spectral resolution of the data. For instance, while subtle land use systems (e.g., small-scale swidden agroforestry) can be difficult to detect and measure or most likely be identified as something else (e.g., fallow vegetation), clear cut deforestation may be readily apparent in an image (Brondízio 2004). This renders some aspects of land use of the same farmer visible, and others invisible, possibly leading one to draw very different conclusions from the same data. Likewise, the temporal availability of data (i.e., date of acquisition, quality, and seasonality) may allow one to capture a particular set of activities (e.g., the growing season of a crop) or not (e.g., the fallow season).

Another dimension of the problem relates to the way different land use systems and social groups are classified/named. The categorical nature of land classifications inevitably masks some degree of internal variability (e.g., a general class of "forest" may actually encompass several forest types). Nested classification systems and/or continuous indices of land cover, as discussed earlier, are important to address such problems. A related challenge in the development of classification systems is the mismatch between technical definitions of land use and cover classes (e.g., using parameters from vegetation ecology, forestry, and agronomy) and the definition and conceptualization used by local stakeholders. Local populations tend to use multiple ecological and/or social criteria to describe landscape features, and are usually more cognizant of their heterogeneity. Robbins and Maddock (2004), for instance, demonstrate empirically how the selection of externally imposed expert classification versus in-situ cover categories derived from local knowledge result in fundamentally different depictions of land cover in Rajasthan, India. They argue persuasively for recognizing the socially constructed nature of land covers, and that "categories are theory-laden metaphors and occur epistemologically prior to any clustering algorithm" (Robbins and Maddock 2004).

Additional ethical issues pertain to the sharing of data and knowledge, and the publication of sensitive information of high spatial/temporal detail. These challenges extend to broader uses of geospatial data, as highlighted in a publication of the National Research Council of the National Academy of Sciences (NAS 2007). Images and maps represent a form of power: selected sectors have access to that power (e.g., datasets), and fewer still have the ability to manipulate it (e.g., represent or transform them). Geospatial data can be used to assert one's territory over another, to formalize ownership, to show the distribution of valuable resources revealed by local knowledge, or to portray illegal activities or settlements which may endanger local people directly or indirectly. Thus, anthropologists and other professionals need to carefully consider their choices depicting and/or describing thematic classes, locations of particular features and social-ecological relationships. As maps and images can serve to assert power or as incriminatory "evidence," there is growing attention to the ethics of their publication.

To some extent, and for some areas, Google Earth and other internet sources may have rendered moot concerns over spatial data privacy. Anthropologists cannot assume that these data have a neutral quality, however. In the 1990s, a period of heated debate ensued between GIS practitioners and critics over the ethics of geographic information technologies and positivism in general (Schuurman 2000). This eventually led to improved collaboration between the two groups, more nuanced critiques, and the inception of Initiative 19 of the National Center for Geographic Information and Analysis (NCGIA) focused on the social and ethical dimensions of geographic information technology. Both Initiative 19 and the NAS report cited above provide valuable guidelines regarding ethical issues in geospatial technologies and GIS/RS research (NAS 2007), emphasizing, among other factors, data sharing and the protection of vulnerable subjects. The sharing of data should be an essential part of all phases of a research project using RS and GIS. Research questions should design participatory elements for greater local relevance, applicability, and salience. Whenever possible, researchers should provide copies of relevant GIS databases as well, thus aiding local applications, management and empowerment. Wherever data sharing or publication are involved, professional guidelines pertaining to the protection of human subjects should be strictly adhered to[5] to protect the confidentiality and security of sensitive information embedded in the data or at any level of analysis.

Finally, it is important that users understand clearly the trade-offs embedded in the type, use and manipulation of spatial data. This chapter provided an introductory overview of their use in environmental anthropology. This process requires collaboration and commitment

[5] Among many techniques used to protect human subjects and hinder the manipulation of sensitive datasets are: data aggregation, substitution of names by IDs, protection of sensitive locations and association between personal data and location, purposely misrepresenting location and sampled units, among others.

to overcome the often steep learning curve involved with each stage of expertise development. The rewards, however, are worth the effort. In the context of global environmental change and the growing spatial and functional connectivity of landscapes, resource use systems, economies, and social groups, RS and GIS will continue to assume a central role in human–environmental research.

APPENDIX

Sites of interest

ACT (Anthropological Center for Training and Research on Global Environmental Change), http://www.indiana.edu/~act

Basic Science and Remote Sensing Initiative, Michigan State University, http://www.bsrsi.msu.edu

Center for Spatially Integrated Social Sciences (CSISS), http://www.csiss.org

CIPEC, Indiana University, http://www.cipec.org

Earth Explorer, http://edcsns17.cr.usgs.gov/EarthExplorer/

Earth Science data on the Global land information system, http://earthexplorer.usgs.gov

ERDAS IMAGINE, http://www.erdas.com/

FAO, http://WWW.fao.org/

Global Observation Information Network (GOIN) Project, http://www.nnic.noaa.gov/GOIN/GOIN.html

INPE (Instituto Nacional de Pesquisas Espaciais, Brasil), http://www.inpe.br

Multispec (Purdue/LARS), http://dynamo.ecn.purdue.edu/~biehl/MultiSpec/

NASA Remote Sensing Tutorial, Nicholas Short, http://rst.gsfc.nasa.gov/ http://www.Landsat.org

National Spatial Data Infrastructure, http://www.cas.sc.edu/geog/rslab/Rscc/mod3/3-3/3-3.html

Spot Image, French SPOT Satellite Images, http://www.spot.com/

UNEP/GRID, http://www.grida.no/

Selected list of specialized remote sensing and GIS journals

Photogrammetric Engineering and Remote Sensing; International Journal of Remote Sensing; Remote Sensing of Environment; Geocarto International; Canadian Journal of Remote Sensing; Remote Sensing Review; GIScience and Remote Sensing;

Cartography and Geographic Information Systems; International Journal of Geographical Information Science; Transactions in GIS; Journal of Geographical Systems; GeoInformatica.

REFERENCES

Aldenderfer, M. and H. Maschner, eds. 1992. *The Anthropology of Human Behavior Through Geographic Information Analysis.* Proceedings of conference held at the University of California at Santa Barbara, February 1–2, 1992.

Anderson, J., E. E. Hardy, J. T. Roach and R. E. Witmer 1976. *A land use and land cover classification system for use with remote sensor data.* Washington: Geological Survey Professional Paper 964.

Behrens, C. 1992. A formal justification for the application of GIS to the culture ecological analysis of land use intensification and deforestation in the Amazon. In M. Aldenderfer and H. Maschner, orgs., *The Anthropology of Human Behavior Through Geographic Information Analysis.* University of California at Santa Barbara, February 1–2, 1992.

Behrens C. A., ed. 1994. Recent advances in the regional analysis of indigenous land use and tropical deforestation, special issue of *Human Ecology* **22**(3): 243–247.

Boucek, B. and E. F. Moran 2004. Inferring the behavior of households from remotely sensed changes in land cover. Current methods and future directions. In M. F. Goodchild, and D. G Janelle, eds., *Spatially Integrated Social Science.* Oxford, UK: Oxford University Press, 23–47.

Brondízio, E. S. 2004. Agriculture intensification, economic identity, and shared invisibility in Amazonian peasantry: Caboclos and colonists in comparative perspective. *Culture and Agriculture* **26**(1 and 2): 1–24.

Brondízio, E. S. 2005. Intraregional analysis in the Amazon. In E. F. Moran, and E. Ostrom, eds., *Seeing the Forest and the Trees: Human–Environment Interactions in Forest Ecosystems.* Cambridge, MA: MIT Press, pp. 223–252.

Brondízio, E. S. 2006. Landscapes of the past, footprints of the future: historical ecology and the analysis of land use change in the Amazon. In W. Balée and C. Erikson, eds., *Time and Complexity in Historical Ecology: Studies in the Neotropical Lowlands.* New York: Columbia University Press, pp. 365–405.

Brondízio, E. S. 2008. *The Amazonian Caboclo and the Açaí palm: Forest Farmers in the Global Market.* New York: New York Botanical Garden Press

Brondízio, E. S., S. Fiorini, and R. Adams n.d. Environmental Anthropology. In UNESCO *Encyclopedia of Life Support Systems, Cultural Anthropology.* Paris, France: UNESCO. Available online: http://www.eolss.net/eolss_sitemap.aspx.

Brondízio, E. S., E. F. Moran, P. Mausel, and Y. Wu, 1994. Land use change in the Amazon estuary: patterns of Cabloco settlement and landscape management. *Human Ecology* **22**(3): 249–278.

Brondízio, E. S., E. Ostrom, and O. Young 2009. Connectivity and the governance of multilevel socio-ecological systems: the role of social capital. *Annual Review of Environment and Resources.* **34**: 253–78.

Conant, F. P. 1978. The use of Landsat data in studies of human ecology. *Current Anthropology* **19**: 382–384.

Conant, F. P. 1984. Remote sensing, discovery and generalizations in human ecology. In E. F. Moran, ed., *The Ecosystem Concept in Anthropology.* Boulder, CO: Westview Press.

Conant, F. P. 1994. Human ecology and space age technology: some predictions. *Human Ecology* **22**(3): 405–413.

Conklin, H. C. 1980. *Ethnographic Atlas of Ifugao: A Study of Environment, Culture and Society in Northern Luzon*. New Haven, CN: Yale University Press.

Cultural Survivor 1995. *Geomatics. Cultural Survival Quartely*, Winter 1995.

D'Antona, A. O., A. D. Cak, and L. VanWey. 2008. Collecting sketch maps to understand property land use and land cover in large surveys. *Field Methods* **20**(1): 66–84.

DeCastro, F., M. C. Silva-Fosberg, W. Wilson, and E. Brondízio, E. Moran 2002. The use of remotely sensed data in rapid rural assessment. *Field Methods* (formerly *Cultural Anthropology Methods*) **14**(3): 243–269.

Di Gregorio, A. and L. J. M. Jansen 2000. *Land Cover Classification System [LCCS]: Classification Concepts and User Manual*. Rome: Food and Agriculture Organization of the United Nations.

Eastman, J. R. and M. A. Fulk 1993. Long sequence time series evaluation using standardized principal components. *Photogrammetric Engineering and Remote Sensing* **59**(8): 1307–1312.

Evans, T. P. and E. F. Moran 2002. Spatial integration of social and biophysical factors related to landcover change. In W. Lutz, A. Frskawetz, and W. C. Sanderson, eds., *Population and Environment: Methods of Analysis* (A Supplement to Vol. 28, Population and Development Review), pp. 165–186.

Fairhead, J. and M. Leach 1995. Reading forest history backwards: the interaction of policy and local land use in Guinea's forest-savanna mosaic. *Environment & History* **1**(1): 55–92.

Fisher, C. and G. Feinman 2005. Introduction to "landscapes over time." *American Anthropologist*, **107**(1): 62–69.

Fox, J., V. Mishra, R. Rindfuss, and S. Walsh, eds. 2003. *People and the Environment: Approaches to Linking Household and Community Surveys to Remote Sensing and GIS*. Amsterdam: Kluwer Academic Press, pp. 223–240.

Galvin, K. A., R. B. Boone, N. M. Smith, and S. J. Lynn 2001. Impacts of climate variability on east African pastoralists: linking social science and remote sensing. *Climate Research* **19**: 161–172.

Geertz, C. (1963). *Agricultural Involution : The Process of Ecological Change in Indonesia*. Berkeley, CA: Published for the Association of Asian Studies by University of California Press.

Gibbons, A. 1991. A "new look" for archeology. *Science* **252**: 918–252.

Goodchild, M. F. and D. G. Janelle, eds. 2004. *Spatially Integrated Social Science*. Oxford, UK: Oxford University Press.

Green, G. M., C. M. Schweik, and J. C. Randolph 2005. Retrieving land-cover change information from Landsat satellite images by minimizing other sources of reflectance variability. In E. F. Moran, and E. Ostrom, eds., *Seeing the Forest and the Trees: Human-Environment Interactions in Forest Ecosystems*. Cambridge, MA: MIT Press, pp. 131–160.

Guyer J. I., E. F. Lambin, L. Cliggett, *et al* 2007. Temporal heterogeneity in the study of African land use interdisciplinary collaboration between anthropology, human geography and remote sensing. *Human Ecology* **35**: 3–17.

Heckenberger, M. J., A. Kuikuruo, U. T. Kuikuro, *et al.* 2003. Amazônia 1492: Pristine forest or cultural parkland? *Science*, **301**: 1710–1713.

Herlihy, P. H. and G. Knapp, eds. 2003. Maps of, by, and for the Peoples of Latin America. *Human Organization* **62**(4).

Hirsch, E. and M. O'Hanlon 1995. *The Anthropology of Landscape: Perspectives on Place and Space*. Oxford, UK: Oxford University Press.

Hunt, R. C. 1995. Agrarian data sets: the comparativist's view. In E. F. Moran, ed., *The Comparative Analysis of Human Societies: Toward Common Standards for Data Collection and Reporting*. Boulder, CO.: Lynne Rienner Publishers, pp. 173–189.

Janssen, L. L. F. and F. J. M. van der Wel 1994. Accuracy assessment of satellite derived land-cover data: a review. *Photogrammetric Engineering and Remote Sensing* 60(4): 419–426.

Jensen, J. 1996. *Introductory Digital Image Processing: A Remote Sensing Perspective*. Upper Saddle River, NJ: Prentice Hall (see online abbreviated version at http://www.r-s-c-c.org/).

John, C., ed. 1990. Proceedings of the symposium *Applications of Space-Age Technology in Anthropology*, John C. Stennis Space Center: NASA.

Jordan, C. F. 1969. Derivation of leaf-area index from quality of light on the forest floor. *Ecology* **50**: 663–666.

Kroeber, A. L. 1939. *Cultural and Natural Areas of Native North America*. Berkeley, CA: University of California Press.

Lambin, E. F. 2003. Linking socioeconomic and remote sensing data at the community or at the household level : two case studies from Africa. In J. Fox, V. Mishra, R. Rindfuss, and S. Walsh, eds., *People and the Environment: Approaches to Linking Household and Community Surveys to Remote Sensing and GIS*. Amsterdam: Kluwer Academic Press, pp. 223–240.

Lambin, E. F. and A. Strahler. 1994. Indicators of land-cover change for change-vector analysis in multitemporal space at coarse spatial scales. *International Journal of Remote Sensing* **15**(10): 2099–2119.

Lawrence, R. L. and W. J. Ripple 1998. Comparisons among vegetation indices and bandwise regression in a highly disturbed, heterogeneous landscape: Mount St. Helens, Washington. *Remote Sensing of Environment* **64**: 91–102.

Lillesand, T. and R. Keifer 1987. *Remote Sensing and Image Interpretation*. New York: John Wiley & Sons.

Liverman, D., E. Moran, R. Rindfuss and P. Stern, eds. 1998. *People and Pixels: Linking Remote Sensing and Social Science*. Washington DC: National Academy Press.

Lu, D., P. Mausel, E. Brondízio, and E. F. Moran. 2004a. Change detection techniques. *International Journal of Remote Sensing* **25**(12): 2365–2407.

Lu, D., P. Mausel, E. Brondízio, and E. F. Moran. 2004b. Relationships between forest stand parameters and Landsat TM spectral responses in the Brazilian Amazon Basin. *Forest Ecology and Management* **198**: 149–167.

Lyons, T. R. and T. E. Avery 1977. *Remote Sensing: A Handbook for Archeologists and Cultural Resource Managers*. Washington: Cultural Resources Management Division, National Park Service.

McCracken, S., E. Brondízio, D. Nelson, *et al* 1999. Remote sensing and GIS at farm property level: demography and deforestation in the Brazilian Amazon. *Photogrammetric Engineering and Remote Sensing* **65**(11): 1311–1320.

McIver, D. K. and M. A. Friedl. 2002. Using prior probabilities in decision-tree classification of remotely sensed data. *Remote Sensing of Environment* **81**(2–3): 253–261.

Maselli, F., C. Conese, A. Rodolfi, T. De Filippis, and L. Petkov 1994. Definition of multi-source prior probabilities for maximum likelihood classification of remotely sensed data. *Proceedings of the SPIE – The International Society for Optical Engineering* **2315**: 711–718.

Miller. D., N. Vogt, M. Nijnik, E. Brondízio, and S. Fiorini 2009. Integrating analytical and participatory techniques for planning the sustainable use of land resources and landscapes. In S. Geertman and J. Stillwell, eds., *Participatory Social Sciences*. Dordrecht, Netherlands: Springer Publishers, pp. 317–345.

Morain, S. 1998. A brief history of remote sensing applications, with emphasis on Landsat. In D. Liverman, E. Moran, R. Rindfuss, and P. Stern, eds., *People and Pixels: Linking Remote Sensing and Social Science*. Washington DC: National Academy Press, pp. 28–50.

Moran, E. and E. Brondízio 2001. Human ecology from space: ecological anthropology engages the study of global environmental change. In M. Lambek and E. Messer, eds., *Ecology and the Sacred: Engaging the Anthropology of Roy Rappaport*. Ann Arbor: University of Michigan Press, 64–87.

Moran, E. F. 1990. Levels of analysis and analytical level shifting: examples from Amazonian ecosystem research. In E. F. Moran, ed., *The Ecosystem Concept in Anthropology*. Ann Arbor, MI: Michigan University Press.

Moran, E. 1998. Remote sensing as a tool. *AAA Anthropology Newsletter*. November 1998.

National Academy of Sciences (NAS) 2002. *Earth Observations from Space: History, Promise, and Reality*. Washington, DC: National Academy Press.

National Academy of Sciences (NAS) 2007. Putting people on the map: Protecting confidentiality with linked social-spatial data. Washington, DC: National Academy Press.

Nyerges, E. A. and G. M. Green 2000. The Ethnography of Landscape: GIS and Remote Sensing in the Study of Forest Change in West African Guinea Savana. *American Anthropologist*. v. 102, n. 2, pp. 1–19 (for color figures see: http://www.cipec.org/publications/nyerges_and_green2000.html).

Ostrom, E. and H. Nagendra 2006. Inaugural Article: Insights on linking forests, trees, and people from the air, on the ground, and in the laboratory *Proceedings of the National Academy of Sciences* **103**: 19224–19231.

Pedroni, L. 2003. Improved classification of Landsat Thematic Mapper data using modified prior probabilities in large and complex landscapes. *International Journal of Remote Sensing* **24**(1): 91–113.

Pickles, J. 1995. *Ground Truth: The Social Implications of Geographic Information Systems*, New York: Guilford Press.

Pinedo-Vasquez, M., J. B Pasqualle, D. Del Castillo Torres, and K. Coffey 2002. A tradition of change: The dynamic relationship between biodiversity and society in sector Muyuy, Peru. *Environmental Science and Policy* **221**: 1–11.

Porro, R. 2000. *Reflections on the promises and perils of integrating remote sensing in anthropological research*. Paper awarded the R. Rappaport Prize in Ecological Anthropology by the "Anthropology and Environment" session of the American Anthropological Association.

Reining, P. 1979. *Challenging Desertification in West Africa: Insights from Landsat into Carrying Capacity, Cultivation, and Settlement Sites in Upper Volta and Niger*. Athens, GA: Center for International Studies, Ohio University.

Rindfuss, R. and P. Stern 1998. Linking remote sensing and social sciences: the need and the challenges. In D. Liverman, E. Moran, R. Rindfuss, and P. Stern, eds., *People and Pixels: Linking Remote Sensing and Social Science*. Washington DC: National Academy Press, pp. 1–27.

Robbins, P. and T. Maddock 2004. Interrogating land cover categories: metaphor and method in remote sensing. *Cartography and Geographic Information Science* **27**(4): 295–309.

Rondeaux, G., M. Steven, and F. Baret 1996. Optimization of soil-adjusted vegetation indices. *Remote Sensing of Environment* **55**: 95–107.

Rouse, J. W., R. H. Haas, J. A., Schell, D. W. Deering and J. C. Harlan 1973. Monitoring the vernal advancement and retrogradation (greenwave effect) of natural vegetation, NASA/GSFC Type III Final Report, Greenbelt, MD.

Roy Chowdhury, R. 2006. Landscape change in the Calakmul Biosphere Reserve, Mexico: modeling the driving forces of smallholder deforestation in land parcels. *Applied Geography* **26**(2): 129–152.

Roy Chowdhury, R. and L. C. Schneider. 2004. Land-cover/use in the southern Yucatán peninsular region, Mexico: classification and change analysis. In B. L. Turner II, J. Geoghegan, and D. Foster, eds. *Integrated Land-Change Science and Tropical Deforestation in the Southern Yucatán: Final Frontiers.* Oxford, UK: Clarendon Press, pp. 105–141.

Sader, S. A., T. Server, J. C. Smoot, and M. Richards. 1994. Forest change estimates for the Northern Peten region of Guatemala: 1986–1990. *Human Ecology* **22**(3): 317–332.

Schuurman, N. 2000. Trouble in the heartland: GIS and its critics in the 1990s. *Progress in Human Geography* **24**(4): 569–590.

Server, T. and J. Wiseman 1984. *Remote sensing and archeology: potential for the future.* Report on a Conference, March 1–2, 1984. Mississipi: Earth Resources Laboratory, NASA.

Singh, A. 1989. Digital change detection techniques using remotely sensed data. *International Journal of Remote Sensing* **10**(6): 989–1003.

Sirén, A. H. and E. S. Brondízio. 2009. Detecting subtle change in small-scale tropical forest shifting cultivation systems: methodological contributions integrating field and remotely-sensed data. *Applied Geography* **29**(2): 201–211.

Sirén, A. 2007. Population growth and land use intensification in a subsistence-based indigenous community in the Amazon. *Human Ecology* **35**: 669–680.

Steward, J. H. 1955. *Theory of Culture Change; The Methodology of Multilinear Evolution.* Urbana, IL: University of Illinois Press.

Stone, G. 1993. *Settlement Ecology.* Tucson, AZ: University of Arizona Press.

Tucker, C. 2005. Introduction to case studies. In E. F. Moran, and E. Ostrom, eds., *Seeing the Forest and the Trees: Human–Environment Interactions in Forest Ecosystems.* Cambridge, MA: MIT Press, pp. 215–222.

Turner, M. D. and P. J. Taylor 2003. Critical reflections on the use of remote sensing and GIS Technologies in human ecological research. *Human Ecology* **31**(2): 177–182.

Vayda, A. P., and B. J. McCay 1975. New directions in ecology and ecological anthropology. *Annual Review of Anthropology* **4**: 293–306.

Vayda, A. P. and Rappaport, R. 1968. Ecology, cultural and noncultural. In J. A. Clifton, ed., *Introduction to Cultural Anthropology: Essays in the Scope and Methods of the Science of Man.* Boston, MA: Houghton Mifflin, pp. xii, 564.

Walker P. A. and P. E. Peters 2007. Making sense in time: remote sensing and the challenges of temporal heterogeneity in social analysis of environmental change – cases from Malawi. *Human Ecology* **35** :69–80.

Wilkie, D. 1987. Cultural and ecological survival in the Ituri Forest: the role of accurately monitoring natural resources and agricultural land use. *Cultural Survival Quarterly* **11**(2): 72–74.

Wilkie, D. 1990. Protecting rain forests and forager's rights using Landsat imagery. In C. John, ed., Conference Proceedings *Applications of Space-Age Technology in Anthropology.* John C. Stennis Space Center.

Wilkie, D. 1996. *Remote Sensing Imagery for Natural Resources Monitoring: A Guide for First-time Users.* New York: Columbia University Press.

13

Deep time, diachronic change, and the integration of multi-scalar data: archaeological methods for exploring human–environment dynamics

EMILY LENA JONES

INTRODUCTION

Over the past 25 years, the environmental science literature has increasingly affirmed that contemporary environments are a product of their long-term histories (e.g., Foster 2000). This growing realization in the ecological community has led to a corresponding interest in histories of human–environment interaction, and thus, archaeological data (Hayashida 2005; Kirch 2005). Archaeologists have long been interested in connections between environment and society; the sub-field known as "environmental archaeology" is entirely devoted to this area of research. Environmental studies and archaeology are a natural fit: archaeological studies provide diachronic data on environmental change, and can be critical for evaluating claims of human response to or influence on these changes. Likewise, the focus of archaeology on the material components of human–environment interaction provides a perspective often missing in more ideological studies of society and environment. Archaeologists have long argued the relevance of archaeological data for environmental studies (Fritz 1973; Lyman and Cannon 2004; Wintemberg 1919); in recent decades, collaborations between archaeologists and environmental scientists have become

Environmental Social Sciences: Methods and Research Design, ed. I. Vaccaro, E. A. Smith and S. Aswani. Published by Cambridge University Press. © Cambridge University Press 2010.

increasingly common (Burgi and Russell 2001; Schimmelmann, Lange, and Meggers 2003). Current areas of interest within archaeology, such as niche construction (Banks *et al.* 2008; Smith 2007) and the impact of abrupt environmental change (i.e., Dansgaard *et al.* 1993) should facilitate such collaborations.

This chapter summarizes archaeological methods relevant to the study of human–environment dynamics, and then turns to examples of the use of archaeological data to address environmental questions.

"ENVIRONMENTAL ARCHAEOLOGY": THE ARTIFACT-BASED METHODS

Though archaeological interest in human–environment dynamics goes back to the origins of the discipline, the term "environmental archaeology" is relatively new, and somewhat problematic. In its broadest use, the term is methodological: it refers to the development and application of techniques for extracting and interpreting data from archaeological remains related to the environment, especially plant remains, animal bones, and archaeological soils (e.g., Albarella 2001; Reitz, Scarry, and Scudder, 2008); I follow this usage here.

Methodological environmental archaeology is generally split into subfields, based on the particular type of artifact or "ecofact" under consideration. The fields of paleoethnobotany (study of plant remains from archaeological sites), geoarchaeology (study of archaeological sediments), and zooarchaeology (study of animal remains from archaeological sites) are all subfields of environmental archaeology. In addition to the analysis of remains from archaeological sites, these specialists also frequently use data from off-site contexts to obtain a more accurate understanding of human decision-making within the wider environment. The environmental archaeology subdisciplines have followed parallel trajectories over the past quarter century, gradually moving from an appendix in excavation reports to center stage.

Though their histories and position within the larger discipline of archaeology are similar, the differences between the subdisciplines make integration of the data generated from them awkward at best and impossible at worst. The environmental archaeology subdisciplines can be lumped together as analytical methods that can be used within archaeology to pursue questions pertaining to human–environment dynamics, but they are distinct from each other in at least two ways. First, the skills needed for analysis in each of these subdisciplines are fundamentally different. A zooarchaeologist, for example, needs to be well-versed in skeletal biology, zoology, and archaeology, while a paleoethnobotanist needs detailed botanical knowledge. Though some methods cross-cut these subdisciplines – notably, stable carbon isotope analysis is used on animal bone to investigate human subsistence practices (Szpak, Orchard, and Grocke 2009), and on soils to investigate landscape use (Wright, Terry, and Eberl 2009) – the application of such methods varies with the subject of analysis. As a result, though all can be termed "environmental archaeologists," geoarchaeologists, paleoethnobotanists, and zooarchaeologists have undergone fundamentally different training, and produce data with different units of measurement and from different temporal scales (Papagianni, Layton, and Maschner 2008).

The subdisciplines also frequently differ in their goals. Each has goals (as well as theories and methods) drawn from sister disciplines in the natural sciences as well as from archaeology and anthropology. The changing role of the subdisciplines in archaeological research is affected not only by shifts in archaeological research trends but by shifts in anthropology and in the natural sciences (Holliday 2001; Pearsall 2000; Reitz and Wing 2008).

GEOARCHAEOLOGY

Geoarchaeology is arguably the environmental archaeology subdiscipline most integrated with archaeology as a whole. Most archaeologists have some training in the application of geological methods to archaeological contexts, as most subjects of archaeological study are recovered from sediments. Certain types of paleoethnobotanical and zooarchaeological research are sometimes considered geoarchaeological methods, because the remains are recovered from soil samples. Geoarchaeology is also the broadest of the environmental archaeology subdisciplines; Rapp and Hill, for example, define geoarchaeology as "the application of any earth science concept, technique, or knowledge base to the study of artifacts and the processes involved in the creation of the archaeological record" (Rapp and Hill 2006: 1). This discussion will focus on two aspects of geoarchaeological research: sedimentary contexts and geochemical analyses. Many other techniques are excluded here to conserve space and because they are less directly applicable to analyses of human–environment interactions.

Sedimentary analyses in geoarchaeology focus on using the attributes of archaeological sediments to infer environments. By analyzing the attributes of sediments (color, grain size and shape, composition, etc.), geoarchaeologists can provide information about the conditions under which those sediments were deposited. Brown (2009), for example, uses an auger survey (a technique which involves systematically coring an area and describing the sediments returned from those cores) to describe soil variation in the Midlands of England; by comparing these data with archaeological and documentary data on agricultural practices, he draws conclusions about the impact of medieval land use on floodplain development. Sedimentary analyses and description have likewise been used to identify archaeological responses to El Niño events in prehistoric Peru (Sandweiss *et al.* 2009). Micromorphology, or the study of sediments in thin-section, assisted by magnification, is particularly useful in identifying anthropogenic disturbances (Courty 2001; Davidson, Carter, and Quine 1992).

Geochemical analyses rely on the fact that human activities alter the presence of particular elements in soil. In this type of study, the area of interest is typically cored in a systematic manner, and the chemical profiles of these cores are compared with those from nearby off-site profiles. Human activity might be indicated in a number of ways: wood burning, for instance, raises the amount of magnesium in the soil, while elevated levels of phosphates, barium, and manganese can indicate refuse areas (Rapp and Hill 2006). These methods have been used extensively in site prospection, but can also be used to identify human impacts on soils (Oonk, Slomp, and Huisman 2009; Spangenberg *et al.* 2008).

PALEOETHNOBOTANY

As with geoarchaeology, the term paleoethnobotany – generally used to mean the study of plant remains from archaeological sites – covers a large number of techniques. Plant remains in archaeological sites include macroremains, phytoliths, and pollen.

Macroremains are botanical remains large enough to be visible to the naked eye, such as charcoal, plant seeds, and shells. They are either recovered during excavation (in situ or through screening) or through flotation (the separation of organic remains from archaeological soils using water), and are then identified using magnification. Both preservation and recovery issues significantly affect interpretations of plant macroremains, but despite this, these remains can be extraordinarily helpful in addressing questions of human–environment interactions. Charcoal, for example, has been used to identify the prehistoric management of olive trees (Terral 2000); plant macrofossils are critical components of arguments for anthropogenically induced landscape transformation, particularly on islands (Burney *et al.* 2001; Hannon and Bradshaw 2000); and the study of tree rings from wood samples (dendroarchaeology) are used to investigate climate variability and human response in a number of regions (Simchoni and Kislev 2009; Towner 2002).

Both phytolith (plant silicate) analysis and palynology (or pollen analysis) are sometimes grouped in geoarchaeology, because these plant remains are typically recovered from soil samples. Phytoliths are rigid, microscopic bodies produced by many plants, especially grasses. Once recovered from soil samples, these can be identified to species. Phytoliths preserve well, particularly in soils that are unfavorable for pollen preservation; they are typically used to help reconstruct paleoenvironments, though the bias towards grasses means that phytoliths cannot be used to obtain a broad overview of vegetation (Neumann *et al.* 2009). The persistence of phytoliths, however, allows for reliable insight into the relative abundance of particular species through time.

Although there are biases towards specific plant families in the pollen record, these are not as severe as in phytolith analysis; thus pollen is more commonly used to obtain the "whole flora" of a particular time period. Pollen can be recovered either from archaeological sites or from contexts with accumulating sediments (i.e., bogs or lakes; this is known as stratigraphic palynology). Stratigraphic palynology is widely used in environmental reconstruction, to establish both the relative frequency of different types of vegetation and the presence of landscape disturbances, such as burning. Archaeological palynology is subject to a wide variety of problems (for a detailed discussion, see Pearsall 2000); however, the recovery of archaeological pollen from human coprolites (preserved feces) has provided direct evidence of human–plant interaction (Horrocks *et al.* 2004). Coprolites can be sources of both macroremains and phytoliths for analysis as well.

Finally, starch residue analysis (Barton 2007; Piperno *et al.* 2000; Piperno *et al.* 2004) is a promising research direction within paleoethnobotany; this technique identifies microscopic starch grains on the surfaces of widely preserved archaeological remains such as ceramics and tools.

ZOOARCHAEOLOGY

Of the methodologically oriented subdisciplines, zooarchaeology has arguably been the most successful at integrating a variety of data in the service of larger questions about environment and society. A search of articles related to archaeology published in the last 10 years in the journal *Conservation Biology* turned up 10 results; of these, all referred either directly or indirectly to zooarchaeological data, while only one discussed paleoethnobotanical data. Geoarchaeological, paleoethnobotanical, and other environmental archaeology methods are by no means unrepresented (see review in Hayashida 2005), but the volume of the zooarchaeological literature dwarfs other contributions.

Zooarchaeologists count the number of identifiable osseous remains in an assemblage, resulting in the NISP, or number of individual identifiable specimens, in each taxonomic group identified. Ideally this would produce the NISP per species, but often specimens can only be identified to genus, or sometimes only to size class (e.g., "small mammal"). Other measures, such as MNI (minimum number of individuals) may be derived from the initial NISP counts. Although various factors may influence which measure a zooarchaeologist uses in a particular analysis, none of these measures reliably estimate the number of individual animals per species or even the estimated contribution of a particular species to the overall diet (Grayson 1984b; Reitz and Wing 2008). For this reason, zooarchaeologists often conduct analyses based on measures of relative abundance, and focus on the ways in which the representation of different species change through time. Figure 13.1, for example, shows the changing representation of wild European rabbit (*Oryctolagus cuniculus*) through time at the archaeological site of Pont d'Ambon (after Jones 2006).

Data such as shown in Figure 13.1 are generally included in a larger analysis, designed to answer an overarching question. Zooarchaeological data have been used to provide paleoenvironmental information (e.g., Delpech 1999); to show how humans intensified use of particular taxa in response to exogenous (Jones 2009; Munro 2004) or anthropogenically induced (Butler and Campbell 2004; Jones *et al.* 2008b) change; and to identify the presence of domesticated animals and associated changes in human subsistence and land use (Frachetti and Mar'yashev 2007; Marom and Bar-Oz 2009; Pavao-Zuckerman 2007), among others.

An extremely productive line of zooarchaeological research has resulted from the use of foraging models drawn from human behavioral ecology. Human behavioral ecology uses models, originally developed to analyze the behavior of non-human animals, to study human behavioral diversity (Winterhalder and Smith 2000). These models have been successfully adapted to address issues of prey choice, dietary

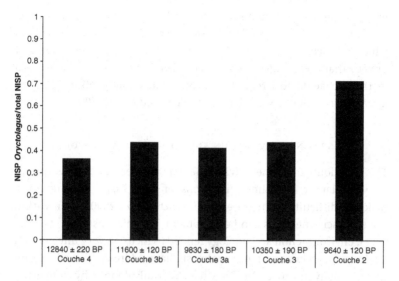

Figure 13.1   Relative abundance of the wild European rabbit (*Oryctolagus cuniculus*) at the archaeological site of Pont d'Ambon, southwestern France (Jones 2006).

shifts, and responses to exogenous environmental change, among other topics (Bird, Bliege Bird, and Codding 2009; Bliege Bird and Bird 2008; Hawkes and O'Connell 1992; Koster 2008; Smith 1991).

Archaeological work on human behavioral ecological topics has grown steadily since the 1970s (Lupo 2007; Winterhalder and Smith 2000). This approach has brought robust theory and an ecological approach to a wide variety of classic archaeological questions: for example, residential mobility and settlement patterns (Waters 2006; Zeanah 2000), transport costs (Metcalf and Barlow 1992), resource intensification (James 2004; Nagaoka 2005), domestication and agriculture (Cannon 2000; Kohler 2004), trade and resource sharing (O'Connell, Hawkes, and Jones 1999; Rautman 1996), and "showing off" and the sexual division of labor (Broughton and Bayham 2003; Hildebrandt and McGuire 2003). Human behavioral ecology has provided a perspective from which zooarchaeologists have been able to explore prehistoric conservation, impacts on the environment, and landscape management.

Optimal foraging theory has been especially productive in supporting investigations of impacts of prehistoric peoples on their environments (Lupo 2007), providing both a theoretical framework and allowing the development of testable hypotheses about how humans

might impact environments (Grayson and Cannon 1999). Many archaeologists have demonstrated that resource depression, or a situation in
which the activities of a predator result in reduced capture rates of
prey by that predator (Charnov, Orians, and Hyatt 1976), is widespread
in the archaeological record (e.g., Butler and Campbell 2004; Dean
2007; Grayson 2001; Nagaoka 2006; Stiner and Munro 2002).

INTEGRATING DATA WITHIN ENVIRONMENTAL ARCHAEOLOGY

The positioning of the environmental archaeology subdisciplines
between larger disciplines, in terms of both goals and methods,
makes it difficult to integrate data sets (Dincauze 2000). Even within
the subdisciplines, this can be a problem. For this reason, in its early
years, environmental archaeology tended to focus on very fine-grained
analysis. Environmental archaeologists have addressed broader questions in many instances, but they have typically done so by comparing
results from their particular specialty to larger-scale environmental
data, rather than by integrating data from across the subdisciplines.

Despite this difficulty, in at least some cases, environmental
archaeologists have found ways to integrate a variety of data in service of a larger research question. For example, in a zooarchaeological study identifying a decline in sooty shearwater (*Puffinus griseus*)
remains at the Minard Site on the southern Washington coast, Bovy
considered data on changing representation of species (drawn from
her own zooarchaeological study), climate, earthquake, land surface,
and sea-level history (drawn from separate geoarchaeological studies)
together (Bovy 2007). This allowed for an investigation of whether climate change, human predation, or some other factor was responsible
for the decline.

Such integration of data is easier when the data are all drawn
from a single site. The archaeological record is formed through a combination of cultural activity and post-depositional processes. Teasing
out the effects of these processes on the archaeological record is
fundamental to the analysis of past human behavior; without understanding the impacts of post-depositional processes, it is impossible to
identify which patterns are due to human behavior. Though post-depositional processes can vary considerably even within an archaeological
site, these differences are magnified across sites, thus hampering the
integration of multi-site data.

When considering change through time at a particular site, the
basic unit of time used in analysis is almost always the stratigraphic

layer. Except in rare cases, each layer in an archaeological site is a palimpsest, a time-averaged deposit that represents separate and repeated episodes of occupation. Layers thus represent variable amounts of time.

Despite these problems, some environmental archaeologists have managed to integrate data across sites and regions in specific, well-dated circumstances. Grayson and colleagues, for instance, correlated increased dominance of reindeer at the Paleolithic site of Grotte XVI, in southwestern France, with reconstructed temperatures based on pollen analyses from eastern France (Grayson *et al.* 2001). This sort of integration can only be done with extreme care, as the authors discuss:

> We could not be more aware of the hazards involved in correlating the Grotte XVI Upper Paleolithic faunal sequence with Guiot's temperature curve in this fashion. This is especially true since Guiot's curve has been dated in very much the same way. We are, in essence, comparing one set of age estimates with another. Nonetheless, we observe that if temperature extremes are driving the evenness decline at Grotte XVI, we expect to see that the assemblages involved intersect the temperature curve at ever-decreasing values ... [T]hey do exactly that. (Grayson *et al.* 2001: 122)

In other words, though integration of data is sometimes possible, problems in either dataset can be compounded when datasets are integrated.

MOVING BEYOND THE SITE: LANDSCAPE ARCHAEOLOGY

Though research in environmental archaeology sometimes integrates different types of data to answer questions about environment and society, these data generally derive from an individual site, or sometimes a group of sites. In contrast, landscape studies attempt to reconstruct human–environment interactions on a scale comparable to how prehistoric people would have experienced their environment; the difference in scale is why landscape archaeology is typically considered separate from environmental archaeology. Many researchers who are involved in landscape archaeology are also specialists in one of the "environmental archaeology" subdisciplines (Jones 2007; Roos, Sullivan III, and McNamee, 2010); paleoethnobotanists have been especially active in landscape-oriented research (Dean 2004; Delcourt and Delcourt 2004; Newsom and Pearsall 2003). These studies are set apart from work in the environmental archaeology subdisciplines by their use of multiple types of data (for instance, zooarchaeology, settlement analysis, palynology) and their synthetic goals (i.e., Doolittle 2006; Gunn *et al.* 2004).

Quantitatively oriented landscape archaeology studies often start with a database of archaeological deposits, dates, and attributes (such as the presence/absence of particular pollen types, animal or plant species, or artifacts). A researcher interested in the role of fire in shaping a particular landscape, for instance, might construct a database containing information on site locations, any dated material associated with those sites, and the presence/absence of charcoal in the palynological profile. GIS software might be used to display the spatial extent of sites containing palynological charcoal in particular time periods and across a particular region. Roos Sullivan and McNamee (2010) used this approach in their study of relationships between prehistoric indigenous societies, climate change, and fire regimes in Southwestern ponderosa pine forests; the combination of geoarchaeological and paleoethnobotanical data with spatial analysis provided a powerful tool for understanding the sustainability of indigenous burning regimes in this environment.

Zooarchaeological data can likewise be incorporated into larger studies of landscape use. Researchers have for years postulated a population crash at the Pleistocene-Holocene transition in the Dordogne region of southwestern France, as the reindeer population in this region (presumed to be the dietary base of the prehistoric hunter-gatherers of the Dordogne) was extirpated. A comparison of the shifting location and faunal composition of archaeological sites during this time period, however, suggests that this was not the case (Jones 2007). Instead of following the reindeer herds north, the combined site location and zooarchaeological data suggest that people switched their resource base.

These two examples both highlight the contributions of quantitatively oriented landscape archaeology to the study of human–environment interactions. It is important to note that a more qualitative school of landscape archaeology is active as well, particularly in Great Britain. These cognitive landscape archaeologists aim to reconstruct people's experience of prehistoric landscapes through techniques such as viewshed analysis and virtual reality (Darvill 2008). Both the qualitative and quantitative schools of landscape archaeology have provided important insights into the way in which prehistoric peoples experienced their environments.

INTEGRATING DATA TO ANSWER LARGER QUESTIONS

Though both the environmental archaeology subdisciplines (Kuijt 2001; Sandweiss *et al.* 2009; Schmitt 2004; Terral 2000) and landscape archaeology (Buchanan, Collard, and Edinborough 2008; Diaz-Maroto and Vila-Lameiro 2008; List *et al.* 2007; Waters 2006) have been applied to questions of environment and society, the strengths of archaeological data can best be seen when integrated with other data sources. By combining various sorts of data – both archaeological and environmental – archaeology can contribute to larger questions about environment and society.

ANTHROPOGENICALLY DRIVEN EXTINCTIONS

Anthropogenically driven extinctions have been of interest for more than two centuries (Grayson 1984a), and the popularity of this topic shows no signs of abatement (Firestone *et al.* 2007; Grayson 2007, 2008; Haynes 2007; Jones *et al.* 2008a). Though anthropogenically induced extinctions and extirpations have been demonstrated in a variety of times and places (Morwood *et al.* 2008; Simmons 1999; Steadman, White, and Allen 1999; Wolff 2000), the larger and more enduring questions concerning extinctions are multi-faceted: under what circumstances do humans cause extinctions? Are extinctions more likely in island or continental settings? When faced with prey not adapted to human predation (i.e., large, flightless landbirds), will human hunting inexorably cause extinction, or is a combination of effects (such as landscape modification and impacts on other fauna) required for extinctions to take place? These questions are most commonly addressed in the most enduring debate on extinctions: that concerning the extinction of North American megafauna at the end of the Pleistocene.

Even prior to the widespread acceptance of human antiquity, researchers suggested that human hunting could be responsible for the extinctions of the suite of mammals that died out at the end of the Pleistocene. Once the scientific community was largely in accord that humans and the Pleistocene fauna had co-existed, this suggestion was widely accepted. Grayson writes:

> [T]he overkill hypothesis gained adherents because other hypotheses seemed inadequate. At the same time, a human role in the extinctions helped lessen the impact of the new realization that people had coexisted with Pleistocene mammals: extinction due to human

> activities was very clearly a part of the modern world … Those who remained convinced that the vicissitudes of the earth's surface had been of sufficient magnitude to account for the extinctions continued to reject the overkill hypothesis. (Grayson 1984a: 34)

The overkill hypothesis remains active (Haynes 2007), as does the hypothesis that climate change associated with the Pleistocene-Holocene transition was the responsible agent (Ugan and Byers 2008). These two standpoints have recently been joined by the extraterrestrial impact hypothesis, which posits that the extinctions resulted from the impact of one or more extraterrestrial objects (Firestone *et al.* 2007; but see Surovell *et al.* 2009). The publication of the extraterrestrial impact hypothesis has inspired new investigations considering how such an event might have combined with human hunting, landscape modification, and demography to impact Pleistocene biotas (Buchanan, Collard, and Edinborough 2008; Stewart and Cooper 2008).

I will not review the Pleistocene extinctions argument here (see Beck 1996; Grayson 2007, 2008; Martin 1967); however, this debate has been of great importance in the development of archaeology as a part of conservation biology. This was one of the first arguments since the development of ecology as a field of research that involved archaeological data in a discussion of significance to environmental science. It also is an early example of the use of archaeological data (particularly zooarchaeological and geoarchaeological data) in tandem with landscape-level archaeological analysis, paleontological data, and ecological theory. Arguments concerning Pleistocene extinctions may involve data on the presence/absence of species drawn from zooarchaeological and paleontological investigations; ecological information about the probable life history and behavior of those species; anthropological data about human hunting behavior; a consideration of the spatial distribution of the archaeological/paleontological assemblages in which the relevant species have been found; stratigraphic and other geoarchaeological contextual information; and a discussion of dates and the techniques through which the assemblages have been dated.

CULTURAL DIVERSITY AND OLD WORLD DOMESTICATES
IN THE AMERICAN SOUTHWEST

The Pleistocene extinctions debate is primarily an example of the integration of archaeological and ecological data; though ethnographic data on human hunting patterns is sometimes involved, it is generally

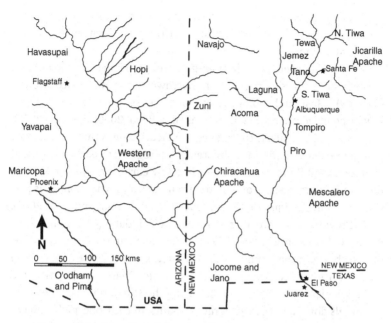

Figure 13.2   Ethnolinguistic groups in the American Southwest.

a minor component. Archaeological, historical and ethnographic data, however, can work well together to explore questions of subsistence decisions and transitions in more recent times (Pavao-Zuckerman 2007; Spielmann *et al.* 2009). An ongoing project investigating cultural diversity and subsistence choices in the American Southwest during the protohistoric is one example (Jones, Taylor, and Toland 2009). The Southwest has long been known as an area of exceptional diversity, in terms of both ethnolinguistic groups and subsistence adaptations (Figure 13.2; Jorgensen, 1983). Although Puebloan farming receives much of the attention in the literature, diverse foodways have been documented both among Puebloan groups and their less agriculturally oriented neighbors (Opler 1972; Thompson and Tsosie 2008).

Prior to AD 1350, the Four Corners was the domain of Ancestral Puebloans, who were primarily maize agriculturalists. Depopulation of the Four Corners, and concentration of Puebloan sites along the Rio Grande and other permanent water sources, began around AD 1280 and continued over the next 75 years. The reasons for this migration are complex: climate, and the end of an unusually wet period, certainly had something to do with it, but an increase in human population, deforestation, and other anthropogenically induced environmental impacts, such as erosion, and social factors may also have played a role. Regardless, by 1380 it appears that the Four Corners region was largely abandoned.

Sites that seem to be hunter–gatherer in origin start showing up in the Four Corners, particularly in northwestern New Mexico, around AD 1450. Most archaeologists attribute these sites to Athabaskan-speaking newcomers (Reed, Baugh, and Reed 2000; Towner 2000). Regardless of ethnicity, these sites are clearly the remains of people practicing a very different subsistence strategy from earlier ancestral Puebloans. While maize is present in a few early "Navajo" sites, most have a higher frequency of wild food remains, and where maize is present the maize ubiquity indices are low (Reed, Baugh, and Reed 2000).

Previously recorded zooarchaeological data (Goodman 2003; Hovezak, Sesler, and Fuller 2002) and data from an ongoing reanalysis of vertebrate fauna from Navajo-affiliated sites, suggest a change in resource use between Dinetah and Gobernador Phase Navajo-attributed archaeological sites (Figure 13.3). During the Dinetah phase, the small mammals dominate the vertebrate remains. In the Gobernador phase, large mammals are dominant. Despite the fact that the Navajo population was likely growing during this time period, there appears to have been an increase in the exploitation of large ungulates during the seventeenth century.

There are several possible explanations for this shift in dominance. The period between AD 1450 and 1650 was a turbulent one in the Southwest; it is possible that there was an increased availability of larger ungulates, due to a decreased Native American population as a result of introduced Spanish diseases, or to some other factor such as climate change. Historical records certainly suggest that disease may have played a role, though the impacts of disease in the less-populated parts of the Southwest are not well known (Barrett 2002). Ethnographic evidence might suggest that this shift is capturing the adoption of Old World domesticates, especially sheep, introduced by the Spanish but soon adopted by the Navajo and made central to Navajo subsistence (Thompson 2009; Weisiger 2004). The question of when, and to what degree, the Navajo adopted sheep herding remains under debate, as relatively few relevant faunal assemblages have been analyzed, and of those that have, the remains are heavily fragmented, making identification to the species level difficult. As sheep were left in the Southwest by Coronado in 1541, however, it is certainly plausible that the increase in large mammals reflects the growth of Navajo sheep herding.

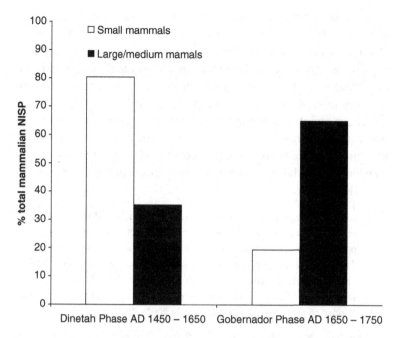

Figure 13.3   Relative abundance of large and small mammals in
Dinetah and Gobernador phase sites (Jones, Taylor, and Toland 2009).

Questions about sheep herding, its origins among the peoples
of the American Southwest, and its impact on landscapes are critical
to modern-day environmental management (Flanders 1998; Schelhas
2002). We are pursuing further zooarchaeological analysis of this question, focusing on the refitting of fragmented assemblages to aid in
identification to the species level. This work will allow us to assess the
hypotheses discussed above. Even at this stage, however, this example
shows how ethnographic and historical data related to human–environment interaction can be used to inform archaeological research
and suggests how archaeological data can be used to distinguish
among various hypotheses suggested by the ethnographic record.

ARCHAEOLOGICAL DATA AND STUDIES OF SOCIETY
AND ENVIRONMENT

While archaeological studies of the environment have a history that
goes back to the founding of the discipline, many archaeologists regard
archaeological data as underutilized by environmental scientists

(Etnier 2007; Lyman and Cannon 2004) and social scientists interested in society and environment (van der Leeuw and Redman 2002) alike. Much of this exclusion may be due to archeologists' traditional preoccupation with method: while formation studies and time-averaging are important issues to archaeologists, they are both hard to explain and not very interesting to non-archaeologists. Difficulties with explaining all the caveats implicit in the interpretation of archaeological data may also play a role, as archaeological studies on past environments have been used to support modern policy decisions with which those who published the studies would not necessarily agree (Hayashida 2005). Hayashida argues

> As archaeologists take a larger role in research relevant to current environmental and land-use issues, the intersection of research and public policy debate is inevitable. Others will use archaeological findings in ways we had not anticipated, in many cases misinterpreting or deliberately misusing them. Only by taking active roles can we shape how our research results are interpreted in public discourse and applied to policy outcomes. (Hayashida 2005: 57)

Archaeology has a long history of existing between disciplinary boundaries. If, however, archaeologists' vision of a discipline integral to environmental studies is to come to fruition, archaeologists need to learn to speak across those disciplinary boundaries, not just in the margins between them.

ACKNOWLEDGMENTS

Thanks to the editors of this volume for the invitation to participate and for critical feedback along the way, to an extremely helpful anonymous reviewer, and to Kerry Thompson and Richard Wilshusen for inspiring conversations about Navajo subsistence. The Navajo Nation and the New Mexico Museum of the American Indian/Laboratory of Anthropology allowed the reanalysis of Navajo faunal collections.

REFERENCES

Albarella, U., ed. 2001. *Environmental Archaeology: Meaning and Purpose.* Dordrecht: Kluwer.

Banks, W. E., F. d'Errico, A. T. Peterson, *et al.* 2008. Human ecological niches and ranges during the LGM in Europe derived from an application of eco-cultural niche modeling. *Journal of Archaeological Science* **35**: 481–491.

Barrett, E. M. 2002. The geography of the Rio Grande Pueblos in the seventeenth century. *Ethnohistory* **49**: 123–169.

Barton, H. 2007. Starch residues on museum artefacts: implications for determining tool use. *Journal of Archaeological Science* **34**: 1752–62.

Beck, M. W. 1996. On discerning the cause of late Pleistocene megafaunal extinctions. *Paleobiology* **22**: 91–103.

Bird, D. W., R. Bliege Bird, and B. F. Codding 2009. In pursuit of mobile prey: Martu hunting strategies and archaeofaunal interpretation. *American Antiquity* **74**: 3–29.

Bliege Bird, R. and D. W. Bird 2008. Why women hunt: risk and contemporary foraging in a Western Desert aboriginal community. *Current Anthropology* **49**: 655–693.

Bovy, K. M. 2007. Global human impacts or climate change? Explaining the sooty shearwater decline at the Minard site, Washington State, USA. *Journal of Archaeological Science* **34**: 1087–1097.

Broughton, J. M. and F. E. Bayham 2003. Showing off, foraging models, and the ascendance of large-game hunting in the California Middle Archaic. *American Antiquity* **68**: 783–9.

Brown, A. G. 2009. Colluvial and alluvial response to land use change in Midland England: an integrated geoarchaeological approach. *Geomorphology* **108**: 92–106.

Buchanan, B., M. Collard, and K. Edinborough 2008. Paleoindian demography and the extraterrestrial impact hypothesis. *Proceedings of the National Academy of Sciences of the United States of America* **105**: 11651–11654.

Burgi, M. and E. W. B. Russell 2001. Integrative methods to study landscape changes. *Land Use Policy* **18**: 9–16.

Burney, D. A., H. F. James, L. P. Burney, *et al.* 2001. Fossil evidence for a diverse biota from Kaua'i and its transformation since human arrival. *Ecological Monographs* **71**: 615–641.

Butler, V. L. and S. K. Campbell 2004. Resource intensification and resource depression in the Pacific Northwest of North America: a zooarchaeological review. *Journal of World Prehistory* **18**: 327–405.

Cannon, M. D. 2000. Large mammal relative abundance in Pithouse and Pueblo period archaeofaunas from southwestern New Mexico: resource depression among the Mimbres-Mogollon? *Journal of Anthropological Archaeology* **19**: 317–347.

Charnov, E. L., G. H. Orians, and K. Hyatt 1976. Ecological implications of resource depression. *The American Naturalist* **110**: 247–259.

Courty, M.-A. 2001. Microfacies analysis assisting archaeological stratigraphy. In P. Goldberg, V. T. Holliday, and C. R. Ferring, eds., *Earth Sciences and Archaeology*. New York: Kluwer Academic/Plenum, pp. 205–239.

Dansgaard, W., S. J. Johnsen, and H. B. Clausen, *et al.* 1993. Evidence for general instability of past climate from a 250-kyr ice-core record. *Nature* **364**: 218–220.

Darvill, T. 2008. Pathways to a panoramic past: a brief history of landscape archaeology in Europe. In B. David and J. Thomas, eds., *Handbook of Landscape Archaeology*. Walnut Creek, CA: Left Coast Press, pp. 60–76.

Davidson, D. A., S. P. Carter, and T. A. Quine 1992. An evaluation of micromorphology as an aid to archaeological interpretation. *Geoarchaeology* **7**: 55–65.

Dean, J. S. 2004. Anthropogenic environmental change in the Southwest as viewed from the Colorado Plateau. In C. L. Redman, S. R. James, P. R. Fish, and J. D. Rogers, *The Archaeology of Global Change: the Impact of Humans on their Environment*. Washington, DC: Smithsonian, pp. 191–207.

Dean, R. M. 2007. Hunting intensification and the Hohokam "collapse". *Journal of Anthropological Archaeology* **26**: 109–132.

Delcourt, P. A. and H. R. Delcourt 2004. *Prehistoric Native Americans and Ecological Change: Human Ecosystems in Eastern North America Since the Pleistocene.* Cambridge, UK: Cambridge University Press.

Delpech, F. 1999. Biomasse d'ongulés au Paléolithique et inférences sur la démographie. *Paléo* **11**:19–42.

Diaz-Maroto, I. J. and P. Vila-Lameiro 2008. Historical evolution and land-use changes in natural broadleaved forests in the north-west Iberian Peninsula. *Scandinavian Journal of Forest Research* **23**: 371–379.

Dincauze, D. F. 2000. *Environmental Archaeology: Principles and Practice.* Cambridge, UK: Cambridge University Press.

Doolittle, W. E. 2006. Agricultural manipulation of floodplains in the southern Basin and Range Province. *Catena* **65**: 179–199.

Etnier, M. A. 2007. Defining and identifying sustainable harvests of resources: archaeological examples of pinniped harvests in the eastern North Pacific. *Journal for Nature Conservation* **15**: 196–207.

Firestone, R. B., A. West, J. P. Kennett, *et al.* 2007. Evidence for an extraterrestrial impact 12,900 years ago that contributed to the megafaunal extinctions and the Younger Dryas cooling. *Proceedings of the National Academy of Sciences of the United States of America* **104**: 16016–16021.

Flanders, N. E. 1998. Native American sovereignty and natural resource management. *Human Ecology* **26**: 425–449.

Foster, D. R. 2000. From bobolinks to bears: interjecting geographical history into ecological studies, environmental interpretation, and conservation planning. *Journal of Biogeography* **27**: 27–30.

Frachetti, M. D. and A. N. Mar'yashev 2007. Long-term occupation and seasonal settlement of eastern Eurasian pastoralists at Begash, Kazakhstan. *Journal of Field Archaeology* **32**: 221–242.

Fritz, J. M. 1973. Relevance, archeology, and subsistence theory. In C. L. Redman, ed., *Research and Theory in Current Archeology.* New York: Wiley, pp. 59–82.

Goodman, J. D., II. 2003. Vertebrate faunal remains. In D. D. Dykeman, ed., *The Morris Site 1 Early Navajo Land Use Study: Gobernador Phase Community Development in Northwestern New Mexico.* Window Rock, AZ: Navajo Nation Archaeology Department, pp. 191–232.

Grayson, D. K. 1984a. Nineteenth-century explanations of Pleistocene extinctions: a review and analysis. In P. S. Martin and R. G. Klein *Quaternary Extinctions: A Prehistoric Revolution.* Tucson, AZ: University of Arizona Press, pp. 5–39.

Grayson, D. K. 1984b. *Quantitative Zooarchaeology.* New York: Academic Press.

Grayson, D. K. 2001. The archaeological record of human impacts on animal populations. *Journal of World Prehistory* **15**: 1–68.

Grayson, D. K. 2007. Deciphering North American Pleistocene extinctions. *Journal of Anthropological Research* **63**: 185–213.

Grayson, D. K. 2008. Holocene underkill. *Proceedings of the National Academy of Sciences of the United States of America* **105**: 4077–4078.

Grayson, D. K. and M. D. Cannon 1999. Human paleoecology and foraging theory in the Great Basin. In C. Beck, D. Rhode, and R. Elston, eds., *Models for the Millennium: Great Basin Anthropology Today.* Salt Lake City, UT: University of Utah Press, pp. 141–151.

Grayson, D. K., F. Delpech, J. -P., Rigaud, and J. F. Simek 2001. Explaining the development of dietary dominance by a single ungulate taxon at Grotte XVI, Dordogne, France. *Journal of Archaeological Science* **28**: 115–125.

Gunn, J., C. L. Crumley, E. Jones, and B. K. Young 2004. A landscape analysis of Western Europe during the Early Middle Ages. In C. L. Redman, S. R. James, P. R. Fish, and J. D. Rogers, eds., *The Archaeology of Global Change: The Impact of Humans on their Environment.* Washington, DC: Smithsonian Books, pp. 165–185.

Hannon, G. E. and R. H. W. Bradshaw 2000. Impacts and timing of the first human settlement on vegetation of the Faroe Islands. *Quaternary Research* **54**: 404–413.

Hawkes, K. and J. F. O'Connell 1992. On optimal foraging models and subsistence transitions. *Current Anthropology* **33**: 63–66.

Hayashida, F. M. 2005. Archaeology, ecological history, and conservation. *Annual Review of Anthropology* **34**: 43–65.

Haynes, G. 2007. A review of some attacks on the overkill hypothesis, with special attention to misrepresentations and doubletalk. *Quaternary International* **169**: 84–94.

Hildebrandt, W. R. and K. R. McGuire 2003. Large-game hunting, gender-differentiated work organization, and the role of evolutionary ecology in California and Great Basin prehistory: a reply to Broughton and Bayham. *American Antiquity* **68**: 790–792.

Holliday, V. T. 2001. Quaternary geoscience in archaeology. In P. Goldberg, V. T. Holliday, and C. R. Ferring, *Earth Sciences and Archaeology.* New York: Plenum, pp. 3–35.

Horrocks, M., G. Irwin, M. Jones and D. Sutton 2004. Starch grains and xylem cells of sweet potato (*Ipomoea batatas*) and bracken (*Pteridium esculentum*) in archaeological deposits from northern New Zealand. *Journal of Archaeological Science* **31**: 251–258.

Hovezak, T. D., L. M. Sesler, and S. L. Fuller 2002. *Archaeological Investigations in the Fruitland Project Area: Late Archaic, Basketmaker, Pueblo I, and Navajo Sites in Northwestern New Mexico.* Dolores, CO: La Plata Archaeological Consultants.

James, S. R. 2004. Hunting, fishing, and resource depression in prehistoric Southwest North America. In C. L. Redman, S. R. James, P. R. Fish, and J. D. Rogers, eds., *The Archaeology of Global Change: The Impact of Humans on Their Environment.* Washington, DC: Smithsonian, pp. 28–62.

Jones, E. L. 2006. Prey choice, mass collecting, and the wild European rabbit (*Oryctolagus cuniculus*). *Journal of Anthropological Archaeology* **25**: 275–289.

Jones, E. L. 2007. Subsistence change, landscape use, and changing site elevation at the Pleistocene-Holocene transition in the Dordogne of Southwestern France. *Journal of Archaeological Science* **34**: 344–353.

Jones, E. L. 2009. Climate change, patch choice, and intensification at Pont d'Ambon (Dordogne, France) during the Younger Dryas. *Quaternary Research* **72**: 371–376.

Jones, E. L., E. J. Taylor, and H. C. Toland 2009. Diversity, niche partitioning, and Navajo ethnogenesis in the protohistoric Southwest. Poster presented at the 74th Annual Meeting of the Society for American Archaeology, Atlanta, Georgia.

Jones, T. L., J. F. Porcasi, J. M. Erlandson, *et al.* 2008a. The protracted Holocene extinction of California's flightless sea duck (*Chendytes lawi*) and its implications for the Pleistocene overkill hypothesis. *Proceedings of the National Academy of Sciences of the United States of America* **105**: 4105–4108.

Jones, T. L., J. F. Porcasi, J. W. Gaeta, and B. F. Codding 2008b. The Diablo Canyon fauna: a coarse-grained record of trans-Holocene foraging from the central California mainland coast. *American Antiquity* **73**: 289–316.

Jorgensen, J. G. 1983. Comparative traditional economics and ecological adaptations. In A. Ortiz, ed., *Southwest*. Washington, DC: Smithsonian Institution, pp. 684–710.

Kirch, P. V. 2005. Archaeology and global change: the Holocene record. *Annual Review of Environment and Resources* **30**: 409–440.

Kohler, T. A. 2004. Pre-Hispanic human impact on upland North American Southwestern environments: evolutionary ecological perspectives. In C. L. Redman, S. R. James, P. R. Fish, and J. D. Rogers, eds., *The Archaeology of Global Change: the Impact of Humans on Their Environment*. Washington, DC: Smithsonian, pp. 224–42.

Koster, J. M. 2008. Hunting with dogs in Nicaragua: an optimal foraging approach. *Current Anthropology* **49**: 935–944.

Kuijt, I. 2001. Reconsidering the cause of cultural collapse in the Lillooet area of British Columbia, Canada: a geoarchaeological perspective. *American Antiquity* **66**: 692–703.

List, R., G. Ceballos, C. Curtin, *et al.* 2007. Historic distribution and challenges to bison recovery in the Northern Chihuahuan Desert. *Conservation Biology* **21**: 1487–1494.

Lupo, K. D. 2007. Evolutionary foraging models in zooarchaeological analysis: Recent applications and future challenges. *Journal of Archaeological Research* **15**: 143–189.

Lyman, R. L. and K. P. Cannon, eds. 2004. *Zooarchaeology and Conservation Biology*. Salt Lake City, UT: University of Utah Press.

Marom, N. and G. Bar-Oz 2009. Culling profiles: the indeterminacy of archaeozoological data to survivorship curve modelling of sheep and goat herd maintenance strategies. *Journal of Archaeological Science* **36**: 1184–1187.

Martin, P. S. 1967. Prehistoric overkill. In P. S. Martin and H. E. Wright, eds., *Pleistocene Extinctions: The Search for a Cause*. New Haven, CT: Yale University Press, pp. 75–120.

Metcalf, M. D. and K. R. Barlow 1992. A model for exploring the optimal tradeoff between field processing and transportation. *American Anthropologist* **94**: 340–356.

Morwood, M. J., T. Sutikna, E. W. Saptorno, *et al.* 2008. Climate, people and faunal succession on Java, Indonesia: evidence from Song Gupuh. *Journal of Archaeological Science* **35**: 1776–1789.

Munro, N. D. 2004. Zooarchaeological measures of hunting pressure and occupation intensity in the Natufian. *Current Anthropology* **45**: S5–S33.

Nagaoka, L. 2005. Declining foraging efficiency and moa carcass exploitation in southern New Zealand. *Journal of Archaeological Science* **32**: 1328–1338.

Nagaoka, L. 2006. Prehistoric seal carcass exploitation at the Shag Mouth Site, New Zealand. *Journal of Archaeological Science* **33**: 1474–1481.

Neumann, K., A. Fahmy, L. Lespez, A. Ballouche, and E. Huysecom 2009. The Early Holocene palaeoenvironment of Ounjougou (Mali): phytoliths in a multiproxy context. *Palaeogeography, Palaeoclimatology, Palaeoecology* **276**: 87–106.

Newsom, L. A. and D. A. Pearsall 2003. Trends in Caribbean island archaeobotany. In P. E. Minnis, ed., *People and Plants in Ancient Eastern North America*. Washington, DC: Smithsonian, pp. 347–412.

O'Connell, J. F., K. Hawkes, and N. G. B. Jones 1999. Grandmothering and the evolution of *Homo erectus*. *Journal of Human Evolution* **36**: 461–485.

Oonk, S., C. P. Slomp, and D. J. Huisman 2009. Geochemistry as an aid in archaeological prospection and site interpretation: current issues and research directions. *Archaeological Prospection* **16**: 35–51.

Opler, M. E. 1972. Cause and effect in Apachean agriculture, division of labor, residence patterns, and girls' puberty rites. *American Anthropologist* **74**: 1133–1146.

Papagianni, D., R. Layton, and H. Maschner, eds. 2008. *Time and Change: Archaeological and Anthropological Perspectives on the Long-Term in Hunter-Gatherer Societies*. Oakville, CT: Oxbow Books.

Pavao-Zuckerman, B. 2007. Deerskins and domesticates: creek subsistence and economic strategies in the historic period. *American Antiquity* **72**: 5–33.

Pearsall, D. M. 2000. *Paleoethnobotany: A Handbook of Procedures*. San Diego, CA: Academic Press.

Piperno, D. R., A. J. Ranere, I. Holst, and P. Hansell 2000. Starch grains reveal early root crop horticulture in the Panamanian tropical forest. *Nature* **407**: 894–897.

Piperno, D. R., E. Weiss, I. Holst, and D. Nadel 2004. Processing of wild cereal grains in the Upper Palaeolithic revealed by starch grain analysis. *Nature* **430**: 670–673.

Rapp, G. R. and C. L. Hill 2006. *Geoarchaeology: The Earth-Science Approach to Archaeological Interpretation*. 2nd edn. New Haven, CT: Yale University Press.

Rautman, A. E. 1996. Risk, reciprocity, and the operation of social networks. In J. A. Tainter and B. B. Tainter, eds., *Evolving Complexity and Enivronmental Risk in the Prehistoric Southwest*. Redding, MA: Addison-Wesley, pp. 197–222.

Reed, P. F., T. G. Baugh, and L. S. Reed 2000. Melding archaeology and ethnohistory into a contemporary view of the early Navajo. In M. Boyd, J. C. Erwin, M. Hendrickson, eds., *The Entangled Past: Integrating History and Archaeology*. Calgary, Alberta: Archaeological Association of the University of Calgary, pp. 65–77.

Reitz, E. J., C. M. Scarry, S. J. Scudder, eds. 2008. *Case Studies in Environmental Archaeology*. 2nd edn. New York: Springer.

Reitz, E. J. and E. S. Wing 2008. *Zooarchaeology*. 2nd edn. Cambridge, UK: Cambridge University Press.

Roos, C. I., A. P. Sullivan III, and C. McNamee 2010. Anthropogenic fire and long-term landscape management: palaeoecological evidence for systematic indigenous burning in the upland Southwest. In R. Dean, ed., *The Archaeology of Anthropogenic Environments*. Carbondale, IL: Center for Archaeological Investigations, Southern Illinois University.

Sandweiss, D. H., R. S. Solís, M. E. Moseley, D. K. Keefer, and C. R. Ortloff 2009. Environmental change and economic development in coastal Peru between 5,800 and 3,600 years ago. *Proceedings of the National Academy of Sciences* **106**: 1359–1363.

Schelhas, J. 2002. Race, ethnicity, and natural resources in the United States: a review. *Natural Resources Journal* **42**: 723–763.

Schimmelmann, A., C. B. Lange, and B. J. Meggers 2003. Palaeoclimatic and archaeological evidence for a similar to 200-yr recurrence of floods and droughts linking California, Mesoamerica and South America over the past 2000 years. *Holocene* **13**: 763–778.

Schmitt, D. N. 2004. Ecological change in western Utah: comparisons between a Late Holocene archaeological fauna and modern small-mammal surveys. In R. L. Lyman and K. P. Cannon, ed., *Zooarchaeology and Conservation Biology*. Salt Lake City, UT: University of Utah Press, pp. 178–92.

Simchoni, O. and M. E. Kislev 2009. Relict Plant Remains in the "Caves of the Spear". *Israel Exploration Journal* **59**: 47–62.

Simmons, A. H. 1999. *Faunal Extinction in an Island Society: Pygmy Hippopotamus Hunters of Cyprus*. New York: Kluwer Academic/Plenum.

Smith, B. D. 2007. Niche construction and the behavioral context of plant and animal domestication. *Evolutionary Anthropology* **16**: 188–199.

Smith, E. A. 1991. *Inujjuamiut Foraging Strategies: Evolutionary Ecology of an Arctic Hunting Economy.* Hawthorne, NY: Aldine de Gruyter.

Spangenberg, J. E., I. Matuschik, S. Jacomet, and J. Schibler 2008. Direct evidence for the existence of dairying farms in prehistoric Central Europe (4th millennium BC). *Isotopes in Environmental and Health Studies* **44**: 189–200.

Spielmann, K. A., T. Clark, D. Hawkey, K. Rainey, and S. K. Fish, 2009. "... being weary, they had rebelled": Pueblo subsistence and labor under Spanish colonialism. *Journal of Anthropological Archaeology* **28**: 102–125.

Steadman, D. W., J. P. White, and J. Allen 1999. Prehistoric birds from New Ireland, Papua New Guinea: extinctions on a large Melanesian island. *Proceedings of the National Academy of Sciences of the United States of America* **96**: 2563–2568.

Stewart, J. R. and A. Cooper 2008. Ice Age refugia and Quaternary extinctions: an issue of Quaternary evolutionary palaeoecology. *Quaternary Science Reviews* **27**: 2443–2448.

Stiner, M. C. and N. D. Munro 2002. Approaches to prehistoric diet breadth, demography, and prey ranking systems in time and space. *Journal of Archaeological Method and Theory* **9**: 181–214.

Surovell, T. A., V. T. Holliday, J. A. M. Gingerich, *et al.* 2009. An independent evaluation of the Younger Dryas extraterrestrial impact hypothesis. *Proceedings of the National Academy of Sciences* **43**: 18155–18158.

Szpak, P., T. J. Orchard and D. R. Grocke 2009. A Late Holocene vertebrate food web from southern Haida Gwaii (Queen Charlotte Islands, British Columbia). *Journal of Archaeological Science* **36**: 2734–2741.

Terral, J.-F. 2000. Exploitation and management of the olive tree during prehistoric times in Mediterranean France and Spain. *Journal of Archaeological Science* **27**: 127–133.

Thompson, K. F. 2009. They used to live here: an archaeological study of late nineteenth and early twentieth century Navajo Hogan households and federal Indian policy. Unpublished Ph.D. dissertation, Department of Anthropology, University of Arizona, Tucson, AZ.

Thompson, K. F. and N. Tsosie 2008. Measuring culture change: what Navajos are still eating and what's eating Navajos. Poster presented at the 73rd Annual Meeting of the Society for American Archaeology, Vancouver, British Columbia.

Towner, R. H. 2000. Concordance and conflict between dendrochronology and historical records. In S. Nash, ed., *A History of Archaeological Dating in North America.* Salt Lake City, UT: University of Utah Press, pp. 257–274.

Towner, R. H. 2002. Archaeological dendrochronology in the southwestern United States. *Evolutionary Anthropology* **11**: 68–84.

Ugan, A. and D. Byers 2008. A global perspective on the spatio-temporal pattern of the Late Pleistocene human and woolly mammoth radiocarbon record. *Quaternary International* **191**: 69–81.

van der Leeuw, S. and C. L. Redman, 2002. Placing archaeology at the center of socio-natural studies. *American Antiquity* **67**: 597–605.

Waters, M. R. 2006. Prehistoric human response to landscape change in the American Southwest. In D. E. Doyel and J. S. Dean, eds., *Environmental Change and Human Adaptation in the Ancient American Southwest.* Salt Lake City, UT: University of Utah Press, pp. 26–45.

Weisiger, M. 2004. The origins of Navajo pastoralism. *Journal of the Southwest* **46**: 253–282.

Wintemberg, W. J. 1919. Archaeology as an aid to zoology. *Canadian Field Naturalist* **33**: 63–72.

Winterhalder, B. and E. A. Smith, 2000. Analyzing adaptive strategies: human behavioral ecology at twenty-five. *Evolutionary Anthropology* **9**: 51–72.

Wolff, W. J. 2000. Causes of extirpations in the Wadden Sea, an estuarine area in the Netherlands. *Conservation Biology* **14**: 876–885.

Wright, D. R., R. E. Terry, and M. Eberl 2009. Soil properties and stable carbon isotope analysis of landscape features in the Petexbatún region of Guatemala. *Geoarchaeology* **24**: 466–491.

Zeanah, D. W. 2000. Transport costs, central-place foraging and hunter-gatherer land-use strategies. In D. B. Madsen and M. D. Metcalf, eds., *Intermountain Archaeology*. Salt Lake City, UT: University of Utah, pp. 1–14.

14

Comparing trajectories of climate, class, and production: an historical ecology of American yeomen

MICHAEL D. SCHOLL, D. SETH MURRAY
AND CAROLE L. CRUMLEY

INTRODUCTION TO HISTORICAL ECOLOGY

Historical ecology uses interdisciplinary synthesis to trace and evaluate the complex relationships between humans and the environment over the long term, typically traversing the course of centuries
(Crumley 1994, 2007: 16). Its methodological backbone is the synthesis
of long-series data produced by practitioners in diverse fields. Work in
historical ecology is guided by theoretical postulates that recognize
that understanding humans' occupation of nearly every environmental niche and the diversity of human social structures requires broadly
integrative methodologies (Balée 1998). Researchers bring about a difficult union between history and science, pay close attention to the
relations of geographic and temporal scales, embrace human social
complexity, and present findings in ways that are broadly accessible
(Crumley 1994, 1996a, 1996b, 2007).

The methods of historical ecology have been shaped by a rejec-
tion of environmental determinism, an interdisciplinary historical synthesis, and interest in questions concerning the historical trajectories
of the changes in humans' relations with the environment. Because
historical ecology melds data from science and the humanities, the
following review of its methods draws from advances in geography,
biology, ecology, history, sociology, and anthropology. That discussion

Environmental Social Sciences: Methods and Research Design, ed. I. Vaccaro, E. A. Smith and
S. Aswani. Published by Cambridge University Press. © Cambridge University Press 2010.

is followed by examples of questions addressed by practitioners of historical ecology, an illustrative case study, and an evaluation of the future of the approach.

REJECTION OF ENVIRONMENTAL DETERMINISM

A critical flaw in some early efforts to reconcile human and environmental history was an underestimation of humans' ability to manage environmental stresses. It was an argument rooted in antiquity (Vayda and Rappaport 1968). One of the most popular versions saw climate as a determinant of human history (cf. Huntington 1912a, 1912b, 1913, 1917). Distance from an optimal, temperate climate was said to have created racial differences, influenced moral character, and metered physical and mental activities. In favorable climates, the aggregated efficiencies of thought and labor gave rise to civilizations and when the weather changed, those civilizations fell (Huntington 1924: 411). Ecologists in biology concentrated on non-human subjects (Gross 2004) and avoided the difficulties posed by humans and their culture. However, anthropologists in the United States directly challenged these notions by developing a four-field perspective which held biology, culture, language, and history as independent, yet interconnected (Boas 1940; Kroeber 1923).

Despite their early avoidance of determinism, anthropologists were slow to integrate environment and history. Ecological studies were first successful in cultural anthropology (cf. Vayda 1969), but the challenging work of ethnography often meant that a historical dimension remained underdeveloped. In the second half of the twentieth century, ecological studies split between practitioners of cultural ecology who sought to examine the ways in which humans are affected by and modify the environment (Netting 1977: 1-3), and ecological anthropologists who closed ranks with plant and animal ecologists (Vayda and Rappaport 1968; cf. Winterhalder 1994 and this influence in historical ecology). By adopting an ecosystems approach, ecological anthropologists began important interdisciplinary work within the sciences, but moved further away from the qualitative analyses carried out in the humanities. Without an explicit mandate for an historical dimension, ecological anthropology was often carried out within an "ethnographic present" and societies were presented as timeless, internally undifferentiated, and adapted to environment rather than dialectically engaged with it (Balée 2006: 76–77). Nevertheless, cultural ecology remained popular among cultural anthropologists, geographers, and archaeologists whose interest in the processes of cultural change required a well-developed temporal dimension (Hardesty and Fowler 2001; Marquardt 1992).

Although some early researchers were misled by perceived racial and cultural hierarchies, they developed an important methodology for merging climatic reconstructions from tree rings with the cultural histories produced by archaeologists (Douglass 1914, 1919, 1928, 1936; Huntington 1912b: 401–411; Huntington *et al.* 1914). Dendrochronology continues to be a useful chronometer and reliable source of climate history, but limited sources of old wood and the specter of environmental determinism discouraged a generation of researchers from attempting a greater synthesis.

The term "historical ecology" was first used to describe one side of a fissure growing within biology. Practitioners called for renewed unity between a *general ecology*, reliant on laboratory methods, and an *historical ecology*, which draws inference from material evidence collected through fieldwork (Deevey 1964, 1969). Early attempts at reconciling biologists' successions of flora and fauna and archaeologists' cultural sequences were hampered by a lack of a shared chronological yardstick (Deevey 1944: 144–146). A breakthrough came with the development of radiocarbon dating which can accurately date ancient organic matter found in the materials examined by historians, archaeologists, climatologists, and oceanographers (Libby 1961). Importantly, radiocarbon dating provided a common metric which can be used to create an historical synthesis of the sciences and the humanities (Deevey 1964).

A resurgence of the environmental movement in the late 1960s and 1970s supported political action and academic study. The United States enacted comprehensive environmental protection laws and scientists pledged to map the changes in climate over the past 10 000 years in order to plan for the future food supply (Libby 1976). In the humanities, historians discovered a new audience and established the Forest History Society in 1946 and the American Society for Environmental History in 1976. European societies soon followed. Members of the history department of the University of Arkansas at Little Rock organized a lecture series and edited volume entitled *Historical Ecology: Essays on Environment and Social Change* (Bilsky 1980). The authors noted the public's concerns with pollution and resource depletion, and began a dialogue between researchers with expertise in history, human ecology, geography, economics, and archaeology. Common themes in the papers were the import role of social structure and identity, cultural perceptions of nature, and the multiple possible solutions for environmental problems (Moneyhon 1980: 4–5).

Some early environmental history has been criticized for overlooking social theory, focusing on calamity, and paying insufficient attention to ecological relations (McNeill 2003: 5–15, 36–39). However, historians were among the first to cogently discuss the role of the environment in recent human history (Le Roy Ladurie 1971; Sponsel 1998: 376; Winterhalder 1994: 21–23; Worster 1977, 1979), puncture the myth of a pristine New World (Cronon 1983; Crosby 1972, 1986; Whitehead 1998: 34–35), and continue to provide important dialogue with the public.

Nature's role in society remained a part of introductory texts, but sociologists never developed a working relationship with those early geographers whose views tended to reduce society to the product of an all-powerful environment (Gross 2004: 583–588). As sociologists struggled with vestiges of "social Darwinism" (Catton 1994: 84), which was an attempt to validate social inequity as a result of biological evolution, researchers steered clear of the environment (Dunlop and Catton 1979: 245). By the late 1950s, human ecology was regarded as part of sociology's past (Gross 2004: 596). In subsequent decades, the environmental movement revived their interest in parks and recreation, government policy, and fostered the growth of the perspective of rural sociology (Buttel 1987; Dunlap and Catton 1979: 250–265).

QUESTIONS IN HISTORICAL ECOLOGY

Historical ecology's broad approach lends itself to studies of long-term resource use, responses to climate change, and establishing the historical course of human–environment relations. One of the first studies to be carried out within historical ecology was an inquiry into the cause of the dispersal of the Mayan state. Archaeologists combined data from lake sediments, settlement data, and excavations in the Petén District of Guatemala to refute hypotheses that a collapse of urban areas was instigated by faltering food production (Rice and Rice 1984). The region continues to be a site of interest to researchers applying the perspective of historical ecology (Balée and Erickson 2006).

Durable production is also at the heart of an on going study of the Burgundy region of France. Begun in 1975, the project has explored the role of environmental and cultural diversity in a region that has reliably produced foodstuffs since the formation of the Celtic states (Crumley 1995: 1–2; Marquardt and Crumley 1987). Researchers have synthesized evidence of past climate, use of forests, pasture and fields, historical demography, local markets, and political structure to argue that economic forces had only short-term influence. However, over the course of centuries, the resilience of the region's social and economic productivity depended on the Burgundians' use of diverse commercial and agro-pastoral practices which were matched to complementary environmental settings (Crumley 1987a, 1987b, 1995).

Practitioners of historical ecology have spent nearly three decades investigating the causes for the failures of the tenth century Norse colonies. In Greenland, researchers synthesized results from excavations, contemporary texts, deduced climatic variation as suggested by the movement of ice sheets, compiled information on the availability of pasturage or long-distance trade, and analyzed regional political structures to conclude that ecological distress was the result of a disjunction between the decisions of distant managers and local conditions (McGovern 1981, 1994). Currently, a large interdisciplinary team is carrying out a similar study in Northern Iceland. Although still in the preliminary phase of analysis and results, the project has revised the view of Icelandic settlement patterns, exposed the influence of political and religious institutions on ecological practices, and identified Norse attempts at slowing deforestation and soil erosion (McGovern et al. 2007).

Historical ecology is not methodologically or theoretically tied to any particular subsistence strategy. In the Amazon basin, practitioners of historical ecology have examined inventories of nutritive and medicinal plants utilized by horticulturalists within the context of qualitative insights gained through ethnographic work, as well as through quantitative measurements of patterns of biotic dispersion. The methodology is innovative since it predominantly relies on observations collected in the present to expose the ways in which rainforests have been shaped by centuries of indigenous resource management (Balée 1989, 1994: 1–2, 1998, 2006: 85–87).

In recent years, researchers concerned with the management of landscapes, typically those within public land, have gathered together under the appellation "applied historical ecology" (Swetnam, Allen, and Betancourt 1999). The additional descriptor refers to their intention to manage human and environmental interactions in order to preserve landscapes or restore them to a desired earlier condition. A chief concern is the establishment of baseline data which can be used to identify the historical range of variation. Researchers synthesize cultural data like historic maps and oral histories with the results of archaeological excavations, plant surveys, and paleobotanical studies to create detailed historical baselines (Egan and Howell 2001).

METHODS IN HISTORICAL ECOLOGY

The information that practitioners of historical ecology seek to synthesize typically includes quantitative and qualitative data which have been collected at diverse scales. Methodologies are usually explicit about the underlying data, but not the subsequent interdisciplinary synthesis. An analysis in historical ecology includes four tasks: (1) information with a temporal dimension is collected from work in multiple disciplines; (2) the data are expressed in terms which establish one or more common scales of reference; (3) either explicitly or interpretively, the multiple lines of evidence are mapped along a temporal axis and sorted by their historical trajectories in order to suggest potential relationships between ecological factors; and (4) researchers present independent arguments explaining relationships between factors, points of causality, and implications of the findings.

The selection of factors with the most potential importance is aided by an attention to landscape. As the material manifestation of human–environment relations (Marquardt and Crumley 1987: 1), landscape presents a map which can be read for clues to the most relevant ecological factors. In order to reduce the risks of producing overly simplistic explanations, the selection process should sample across a broad spectrum of variables. Human–environment relations are extremely complex and research projects in historical ecology have found that inclusive perspectives do not result in wasted efforts. In order to avoid deterministic conclusions, researchers must not assume supremacy of humans or the environment. Their relations should be regarded as dialectical (Balée 1998: 13; Crumley 1996a), which is to say engaged and having mutual affect. The range of selected factors should be multidimensional and bridge the sciences and humanities (Crumley 1994: 1–2). In short, those seeking to explain the role of the environment in human history must consider an array of social and natural factors without assuming any rankings of importance.

A particular challenge in historical ecology is the reconciliation of information from multiple disciplines. The data must be expressed at a common scale while remaining sensitive to potential differences between local and regional scales, and between short-term and long-term patterns. A pragmatic approach is to use the units of measure, terminology, and environmental methods of the practitioners. This information is often discovered prior to the beginning of data collection and, if viewed critically, can assist in the selection of potentially important factors.

In order to reveal the relationships between the selected ecological factors, they must be mapped to their historical paths and sorted by shared trajectories. With qualitative data, this is very often accomplished through an interpretive argument which pays close attention to the movements of ecological factors in relation to each other. With numerical data, a simple framework is to sort lines of evidence into their shared trends. Those factors which are most likely to be ecologically engaged will follow similar or opposing courses through time. Unrelated phenomena are most likely to follow oblique or erratic paths in relation to the others. Although statisticians sometimes refer to this as "causal analysis," it is important to remember that covariance (i.e., similarities in historical paths) merely suggests potential relationships. Arguments concerning causation are not implied by the similarities of the trajectories, but by the quality of the research design (Denis and Legerski 2006). In historical ecology, this means that it is not sufficient to merely establish similar historical paths, but also an understanding of the processes and agents of change.

CASE STUDY: HISTORICAL ECOLOGY AND
THE AMERICAN YEOMAN

In order to demonstrate historical ecology's ability to draw together diverse data, the following case study examines the ecological underpinnings of the yeoman class as it rose and fell in colonial Pennsylvania. The project emerged out of an interest to advance historical ecology's methodology by considering a particularly large number of quantified factors. Researchers have typically relied on qualitative analyses to reconcile the differences in scale and scope among information originating in multiple disciplines. It was hoped that the use of numeric data might present new challenges whose solutions would advance our understanding of interdisciplinary methods.

A disciplinary goal was to create an ecological context for the British colonial period in the Delaware Valley of the eastern United States. Colonists wrote little about such mundane tasks. With some notable exceptions, the agricultural literature was authored by nineteenth century reformers who typified colonial practices as backward, or at best, stuck in time. However, that conclusion is at odds with the region's role as "bread basket" of British America, and as an exporter of foodstuffs to Europe and the Caribbean Islands. Chester County, Pennsylvania, a predominantly rural county adjacent to Philadelphia on the Delaware River, was selected for the completeness of its archives, excellent historical literature, and available environmental data. The final interest was a political concern that industrialized agriculture's great profitability may mask problems with food security and result in undesired social effects. It was hoped that research into the roots of that system might help map its historical trajectory and contribute to a clearer picture of where food production is headed.

When European colonists arrived in the seventeenth century, they found that Native Americans had created park-like conditions of grasses and old hardwoods by managing underbrush with controlled burns. As the British occupation of the Delaware Valley progressed, agriculturalists divided the relatively homogeneous landscape into a patchwork of open fields, meadows, and wood lots. Their principal ecological endeavors were non-irrigated cultivation of wheat and rye, and free range grazing of cattle, horses, sheep, and swine. Based on what is known about eighteenth century Pennsylvania colonists, it was hypothesized that potentially important factors included measures of the success of their agricultural practices, changing climate, class structure, demographic growth, and choice of settlement locations. Since colonial America was primarily agricultural, seasons and crop cycles are the most relevant unit of time. Households, the smallest social group, were organized by township, and thereby present the most practical political and geographic units. Analysis used bushel and field acreage of grains, head of livestock, and values of goods were recorded in specie, a method of accounting based on the value of Pennsylvania currency in comparison to the metal value of contemporary coinage.

The three primary sources of data are a reconstruction of eighteenth century climate, geographic information system (GIS) data, and probate inventories. Secondary sources included a large body of historical data which includes indexes of market prices of grain, average sizes of land holdings, tax assessments, and social history. Since the focus here is on interdisciplinary analyses, the methods used to generate the supporting data will not be given as thorough a discussion as might be warranted. However, these analytical methods are discussed in other chapters of this volume (Beltran in Chapter 2; Hames in Chapter 3; Jones in Chapter 5; Brondízio and Roy Chowdhury in Chapter 12) and elsewhere (Scholl 2008).

CLIMATE

Pennsylvania is located along an axis of the "westerlies," a prevailing polar jet stream whose movement can cause rapid and unpredictable changes in the weather and long-term alterations in the climate. A long-series of temperature and precipitation for the Philadelphia region was reconstructed by applying linear regressions from twentieth century data to eighteenth century observations made in other colonies (Landsberg, Yu, and Huang 1968). Since the methodology does not account for any fundamental changes in climate, the reconstruction was compared to local observations which were not included in the original analysis. The results suggest that the reconstruction does not capture the full range of variation, but, on average, it agrees to within 1 °F of contemporary observations and accurately captures the general trend.

SETTLEMENT PATTERN AND SOIL QUALITY

Demographic and soil data were consulted in order to see if ecological practices were influenced by the settlement of differing environmental settings. GIS data produced by federal, state, and county agencies were modified to reflect the boundaries of townships in each decade of the eighteenth century as they were represented in contemporary descriptions. The political boundaries were compared with mid-twentieth century soil surveys and the numbers of heads of households in eighteenth century tax assessments. The distribution of meadows, prime agricultural land, and settlement in the county was fairly even and there was no indication that colonists favored certain townships or environmental settings.

PROBATE RECORDS

In Britain and her colonies, county clerks filed a series of records concerning the dispersal of estates. Wills, codicils, and administrative accounts typically included a designation of social class, place of residence, and details about the composition of the deceased's household. The documents which are most revealing about ecological relations are appraisals of moveable estate. Under British law, household furnishings, livestock, bound field laborers, and agricultural produce were the property of the head of the household. Of the 4070 microfilmed probates dated between 1713 and 1789 on file at the Chester County Archives, 3551 include complete and legible inventories of households located within the county. Based on historians' estimates of the size of a typical household, the contents of these inventories represent the labors of more than 20 000 people.

Class

It has been a common practice for students of history to follow the democratized usage of nineteenth century America and refer to anyone from day laborer to corporate head as a "farmer." In eighteenth century Britain and her colonies, farmers were a minority class of entrepreneur who used hired labor on rented farms for short-term profits. Based on their own descriptions of class in probates, the social majority were yeomen who worked their own lands. They represented more than three-quarters of all Chester County men described by class and inventoried between 1713 and 1789 (Figure 14.1). The yeoman class arose in feudal Europe from skilled servants who were compensated with land. Its possession gave them legal rights above peasantry and an ability to pass real estate to their offspring (Campbell 1942). The keeping of probate records is closely tied to the formation of the yeoman class and reflects their desire to protect their freeholder status. Armed with agricultural skills and the price of passage, many early immigrants to Pennsylvania were of the yeoman class, and the ready availability of land meant that other soon joined their ranks.

Grain

Yeomen grew spelt, oats, buckwheat, and Indian corn (maize), but wheat and rye were the principal crops. More than three-quarters of acreage was planted in wheat, rye, or a mix of the two cereals. Using a methodology developed by historians of British agriculture, annual yields were estimated by comparing acres of field crops with bushels of grain inventoried after the subsequent harvest. The accuracy of such estimates is dependent on sample sizes which increase as the century progressed. As a check on the precision of the early decades, the results were compared to the observations of Philadelphia merchants

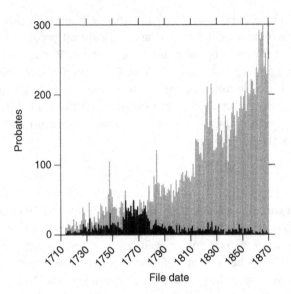

Figure 14.1   Persons described as yeomen (in black) and all other probates (in gray) Chester County, Pennsylvania, 1713–1870 (by file date; Chester County Archives wills and administrations index 2006).

contained in letters to their trading partners. In no cases were there substantial disagreements between the estimated yields and the grain merchants' perceptions.

Livestock

Colonists kept horses, cattle, swine, and sheep, as well as small numbers of beehives, turkeys, and ducks. Much to the dismay of agricultural reformers, most animals ranged free in both summer and winter and yeomen had only a passing interest in specialized breeds. Herd size grew only slowly as the century progressed. They possessed the technology to augment natural grasses with the tops of Indian corn stalks, clover, and English grasses, but only a few chose to invest the necessary labor. The availability of natural grasses was estimated by subtracting acreage in crops, wood lots, and buildings from land holdings recorded in tax assessments. The ratio of grain to grass establishes the number of years that a field might have been in a restorative fallow and the number of animals that might have been fed.

Labor

The agricultural cycle was such that yeomen planted, cut, or threshed in all but the coldest part of winter. The nearby frontier promised inexpensive land so few were willing to labor for others. Many yeomen resorted to bound labor and one-fifth of inventories included an appraisement of one or more slaves, servants, or apprentices. Since rural Pennsylvania was predominantly agricultural, the numbers of bound persons reflect the rate of resource exploitation.

ENVIRONMENTAL RISK

The complaints of agricultural reformers and patterns of land use in probate inventories indicate that yeomen used field scattering, shifting cultivation, and inter-cropping to dilute the effects of environmental hazards. Appraisals of damaged and undamaged fields of grain indicate that yeomen's scattered fields served to spread risk over space and ensured that a localized disaster would not damage an entire crop. The hard labor of breaking land meant that yeomen had a mix of old, mature, and new fields. The grain from freshly broken fields was not always the most valuable and crops on old fields did not always receive the lowest appraisals. The differing conditions may have helped ameliorate the effects of unfavorable weather. For example, a common concern was that early rains in new fields can cause wheat to "lodge" or fall over and become vulnerable to mildew and insects. A field with lower levels of nutrients slows the rate of maturation so that stalks kept pace with the plant's head.

Pennsylvania yeomen did not use crop rotations, but repeatedly planted the same field with the same grain. Only when a plot had become exhausted did yeomen allow it to fall into natural fallow and break a new parcel. A benefit of back-to-back planting is that it reintroduced seeds whose loose husks had allowed the grain to fall from the stalks. Yeomen were free from the labor of gleaning fields, crops needed only light seeding, and the preservation of grain with loose husks aided the threshing and cleaning of grain. Yeomen spread risk over product by mixing wheat and rye in the same field. Rye's faster maturation protected wheat from adverse weather, but it also had a lower market price. In the decades around the middle of the century, yeomen commonly traded higher potential profit for the surety of a good harvest.

MARKET RISK

Its position on the periphery of the world market and Britain's restrict-
ive trade policies meant that yeomen could only react to fluctuations
in the international market. Their best tools were market abstention,
diversification into manufacturing, and investment of their profits
into their local communities. Quantities of grain in inventories indicate that in the early decades of the eighteenth century yeomen grew
wheat to the exclusion of most other grains. Wheat prices increased
as the century progressed, but they also grew more unpredictable.
Individually yeoman grew less and less wheat, but strong immigration
and internal growth meant that they grew more wheat in each subsequent decade.

Yeomen spread risk over product by the adoption of manufacturing trades. One in four households included crafts persons, but manufacturing grew only slowly and craftsmen tended to leave smaller
estates. A common way to insure oneself against market downturn
was to loan agricultural profits at interest to others in the community.
Nearly 70 percent of inventories listed loans which ranged from small
sums for day-to-day bartering to mortgages for large parcels of land.
In total, money on loan was equal to nearly one-half of all inventoried
wealth. This system of social banking provided the means by which
many young people could establish their own places, and in return,
the lender gained interest, status, and the ability to call in debts during times of need.

ANALYSIS BY HISTORICAL TRAJECTORY

The above research provided 26 quantified factors of yeoman ecology
(Table 14.1). The spring, summer, fall, and winter temperatures (A, B,
C, and D) as well as rainfall (E, F, G, and H) are drawn from the climatic
reconstruction for the Philadelphia region. The value of all estates (I)
included every inventory with a class descriptor and the wealth of yeoman estates (J) is a subset of that data. The frequency of probated persons for whom their highest class is yeoman (K) includes male and a
few female-headed households. Landholding (L) is an estimate of the
mean acreage held based on samples collected by Chester County historians. The frequency of wheat producers (M) and Indian corn grow-
ers (O) are percentages of all who grew grain. Average acreage in wheat
(N), Indian corn (P), all grain (Q), and wheat yields (R) are estimated
from the inventory data. Livestock units (S) are the average herd size

reduced to equivalents of size (1 horse = 1 bovine = 5 swine = 7 sheep). Bound laborers (T) are the number of slaves, servants, and apprentices per inventory. Inter-cropped (U) is the proportion of the acreage of wheat and rye sown in a mixed field. The minimum and maximum fallows (V and W) define the range of years for which a field may be left to natural grasses and free range livestock. Social banking (X) is the mean portion of estates that were put out on loan. Wheat's market prices (Y) were drawn from historical studies of colonial prices. The frequency of decedent households containing crafts persons' goods or products (Z) reflects movement away from agriculture. In order to more easily compare their historical trajectories, the 26 factors were expressed on similar numeric scales, normalized to 1750, and sorted into increasing, stable, and decreasing trends (Table 14.2).

The increasing trends suggest that yeomen as well as those of other classes grew wealthier in the context of rising wheat prices, but appear to have played it safe by diversifying their grains, and increasing their production of manufactured goods. In the context of their financial success, yeomen scaled back the size of their holdings, shortened natural fallows, reduced their investment in bound labor, decreased the size of their herds, and wheat yields fell. The proportion of decedents described as yeomen in probate records and the practice of inter-cropping peaked in the 1760s and fell throughout the remainder of the century. These trends appear to explain agricultural reformers' concerns with falling agricultural efficiencies, and yeomen's hesitance to fundamentally change a profitable enterprise.

The weather, percentage of wheat producers, and lending of profits appear to have remained relatively stable throughout the century. However, the clustering of the climatic factors suggests that their historical trajectories may have been masked by their expression on scales different from the other data. In other words, small changes in rain and precipitation may have had larger effects on agricultural practices. A solution to the problem is to carry out a statistical procedure which uses correlation matrices to expose potential relationships within data which are expressed at multiple scales. Statistical analyses are an extremely useful tool, but their use here should not give the impression that they are an ultimate means of analysis in historical ecology.

Principal component analysis (PCA) is a favorite tool of advocates of exploratory data analysis who eschew traditional hypothesis testing and its reliance on confidence intervals in order to pursue pattern recognition (Shennan 1997: 265–307). They are of particular utility to

Table 14.1 *Ecological and historical trends in Chester County, Pennsylvania, inventories and climate data, 1730–1789 (letters are keyed to Figure 14.2).*

	1730–1739	1740–1749	1750–1759	1760–1769	1770–1779	1780–1789
A. Spring temperature °F	55.8	54.7	53.3	52.1	51.3	52.3
B. Summer temperature °F	74.7	74.6	73.4	73.2	72.5	75.0
C. Autumn temperature °F	55.7	56.0	56.4	55.3	56.2	55.9
D. Winter temperature °F	35.4	31.5	36.8	36.4	37.0	31.3
E. Spring precipitation inches	11.0	10.8	10.0	9.7	9.4	10.6
F. Summer precipitation inches	13.4	12.3	13.5	12.1	12.4	12.6
G. Autumn precipitation inches	9.7	9.4	9.3	9.3	9.3	10.1
H. Winter precipitation inches	9.1	9.0	8.7	8.2	7.8	9.0
I. All Estates / £10	21.1	24.3	27.7	36.8	36.9	49.9
J. Yeoman Estates / £10	22.3	24.1	28.6	30.5	34.0	48.8
K. Yeoman Class %	63.0	52.0	61.0	68.0	66.0	48.0
L. Land held / 10 acres	14.5	13.5	12.0	10.5	10.0	9.5
M. Wheat producers %	56.0	62.0	60.0	59.0	68.0	65.0

N. Wheat acres	14.3	13.5	15.0	10.6	10.6	9.6
O. Maize producers %	19.0	22.0	27.0	37.0	41.0	48.0
P. Maize acres	4.3	3.6	8.9	6.0	4.8	19.9
Q. All grain acres	19.7	22.4	25.1	21.2	21.2	28.8
R. Wheat yields bushel / acre	8.1	9.1	8.1	7.0	6.8	5.7
S. Livestock units	18.8	17.2	15.6	13.6	12.7	12.5
T. Bound laborers /10 probates	4.8	4.8	3.1	2.9	2.7	2.0
U. Inter-cropped %	14.0	28.0	22.0	31.0	22.0	13.0
V. Minimum fallow years	5.3	4.5	3.9	3.9	3.5	2.9
W. Maximum fallow years	7.3	6.1	5.0	5.0	4.3	3.3
X. Social banking %	35.0	39.0	44.0	54.0	43.0	46.0
Y. Wheat £ / 10 bushel	1.6	1.8	2.2	2.8	3.4	3.9
Z. Manufacturers %	23.0	22.0	26.0	25.0	31.0	28.0

Table 14.2 *Indices of ecological and historical trends in Chester County, Pennsylvania, inventories and climate data, 1730–1789 and normalized to the 1750s Mean (letters are keyed to Figure 14.2).*

	1730–1739	1740–1749	1750–1759	1760–1769	1770–1779	1780–1789
Increasing Trends						
P. Maize acreage	48	40	100	67	54	224
O. Maize producers number	70	81	100	137	152	178
Y. Wheat market price	73	82	100	127	155	177
I. All classed estates value	76	88	100	133	133	180
J. Yeoman estates value	78	84	100	107	119	171
Q. All grain acreage	78	89	100	84	84	115
Z. Manufacturers	88	85	100	104	119	108
Stable Trends						
G. Autumn precipitation	104	101	100	100	100	108
M. Wheat producers number	93	103	100	98	113	108
C. Autumn temperature	110	108	100	97	94	106
X. Social banking	80	89	100	123	98	105
H. Winter precipitation	105	103	100	94	90	103
A. Spring temperature	102	102	100	100	99	102
B. Summer temperature	99	99	100	98	100	99
E. Spring precipitation	105	103	100	98	96	98
F. Summer precipitation	99	110	100	90	92	93
D. Winter temperature	94	86	100	99	101	85

Decreasing Trends

S. Livestock units	121	110	100	87	81	80
L. Landholding	121	113	100	88	83	79
K. Yeoman class	103	85	100	111	108	79
V. Minimum fallow	136	128	100	100	90	74
R. Wheat yields	100	112	100	86	84	70
W. Maximum fallow	146	122	100	100	86	66
T. Bound laborers	155	155	100	94	87	65
N. Acreage in wheat	95	90	100	71	71	64
U. Inter-cropped	64	127	100	141	100	59

Table 14.3 *Principal component loadings of factors in yeoman ecology, Chester County, Pennsylvania 1730–1789.*

Component	1	2	3	4
A. Spring temperatures	**0.92**	0.37	−0.02	0.06
B. Summer temperatures	0.32	**0.92**	−0.24	0.02
C. Autumn temperatures	−0.04	0.06	**0.87**	−0.48
D. Winter temperatures	0.03	**−0.82**	0.35	0.44
E. Spring precipitation	0.58	**0.79**	−0.15	0.01
F. Summer precipitation	0.46	0.25	**0.71**	0.41
G. Autumn precipitation	−0.24	**0.90**	−0.06	0.30
H. Winter precipitation	0.51	**0.84**	−0.05	0.01
I. All estates value	**−0.96**	0.24	−0.15	0.08
J. Yeoman estates value	**−0.90**	0.43	0.02	0.06
K. Yeoman class size	0.11	**−0.88**	0.03	0.45
L. Landholding size	**0.99**	0.11	0.03	−0.01
M. Wheat producers number	**−0.74**	−0.02	0.24	−0.49
N. Wheat acreage	**0.86**	−0.02	0.41	−0.07
O. Maize producers	**−0.99**	0.06	−0.08	0.07
P. Maize acreage	**−0.66**	**0.69**	0.08	0.15
Q. All grain acreage	−0.58	**0.66**	0.20	−0.17
R. Wheat yields	**0.89**	−0.17	0.04	−0.40
S. Livestock units	**0.99**	0.15	0.04	0.04
T. Bound laborers	**0.96**	−0.02	−0.13	−0.15
U. Inter-cropping	0.07	**−0.68**	−0.48	0.46
V. Minimum fallow	**0.96**	−0.10	−0.09	0.17
W. Maximum fallow	**0.97**	−0.10	−0.10	0.14
X. Social banking	**−0.68**	−0.34	−0.43	0.12
Y. Wheat market	**−0.98**	0.10	0.00	0.05
Z. Manufacturing	**−0.83**	−0.22	0.44	0.07
Variance explained	14.26	6.51	2.41	1.67
Percent of variance	54.84	25.06	9.26	6.43

historical ecologists since PCA presents interpretable maps of covariance, those things which move together through time. Factors which share historical trajectories are bundled into *components* and given *scores* (Table 14.3; Figure 14.2) based on the degree they correlate with others. PCA also calculates *loadings* (Figure 14.3) which reflect the weights given to each decade in the first two principal components. Those factors whose scores approach one (1) are positively related and

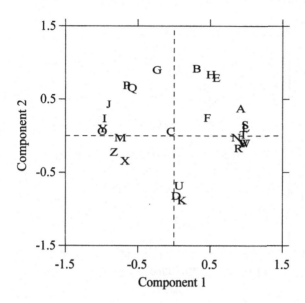

Figure 14.2   Factor scores of the first and second components of the ecological factors of yeoman production, Chester County, Pennsylvania, 1730–1789.

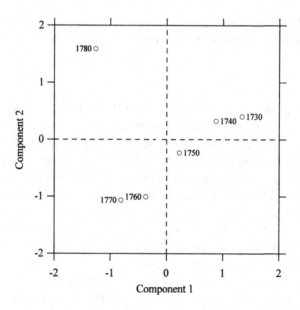

Figure 14.3   Loadings of the first and second principal components of the ecological factors of yeoman production, Chester County, Pennsylvania, 1730–1789.

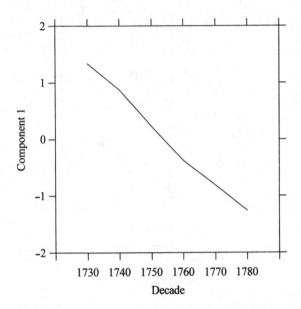

Figure 14.4 Historical trajectory of the first component of the ecological factors of yeoman production, Chester County, Pennsylvania, 1730–1789 (NB The downward trend represents increasing wealth).

scores approaching negative one (–1) are inversely related. Factors with a score around zero (0) are unlikely to be related to the others.

RESULTS

The circular pattern demonstrated by 25 of the 26 factors of yeoman ecology in Figure 14.2 suggests that the factors were well chosen. Only temperatures during autumn, the harvest and planting season, appear to have been ecologically unimportant. The first two principal components indicate very strong patterns and explain 80 percent of the variance within the 26 factors (see Table 14.3), and successfully expose the role of climate in yeoman ecology. The first component (Figure 14.4) describes the inverse relationship between increasing wealth and declining factors of production that were seen in the simple trends analysis. However, a better control of scale reveals that the constriction of agriculture was concurrent with changes in weather. As spring temperatures (A) became colder after 1740, wheat yields fell (R) and yeomen reduced the size of the average plantation (L), acreage in wheat (N), sizes of their herds (S), use of slaves, servants and apprentices (T), and length of regenerative fallows (V and W). A strong market price (Y) increased profitability and demographic growth provided more yeomen to grow wheat (M). The values of estates rose (I and J) and yeomen used that money to invest in local manufacturing (Z) and increase their loans to others (X). As spring temperatures warmed in the 1780s, increasing numbers of cultivators put more acres in Indian corn (O and P).

The relationship between wealth and poor spring weather is a complex one. Using the modern axiom that more food production is inherently more profitable, it might be expected that yeomen's fortunes would have been directly proportional to the size of their herds, numbers of bound laborers, and wheat yields. However, the demand for Delaware Valley foodstuffs was sufficiently strong that producers were increasingly profitable despite falling labor efficiencies from cooler springs and diminishing land holdings. Yeomen were not maximizers, and used the strong markets to diversify their products and maintain high wheat prices, which offered some protection from swings in market price. The counter-intuitive nature of these relationships probably lay at the heart of reformers' puzzlement over yeoman's continued adherence to traditional practices in the face of a strong international market.

As the first component describes yeoman's increasing wealth, the second component describes the relationship between class and risk-management (Figure 14.5). Yeomen grew in numbers (K) and increasingly inter-cropped wheat and rye (U) as summer temperatures fell (B), winters warmed (D), and springs, falls, and winters became drier (E, G, and H). It appears that mixed-cropping winter grains were a means of ameliorating the effects of cooler, drier growing seasons. Rye's fast growth meant that its large roots may have retained water throughout the winter and spring, and attenuated wheat's growth until the arrival of summer rains. The number of yeomen rose and fell with the practice of mixed-cropping, suggesting that the class's low-risk practices may have been an element of a class ideology valuing sustainable landownership over maximizing potential profits. A corollary class value may have been abstention from the volatile wheat market as yeomen planted more Indian corn (maize) (P) and thereby increased total grain output (Q).

These findings give little credence to reformers' complaints that yeomen were stuck in time or resistant to change. Their use of shifting cultivation and inter-cropping were effective responses to climate change and ensured a steady increase of wealth. The first and second components embrace the dual nature of the American yeoman as

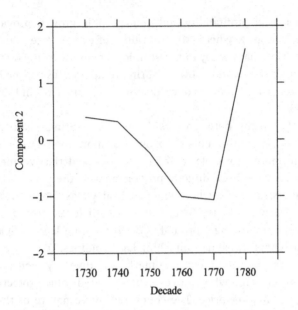

Figure 14.5   Historical trajectory of second principal component of the ecological factors of yeoman production, Chester County, Pennsylvania, 1730–1789 (NB The downward trend represents growth of the yeoman class).

producers for foreign markets and practitioners of time-tested, low-risk strategies which preserved long-term sustainability. Above all other factors, it was the prevalence of risk-reducing strategies that were most closely correlated with the growth and dissolution of the yeoman class. Initially, these practices preserved financial success in the face of inclement weather and waning labor efficiencies. As better weather came in the last two decades of the century, Chester County agrarians abandoned risk-minimizing strategies and the yeomen class ideologies which encouraged them. By the middle of the nineteenth century, the descendants of Chester County yeomen had become gentlemen farmers, inventors of agricultural machinery, and authors of literature advocating reform (Scholl 2008).

CONCLUSION

As this case study of the yeoman class in colonial Pennsylvania demonstrates, the value of methods in historical ecology is their ability to reconcile interdisciplinary data in order to address complex questions about the past. A study focusing solely on wealth and market would have missed the ways in which yeomen responded to climate change and their agricultural practices would have looked as backward as their critics had claimed. As the material aspect of ecological relations, landscape serves as a reliable guide for research design. Attention to scale during data collection and analysis is critical to fitting together properly the pieces of the ecological puzzle without resorting to a preconceived hierarchy of causality.

Historical ecology has no outward limit in terms of the kinds of human societies which can be examined, but it has an important inner limitation posed by insufficiently integrative analyses. Nevertheless, broad synthesis comes at a high cost. A researcher must not only contribute data to their particular disciplinary expertise, but also tackle the methods and theories of others. Building interdisciplinary competence is likely to be at the center of future methodological developments in historical ecology as researchers attempt increasingly complex syntheses within the context of long-term regional research projects.

REFERENCES

Balée, W. 1989. The culture of Amazonian forests. *Advances in Economic Botany* **7**: 1–21.

Balée, W. 1994. *Footprints of the Forest: Ka'apor Ethnobotany: The Historical Ecology of Plant Utilization by an Amazonian People.* New York: Columbia University Press.

Balée, W. 1998. Historical ecology: premises and postulates. In W. Balée, ed., *Advances in Historical Ecology.* New York: Columbia University Press, pp. 13–29.

Balée, W. 2006. The research program of historical ecology. *Annual Review of Anthropology* **35**: 75–98.

Balée, W. and C. Erickson, eds. 2006. *Time and Complexity in Historical Ecology: Studies in the Neotropical Lowlands.* New York: Columbia University Press.

Bilsky, L. J., ed. 1980. *Historical Ecology: Essays on Environment and Social Change.* Port Washington, NY: Kenniket Press.

Boas, F. 1940. *Race, Language, and Culture.* Chicago, IL: University of Chicago Press.

Buttel, F. H. 1987. New directions in environmental sociology. *Annual Review of Sociology* **13**: 465–488.

Campbell, M. 1942. *The English Yeoman: Under Elizabeth and the Early Stuarts.* New Haven, CT: Yale University Press.

Catton, W. R. 1994. Foundations of human ecology. *Sociological Perspectives* **37**(1): 75–95.

Cronon, W. J. 1983. *Changes in the Land: Indians, Colonists, and the Ecology of New England.* New York: Hill & Wang.

Crosby, A. W. 1972. *Ecological Imperialism: The Biological Expansion of Europe, 900–1900.* Cambridge, UK: Cambridge University Press.

Crosby, A. W. 1986. *The Columbian Exchange. Biological and Cultural Consequences of 1492.* Santa Barbara, CA: Greenwood Press.

Crumley, C. L. 1987a. Historical ecology. In C. L. Crumley and W. H. Marquardt, eds. *Regional Dynamics: Burgundian Landscapes in Historical Perspective.* New York: Academic Press, pp. 237–264.

Crumley, C. L. 1987b. Periodic markets in contemporary southern Burgundy. In C. L. Crumley and W. H. Marquardt, eds. *Regional Dynamics: Burgundian Landscapes in Historical Perspective.* New York: Academic Press, pp. 335–360.

Crumley, C. L. 1994. Historical ecology: a multidimensional ecological orientation. In C. L. Crumley, ed., *Historical Ecology: Cultural Knowledge and Changing Landscapes.* Santa Fe, NM: School of American Research Press, pp. 1–16.

Crumley, C. L. 1995. Building an historical ecology of Gaulish polities. In M. Geselowitz and B. Arnold, eds., *Celtic Chiefdoms, Celtic States.* Cambridge, UK: Cambridge University Press, pp. 26–33.

Crumley, C. L. 1996a. Historical ecology. In D. Levinson and M. Ember, eds., *Encyclopedia of Cultural Anthropology.* New York: Henry Holt and Company.

Crumley, C. L. 1996b. Foreword. In W. Balée, ed., *Advances in Historical Ecology.* New York: Columbia University Press, pp. ix-xiv.

Crumley, C. L. 2007. Historical ecology: integrated thinking at multiple temporal and spatial scales. In A. Hornborg and C. Crumley, ed., *The World System and the Earth System: Global Socio-environmental Change and Sustainability Since the Neolithic,* Walnut Creek, CA: Left Coast Press, pp. 15–28.

Deevey, E. S. 1944. Analysis and Mexican archaeology: an attempt to apply the method. *American Antiquity* **10**(2): 135–149.

Deevey, E. S. 1964. General and historical ecology. *BioScience* **14**(7): 33–35.

Deevey, E. S. 1969. Coaxing history to conduct experiments. *BioScience* **19**(1): 40–43.

Denis, D. J. and J. Legerski 2006. Causal modeling and the origins of path analysis. *Theory & Science* **7**(1). Available online: http://theoryandscience.icaap.org/content/vol7.1/denis.html.

Douglass, A. E. 1914. A method for estimating rainfall by the growth of trees. *Bulletin of the American Geographical Society* **46**(5): 321–335.

Douglass, A. E. 1919. *Climatic Cycles and Tree-growth, Volume I.* Philadelphia, PA: Carnegie Institution of Washington and J. B. Lippencott Co.

Douglass, A. E. 1928. *Climatic Cycles and Tree-growth, Volume II.* Philadelphia, PA: Carnegie Institution of Washington and J. B. Lippencott Co.

Douglass, A. E. 1936. *Climatic Cycles and Tree-growth, Volume III.* Philadelphia, PA: Carnegie Institution of Washington and J.B. Lippencott Co.

Dunlap, R. E. and W. R. Catton 1979. Environmental sociology. *Annual Review of Sociology* **5**: 243–273.

Egan, D. and E. A. Howell 2001. *The Historical Ecology Handbook: A Restorationist's Guide to Reference Ecosystems.* Washington DC: Island Press.

Gross, M. 2004. Human geography and ecological sociology: the unfolding of a human ecology, 1890 to 1930 – and beyond. *Social Science History* **28**(4): 575–605.

Hardesty, D. L. and D. D. Fowler 2001. Archaeology and environmental changes. In ed. C. L. Crumley, ed., *New Directions in Anthropology and Environment.* Walnut Creek, CA: AltaMira Press, pp. 72–89.

Huntington, E. 1912a. The fluctuating climate of North America part I: the ruins of Hohokam. *The Geographical Journal* **40**(3): 264–280.

Huntington, E. 1912b. The fluctuating climate of North America (continued). *The Geographical Journal* **40**(4): 392–411.

Huntington, E. 1913. Changes of climate and history. *The American Historical Review* **18**(2): 213–232.

Huntington, E. 1917. Temperature optima for human energy. *Proceedings of the Natural Academy of Sciences of the United States of America* **3**(2): 127–133.

Huntington, E. 1924. *Civilization and Climate.* Rev. of 1915 edn. New Haven, CT: Yale University Press.

Huntington, E., C. Schuchert, A. E. Douglass, and C. J. Kullmer 1914. *The Climatic Factor as Illustrated in Arid America.* Washington, DC: Carnegie Institution.

Kroeber, A. L. 1923. *Anthropology.* New York: Harcourt, Brace and Company.

Landsberg, H. E., C. S. Yu, and L. Huang, 1968. Preliminary reconstruction of a long time series of climatic data for the eastern United States. Technical Notes BN-571. Institution of Fluid Dynamics and Applied Mathematics, University of Maryland.

Le Roy Ladurie, E. 1971. *Times of Feast, Times of Famine: History of Climate Since the Year 1000.* New York: Doubleday Press.

Libby, W. F. 1961. Radiocarbon dating. *Science* New Series **133**(3453): 621–629.

Libby, W. F. 1976. Climatology conference. *Science* New Series **192**(4242): 843.

Marquardt, W. H. 1992. Dialectical archaeology. *Archaeology Method and Theory* **4**: 101–140.

Marquardt, W. H. and C. L. Crumley 1987. Theoretical issues in the analysis of spatial patterning. In C. L. Crumley and W. H. Marquardt, eds. *Regional Dynamics: Burgundian Landscapes in Historical Perspective.* New York: Academic Press, pp. 1–18.

McGovern, T. 1981. The economics of extinction in Norse Greenland. In T. M. L. Wrigley, M. J. Ingram, and G. Farmer, eds., *Climate and History: Studies in Past Climates and Their Impact on Man.* Cambridge, UK: Cambridge University Press, pp. 404–433.

McGovern, T. 1994. Management and extinction in Norse Greenland. In C. L. Crumley, ed., *Historical Ecology: Cultural Knowledge and Changing Landscapes* Santa Fe, NM: School of American Research Press, pp. 127–154.

McGovern, T. H., O. Vesteinsson, A. Fridriksson, *et al.* 2007. Landscapes of settlement in northern Iceland: historical ecology of human impact and climate fluctuation of the millennial scale. *American Anthropologist* **109**(1): 27–51.

McNeill, J. R. 2003. Observations on the nature and culture of environmental history. *History and Theory* **42**(4): 5–43.

Moneyhon, C. H. 1980. Introduction. In L. J. Bilsky, ed., *Historical Ecology: Essays on Environment and Social Change.* Port Washington, NY: Kenniket Press, pp. 3–8.

Netting, R. M. 1977. *Cultural Ecology.* San Francisco, CA: Cummings Publishing.

Rice, D. and P. Rice 1984. Lessons from the Maya. *Latin American Research Review* **19**(3): 7–34.

Scholl, M. D. 2008. The American yeoman: an historical ecology of production in colonial Pennsylvania. Ph.D. Dissertation, Department of Anthropology, University of North Carolina at Chapel Hill.

Shennan, S. 1997. *Quantifying Archaeology.* 2nd edn. Iowa City, IA: University of Iowa Press.

Sponsel, L. 1998. The historical ecology of Thailand: increasing thresholds of human environmental impact from prehistory to the present. In W. Balée, ed., *Advances in Historical Ecology.* New York: Columbia University Press, pp. 376–404.

Swetnam, T. W., C. D. Allen, and J. L. Betancourt 1999. Applied historical ecology: using the past to manage for the future. *Ecological Applications* **9**(4): 1189–1206.

Vayda, A. P., ed. 1969. *Environment and Cultural Behavior: Ecological Studies in Cultural Anthropology*. Garden City, NY: The Natural History Press.

Vayda, A. P. and R. A. Rappaport 1968. Ecology, cultural and noncultural. In J. A. Clifton, ed. *Introduction to Cultural Anthropology: Essays in the Scope and Methods of the Science of Man*, Boston, MA: Houghton Mifflin, pp. 477–497.

Whitehead, N. L. 1998. Ecological history and historical ecology: diachronic modeling versus historical explanation. In W. Balée, ed., *Advances in Historical Ecology*. New York: Columbia University Press, pp. 30–41.

Winterhalder, B. 1994. Concepts in historical ecology. In C. L. Crumley, ed., *Historical Ecology: Cultural Knowledge and Changing Landscapes*. Santa Fe, NM: School of American Research Press, pp. 17–42.

Worster, D. 1977. *Nature's Economy: A History of Ecological Ideas*. Cambridge, UK: Cambridge University Press.

Worster, D. 1979. *Dust Bowl: The Southern Plains in the 1930s*. New York: Oxford University Press.

15

Socioecological methods for designing marine conservation programs: a Solomon Islands example

SHANKAR ASWANI

INTRODUCTION

This concluding chapter provides an example of how the integration of various social and ecological methods, such as the ones presented in this volume, can shape the formulation of successful public environmental policy. Using marine conservation as an example, I elaborate and delineate various integrated methodological approaches for designing conservation areas such as marine protected areas (MPAs) that can be used by anthropologists and natural scientists alike. I also discuss how social scientists are favorably positioned to design conservation programs that are better tailored to the local context and summarize some ideas about how they can achieve the elusive goal of long-term project sustainability.

Most marine biologists agree that sound scientific data are essential when designing MPAs (e.g., Bergen and Carr 2003). Marine biologists have also widely promoted MPAs as enhancing spawning stock biomass, allowing for larval dispersal and the export of adults to adjacent non-protected areas, maintaining species diversity, preserving habitat, and sustaining ecosystem function (Roberts *et al.* 2001; Russ and Alcala 1999). Social scientists, however, have been generally critical of marine and fishery scientists for paying too much attention to biodiversity and stock-recruitment models and neglecting the social dimension of human–marine relations when designing and

Environmental Social Sciences: Methods and Research Design, ed. I. Vaccaro, E. A. Smith and S. Aswani. Published by Cambridge University Press. © Cambridge University Press 2010.

implementing conservation and fishery policies, respectively (Acheson and Wilson 1996; Pollnac, Crawford, and Gorospe 2001).

This appeal is particularly poignant in the context of MPAs, because MPAs are generally designed by natural scientists and, for that reason, social scientists feel that their contributions are given secondary considerations. This sentiment has been expressed in recent appeals for an understanding of the social dimensions of MPAs when they are being designed, implemented, and evaluated (e.g., Charles and Wilson 2009; Christie 2004; Jentoft, van Son, and Bjørkan 2007). This reaction has also been voiced in the context of terrestrial natural resource management (e.g., West and Brockington 2006). Social scientists, however, need to move beyond programmatic statements and provide coherent research tools and policy guidelines for the integrated design and analysis of MPAs and terrestrial and marine conservation areas more generally. In fact, social scientists need to demonstrate how stakeholder-driven conservation programs are likely to be more successful than purely biologically driven ones through the actual design of and/or engagement with conservation programs on the ground. To this end, I draw from my own applied and scientific work in the New Georgia Group in the Western Solomon Islands to illustrate various socioecological methods and integrated approaches for designing and sustaining marine protected areas, respectively. The outlined methods are also relevant for designing terrestrial protected areas.

STUDY SITE

The New Georgia Group in the Western Solomon Islands consists of volcanic islands that stretch from the northwest to the southeast (Figure 15.1). The marine ecosystem consists of coastal and coral atoll lagoons, barrier reefs, grass beds, mangrove forests, river mouths, and mudflats, and it is moderately undamaged by human activities, making this area one of the world's marine biodiversity hotspots (Hughes, Bellwood, and Connolly 2002). Local inhabitants have customary land and sea tenure, which in principle allows inclusive members right of access and use of marine and terrestrial resources and also bars those without tribal entitlements. These rights are contingent upon a member's birthright, spousal affiliation, and location of residence, and chiefs and elders control each district and exercise control over tribal territories. Today, a majority of coastal inhabitants still rely on fishing and horticulture as their means of subsistence, despite extensive social and cultural change over the

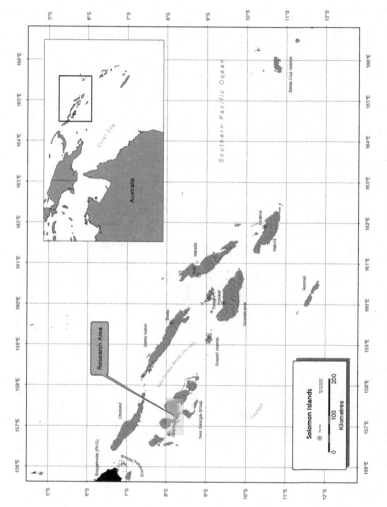

Figure 15.1 The Solomon Islands (research area highlighted in gray).

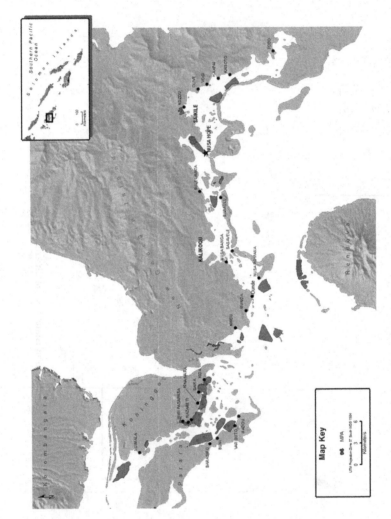

Figure 15.2   Current MPA sites in Roviana and Vonavona Lagoons and Rendova Islands (sites in the Marovo Lagoon are not illustrated).

past two centuries. The most direct threats to coral reefs and marine resources in the Western Solomon Islands are over-fishing due to sustained population growth (around 3 percent per annum), run-off sedimentation from logging, and the likely negative effects of global climate change. These factors are increasingly resulting in environmental degradation and social tensions across many communities.

In 1999, local communities in tandem with my research team established a marine conservation and development program in the Roviana and Vonavona lagoons as a preventive management strategy to address some of these environmental problems. As of 2009, a system of more than 30 "no-take" marine reserves and "spatiotemporal" refugia had been instituted in the New Georgia Group covering over 5000 hectares of diverse marine habitats, including mangroves, sea grasses, and coral reefs of various ecological characteristics (Figure 15.2). We are currently expanding this MPA system across various islands in the Western Solomons (e.g., Marovo, Rendova, and Vella LaVella). The general biological objectives of the reserves are to enhance fishery productivity locally, protect vulnerable species and habitats (biodiversity and ecosystem functioning), and to protect susceptible life-history stages (spawning and nursery grounds). The social objectives are to build upon practices with which the communities are familiar, including customary sea tenure and indigenous ecological knowledge (IEK) to protect peoples' livelihoods.

SOCIOECOLOGICAL METHODS FOR DESIGNING MPAS

Between 1992 and 2009 I conducted a number of biological and social studies to gain understanding of various dimensions of human–environmental relationships (or over 100 months of cumulative fieldwork by the author and team members). The first phase of these socioecological studies used a combination of qualitative and quantitative methods to delineate the dynamics of common-property institutions and various facets of IEK and associated resource exploitation strategies. The results of these studies offered a framework for designing and establishing a number of the marine protected areas. Next, I review some of the socioecological approaches and methods (a mix of ethnographic, geographic, economic, and ecological research methods), some of which have been presented in this volume, used to design the marine protected areas and provide guidelines on how socioecological projects co-led by social and natural scientists can generate conservation programs that are applicable elsewhere in the world.

SEA TENURE: ETHNOHISTORY AND GENEALOGICAL DEMOGRAPHY

History matters when designing conservation programs that incorporate local governance institutions in community-based management. In the Western Solomons, the major bases for current managerial differences between local communities lie in the history of regional patterns of settlement and demographic processes, as well as the way these interplay with the political economy to shape current territorial rights. We asked: Do differences in governance and management practices exist among local communities? And if so, what effects have historical, demographic, economic, and political changes had on the organizational structure and managerial outcomes of each common-property regime today? A combination of ethnohistorical, genealogical demography, and microeconomic methods were used to answer these questions.

Sampling

The first step was to determine the research population through a household census. Once a list of all household heads in each village had been compiled, a random sample at each hamlet was conducted (Pelto and Pelto 1978; Rogers and Schlossman 1990). For small villages containing fewer than 30 households, a complete sample was conducted, while for larger villages of 40 households or more, a 50 to 75 percent sample was taken. Next, a household questionnaire was conducted in each of the randomly selected households. The variables in the questionnaires included basic census data as well as questions on labor history, household income, household expenditures, rough estimates of task and time allocation to productive activities, commonly exploited commercial marine resources, asset ownership, and a series of other important issues. Afterward, structured interviews were conducted with household heads to explore in-depth kinship, tribal history, marine territoriality, and particularly people's current perceptions of resource use and access rules, and their actual behavior within each tribal territory (i.e., tenure regimes).

Ethnohistory

For the ethnohistorical research, the household heads interviewed during the census and by questionnaires were asked to identify key informants (or a snowball sample). Once identified, the informants (mostly elders in their 70s or 80s) were interviewed with in-depth, open-ended, semi-structured, and structured interviews on regional oral history. Note that oral history contrasts with folk tales and myths in that the latter are not generally structured in sequence and duration (Henige 1974: 2). Some ethnohistorians have argued that the boundaries between myth and oral history are often unidentifiable, and any sharp distinction between them is false (Neumann 1992). Nonetheless, Solomon Islands informants do distinctly distinguish between significant historical events and more myth-like episodes, and they more closely relate the temporal and spatial manifestations of oral histories to particular genealogies and archaeological remains. We cross-referenced archaeological data and early historical accounts of Europeans with the oral histories to better understand the historical processes that have impinged upon current territorial configurations. The combined data suggested that inter- and intra-political and economic competition between the sixteenth and nineteenth centuries, which resulted in differential settlement patterns among members of different tribal groups, have shaped the characteristics of current land and sea territorial claims (see Aswani 1999).

Insofar as the conservation program is concerned, the household questionnaires in tandem with the oral history interviews provided: (1) a qualitative review of historical settlement patterns and the identification of different sea tenure regimes within the region, and (2) a quantitative measure of the geographical distribution of households having members with tribal affiliations to the major estates of the region. A simple chi-square test was employed to analyze the distribution of households with at least one member belonging to the major estates, which showed that the observed association between contemporary villages and existing tribal affiliations is significantly non-random. The results illustrated how peoples' asymmetric regional settlement patterns in the recent past have influenced their current capacity to institute cooperation and enforcement mechanisms communally.

Genealogical demography and spatial patterns of settlement

Historical demographic processes can have important repercussions on the social institutions that manage indigenous common property regimes. Population trends in the Western Solomons suggest that populations have steadily increased over the last fifty years (Solomon

Islands Government 1999). We collected data on general regional trends such as fertility, mortality, and population growth from the government's 1986 and 1999 census and our household questionnaire census data to gauge the possible effects of demographic changes on resource management strategies. Also, we used an analysis of "family mapping" and spatial patterns of settlement to fine-tune information on population trends within each identified common-property system in the region (Roviana and Vonavona only).

The family mapping method, based on genealogical demography, was used to identify main family trees for sampling within selected villages of each sea-tenure regime starting with the parents of the older living members of a community (Chun and Means 1997). Once the main lineages had been identified, members of each were asked to identify all children born (dead and alive) to each person in each generation beginning with the parents of the older living generation. As older people found it hard to remember accurate dates, significant historical markers were used to aid people's memory, including World War II (1940s), the rise of the Christian Fellowship Church (1960s), the coming of logging (1980s), and the new millennium (2000s).

Informants were then asked to identify all old and new settlements established over the informant's lifespan to determine changes in spatial settlement patterns for villages within each regime. Informants that had resided at a settlement for 75 years or more were asked to identify new settlements across three points in their lifetime (youth, maturity, old age). To allow for variation in settlement size, informants were asked to rank settlements according to a rough estimate of population size (e.g., single family, extended family, village, etc.). Thereafter, the average distance between settlements at the three temporal points was measured and plotted in a set of aerial photographs. We are now importing this data into a GIS according to estimated year of establishment. This analysis provided a rough measure of population density change patterns over the last century. In sum, these two approaches allowed us to identify population trends within each sea-tenure regime and to extrapolate the possible effects of population growth on the spatial distribution of stakeholders, and consequently, on their territorial strategies.

SEA TENURE: SOCIOECONOMIC TRANSFORMATIONS
AND COPING STRATEGIES

Population changes and spatial settlement need to be articulated with changing consumer demands and economic activities to understand the institutional resilience of each sea-tenure regime to withstand contemporary socioeconomic changes. I asked: does the open-access commons emerge from the breakdown of local institutions caused by changing consumer demands and the market economy?

To elucidate the vulnerability and/or stability of indigenous sea-tenure institutions to changing consumer demands and to the encroachment of the market economy, it was necessary to understand the economic behavior of lagoon dwellers. Existing economic and livelihood differences between villages were recorded across sampling years (1994–5, 1998–2003, 2009) to explain the relationship between economic disparity and control of marine resources. A combination of methods, including income and expenditure analysis, time-allocation studies, food diaries, and structured interviews were employed to provide an understanding of people's livelihoods and food security and to assess their responses to changing economic circumstances. These results, in turn, facilitated the design of MPAs sensitive to local coping strategies.

Income and expenditure analysis

Income and expenditure analysis was conducted to establish each household's participation in the market economy, and a diary method was used to attain a larger sample size. The first step was to improve our survey instrument so that it could be easily comprehended and completed by the selected members in each sampled household. The sampled households in all targeted villages were identified by the censuses carried out during 1994 and 2001. Members of randomly selected households (at least 50 percent of households in 15 villages) were asked to keep a record of all economic activities for a week. The income schedule included questions ranging from day of transaction and goods sold to the member selling the product and the contribution to income by each gender. The expenditure schedules were formulated similarly. Several schedule cycles were conducted to allow for a representative sample within the framework of seasonal variation in economic activities, particularly those concerned with marine resource exploitation. Data were compared across sampling years to examine recent developments and identify any economic and institutional changes associated with sea-tenure regimes. ·

Time-allocation studies

Discerning time-allocation patterns among fishers is crucial to understanding how households meet their subsistence and economic needs. Time-allocation studies focus on people's use of time and their various productive modes. The advantage of analyzing time budgets is that measurements of daily activities can be objectively generated without having to rely on ambiguous descriptions of behavior gathered through interviewing alone. Time allocation to productive activities was extrapolated from the household questionnaires and was ground-truthed with the spot-check method (Johnson 1975), which consists of randomly selecting times and dates to visit households and to record household members' activities as soon as they are observed. Activities of absent members are recorded by asking available individuals. The proportion of observations for each behavior was calculated by dividing the number of observations for any given activity by the total number of spot-check observations (for all activities). Our familiarity with local modes of production in the region allowed for informed coding of the activity categories. To maintain randomness and generality, sampling of behaviors was carried out throughout the year by local research assistants. These measurements allowed us (1) to discern regional differences in the use of time for income-productive activities vis-à-vis subsistence ones, (2) to examine seasonal inter-regional shifting patterns of resource use, and most importantly (3) to observe time-use differentiation across the identified sea-tenure regimes and its relation to changing consumer demands and fishery commercial activities.

Food security

We used various interviewing and food-diary methods to elucidate issues of household food security in communities within each sea-tenure regime. Structured interviews complemented other methods detailed in this chapter by exploring (1) the number of meals prepared daily, (2) dietary diversity, (3) incidence of food shortage, (4) coping strategies for insufficient food, and (5) perceptions of food security and adequacy. We collected these data using a Likert-scale questionnaire design. In addition, food diaries were used to quantify actual household food intake. A member of the household was asked to keep a record for a week of all meals and food per meal consumed by each member. Data (food diaries and kitchen forms) were compared to determine if differences existed between sampling years and villages and to gauge whether different resource-management strategies within each sea-tenure regime had an impact on levels of household food security.

Identifying how people understand their territorial rights (i.e., what is claimed, or property rights) and how this translates into an effective activation of those rights – that is, actual behavior – through the control of participating members and exclusion of interlopers is crucial to understanding current management choices. This requires an understanding of people's differences and similarities in sea tenure cognition (as a proxy for "cultural consensus"), their cultural attitudes regarding interloping, good governance, resource conflicts (as a proxy for "enforcement of access"), and why people may or may not cooperate to protect their natural resources. We used various methods to understand these processes, including cultural consensus analysis, structured interviewing, and the use of experimental economic "public goods games" to provide information about group cohesion, conflict, and likelihood of cooperative behavior. Understanding the mental processes (e.g., cultural consensus) that inform, among other factors, people's current governance and management decisions in local communities is key to successful resource management.

Cultural consensus analysis

In order to gain knowledge of the underlying assumptions that inform people's decisions, cultural knowledge was measured using cognitive anthropological techniques, which are used to investigate the extent of shared knowledge among human communities (D'Andrade 1995). The objective was to develop a cultural model utilized by people of different areas within Roviana Lagoon (e.g., Baraulu and Dunde villages) for understanding the operation of, and threats faced by, their sea-tenure institutions, and to assess whether differences existed among them in their cultural perceptions regarding property rights and management strategies. Standard ethnographic methods of participant observation and informant interviews were paired with cognitive anthropological methods that included agreement questionnaires, free lists, and pile sorts (Bernard 2000). Free listing generated lists of words pertaining to property rights that helped us to identify underlying ideas and notions about sea tenure. In the pile-sorting exercise, informants were given a set of cards inscribed with words in English and Roviana (which were formulated from the free-listing exercise), and they were asked to divide the cards into piles consisting of the most similar concepts. Final groupings were expected to reflect implicit classification elements for a specific cultural domain.

For data analysis, we converted the survey results into an "agree/disagree" format and subjected them to a consensus analysis. This method compares answers to a "test" through a matrix of numerical values within a pair of vectors. The assumption is that agreement among informants implies a degree of shared knowledge. The pile sort results were analyzed using multi dimensional scaling, which transforms a matrix of similarities and dissimilarities into a map with coordinates in Euclidean distances (Bernard 2000). Then, the grouping of terms, or "clusters," allowed identification of the terms that were most frequently associated with one another, which reflect implicit knowledge shared by informants. Results showed that informants, regardless of age, sex, education, etc., were using a single cognized model to answer the survey questions regarding sea tenure. However, further analysis using non-metric, multi dimensional scaling (MDS) revealed that meaningful divergence in cognition existed between communities regarding population size, interloping, and overfishing. These differences, in turn, corresponded with people's notions of positive or negative capacity within each identified sea-tenure regime to manage marine resources (Aswani and Herman unpublished data; Aswani 2005).

Conflict and natural resources

It was crucial to identify whether or not conflict existed across the region as a result of differences in sea-tenure governance. Interview schedules and household questionnaires were conducted to provide an understanding of conflict between participants and between neighboring communities. We tried to identify conflicts among each estate's stakeholders, changes in use and access rules, modifications of boundary delineations, local mechanisms used to enforce management decisions, monitoring capabilities, traditional and legislative conflict-resolution mechanisms, and poaching incidence for each area (carried out by inclusive members or neighboring groups). The interviews and questionnaires also inquired about changes in the number of incidences of illegal fishing practices (as measured by fines levied, fishers caught, etc.). For each measure of interloping and good governance, differences between villages were determined with simple between-groups ANOVA with alpha set at $p < 0.05$ for each comparison.

Cooperation and natural resources

Finally, understanding cooperative behavior between stakeholders living under different tenure regimes is important for designing successful conservation programs. We asked: what individual-level variables (e.g., age, sex, education, ethnicity, etc.), and group-level variables (e.g., governance institutions, group coercive action, etc.), lead to cooperative behavior for managing natural resources? Does ethnic diversity, for instance, enhance (Santos, Santos, and Pacheco 2008) or diminish (Habyarimana et al. 2007) social cohesion and cooperation in public goods situations? And, more generally, what historical, economic, and political circumstances lead people to make greater contributions to public goods, such as engaging in conservation projects? In order to gauge cooperative behavior among stakeholders belonging to different sea-tenure regimes, we used a simplified version of a "voluntary contribution" *public goods game* (PGG) from experimental economics. The game is designed, in part, to understand prosocial behavior (or voluntary actions such as sharing that can benefit others or groups), and it examines people's behavior when individual and group interest conflict with each other (Henrich et al. 2005).

A large portion of men across six Roviana villages and one regional town (Noro) between the ages of 40 and 70 years were asked to participate in the PGG. Each participant was given $15 SDB (Solomon Dollars), and they were told that they could anonymously contribute any portion of their donation to a village common pot. Participants were then instructed that the contributed funds would be doubled and that the total in the common pool would be equally distributed to all participants regardless of their initial contribution. If participants separately cooperated and contributed their $15 SBD, they were expected to receive a payoff of $30 each. The problem is that (depending upon group cohesion and trust), many individuals are expected to "free-ride" and contribute as little as possible independent of other's actions, thus expecting a larger payoff at the cost of others (Henrich et al. 2005). The rational choice, therefore, is to free ride and invest as little as possible or nothing at all. This can result in a situation in which participants (especially in groups where there is mistrust) will sacrifice the public good in an attempt to maximize their own returns. If everyone does the same, this results in a state of shared defection and economic paralysis (Hauert 2006). Our preliminary results suggest that religious and ethnic homogeneity favored prosocial behavior among players in each village and that free-riding was more common in socially heterogeneous hamlets.

SEA TENURE AND ECOLOGICAL ASSESSMENTS

Interest is growing in better understanding of the relationship between remnant customary sea-tenure regimes and ecological sustainability (e.g., Cinner, Marnane, and McClanahan 2005). This is due to the general failure of centralized and science-driven coastal fisheries programs in the Pacific region. In our research, we investigated the relationship between changing fishing intensity and management systems and the abundance of species that play a critical role in the resilience and vulnerability of coral reef ecosystems. For instance, we investigated the ecological impact of localized subsistence and artisanal fishing pressure on parrotfish fisheries in Gizo Town (with weak sea tenure) in the Western Solomon Islands and used this information to conduct a comparative assessment of parrotfish abundance in open-access and customary closed-access coral reefs in nearby Kinda and Nusa Hope villages (with functional sea tenure).

The density and size distributions of parrotfish in Gizo were measured during two years (2004 and 2005) using an underwater visual census (UVC) to determine if artisanal fishing pressure has resulted in localized shifts in parrotfish sizes and abundance over time. Recall diary and creel survey data were collected for the same period of time to independently assess catch-per-unit-effort (CPUE) and the ecological impact of localized subsistence and artisanal fishing pressure on parrotfish populations. Then, we used equivalent unpublished and published UVC data on the abundance and size distribution of parrotfish in open-to-fishing (control) and closed-to-fishing (experimental) sites in Kinda and Nusa Hope to weigh against the Gizo findings. Data for the open-to-fishing sites across these settlements were compared with the closed-to-fishing sites in Kinda and Nusa Hope villages to determine the local effects of moribund (Gizo), vulnerable (Kida), and robust (Nusa Hope) customary fishery management systems. The results suggested that the erosion of customary sea tenure is fostering the rapid decline of already vulnerable fisheries around urbanized regions of the Western Solomon Islands and that functioning customary management systems can positively affect the management and conservation of parrotfish fisheries (see Aswani and Sabetian 2010 for further discussion).

Natural scientists rarely consider the specific characteristics of human foraging strategies when designing marine conservation programs. However, studying fishing behavior affords an understanding of spatio-temporal human resource exploitation patterns (e.g., seasonal changes in fishing gear), human responses to variability in inter- and intra-habitat relative productivity (as determined by catch rates) and the influence of this variability on fishing strategies, and human threats to particular marine habitats. This information can help in the design of permanent and seasonal closures modeled in accordance with human seasonal foraging patterns. Integrating fishing behavioral patterns into program design enhances people's compliance with conservation.

Human behavioral ecology and fishing

Human ecologists have regularly employed optimal foraging theory models to predict various aspects of human foraging behavior (e.g., Smith 1991). In our Roviana research, we tested hypotheses drawn from the patch-choice model and the marginal value theorem (MVT) to study fishers' patch choices and time use across spatiotemporal variation (see Stephens and Krebs 1986). We utilized predictions from these models to analyze the seasonal movements of fishers, to forecast the decisions that fishers make in the types and abundance of fish that they prey on, the use frequency of marine habitats, and the fluctuating intensification of fishing efforts. For example, when using the patch-choice model, we tested the hypothesis that overall time allocation to a habitat type (set of patches) increases when seasonal productivity for that habitat increases and is higher than that of other habitats. Conversely, overall time allocation to a habitat type decreases when seasonal productivity for that set of patches declines and is lower than that of other habitats.

Two related methods were used to test this hypothesis: focal follows and self-reporting diaries. Focal follow analysis involves keeping time–motion records for fishers and measuring their catches. The diary method consists of recruiting randomly selected subjects to keep diaries of their fishing activities. We compiled, through direct observations and self-reporting diaries, seasonal foraging data for a sustained period of 10 years (1994–2004) covering more than 10 000 foraging events and 15 000 hours of fishing activities. These data were used to explore the effects of village and habitat type on mean net return rates and fishing event duration. The mean net return rate measurement is equivalent to the energy gained during fishing (the kcal value of the edible catch) minus the labor input (labor costs incurred during foraging, including travel, search, and handling times) divided by the total residence time at a fishing ground (see Smith 1991).

On the whole, results showed that overall effort was directed to the habitats with the highest yields and that fishers moved between habitat types, fishing grounds, and species assemblages across different seasons to maximize their mean net rate of return. More specifically, the results provided a better understanding of (1) the distribution of fishing methods and the geographical disparities in yield and effort, (2) different habitat productivities across seasonal and spatial variations, and (3) the changes in time use as a response to resource abundance or scarcity. Variance in fishing return rates and effort data for different habitats in regional villages not only showed differences in foraging strategies but also hinted at the effectiveness of each community's resource-management strategies. The research generated data on local foraging patterns that aided in the MPA designation process.

Human foraging patterns and Geographical Information Systems (GIS)

A GIS database can be used to incorporate sociospatial information, such as artisanal fishing data, along with biophysical information to help in the design of conservation programs such as marine protected areas. In our research, we distinctively conceptualized human foraging strategies spatiotemporally by querying our GIS database and then displaying the data derived from the queries. The GIS was used to link our cartographic spatial dataset of indigenously defined resource patches (615 sites collected with GPS receivers) with our nonspatial attribute data (foraging dataset). This permitted an analysis of the spatiotemporal relationships between particular marine habitats and the patches within them, on the one hand, and changes in their relative productivity and associated temporal increases or decreases in foraging effort by fishermen of various regional villages to exploit these resources, on the other.

For instance, we ran a query with the GIS that extracted the fishing events associated with each of the three locally recognized tidal seasons in the region (e.g., Roviana Lagoon). We then used the GIS to factor the proportional mean net return rate and time allocation for each fishing ground of each habitat type for each season. Then we displayed and printed these six maps in juxtaposition to enhance visual interpretation and pattern description. The visual representation of our foraging analysis made details more apparent and consequently gave us a deeper understanding of intra-habitat variability and human responses to and strategies for dealing with this variability. This allowed us to design MPAs that were less disruptive to people's fishing strategies and, therefore, livelihoods (see Aswani and Lauer 2006a).

INDIGENOUS ECOLOGICAL KNOWLEDGE

Incorporating IEK into inshore fisheries management is increasingly being recognized as important by scientists and policy-makers alike (e.g., Acheson and Wilson 1996). Local fishers have first-hand experience and knowledge of the environment that they exploit, including knowledge about the direct assessment of local marine stocks and how they change over time, which is an expertise marine biologists rarely have. The value of local knowledge and practices for marine resource management is not just hypothetical – as we have shown, marine protected areas that integrate IEK into their design can be successful biologically and socially (e.g., Aswani et al. 2007).

We documented local ecological knowledge over the last 17 years (1992–2009) through open-ended and structured interviews conducted with more than 300 young (18–39), middle-aged (40–59), and elderly (>60) men and women from across villages in the lagoons. We elicited information on a number of biological parameters, data which were then matched with corresponding Western information to describe climatic phenomena, habitat composition, and biotic taxonomies. Fishers identified over 50 fishing methods, hundreds of vertebrate and invertebrate marine species, and around 14 major habitat types and 6 minor ones, as well as 615 locally delineated fishing grounds throughout the region. The latter were mapped onto aerial photographs of the Roviana and Vonavona Lagoons manually, thus establishing the spatial foundation for the ensuing GIS visual representation. In our participatory conservation efforts, therefore, socioecological and spatial analyses were fundamental, especially when delimiting the fragmentation and distribution of locally identified habitats across the Roviana, Vonavona, and Marovo lagoons.

Indigenous ecological knowledge and GIS

Habitat mapping serves to catalogue habitat diversity and zonation and identifies sites that incorporate the ecological processes that support biodiversity, including the presence of exploitable species, vulnerable life stages, and interconnectivity among habitats for designing marine protected areas. In our studies, we developed a reliable and participatory way to produce maps of the benthos and associated biological communities. First, we formulated a qualitative definition of benthic communities that incorporated both physical and biological characteristics (Diaz, Solan, and Valente 2004). This allowed for the formulation of an emic classification of benthic habitats commonly found in some of the planned MPAs (Figure 15.3). Next, we used a large-format plotter to print a two-foot by four-foot hard-copy map of the planned MPA with a scale of approximately 1:3500 (one inch equalling about 50 meters). Informants (five men and women), were selected to be the photo interpreters based on their knowledge of the marine environment and their overall fishing experience. Then informants identified the main reefs and predominant benthic characteristics and cooperatively drew the boundaries of abiotic and biotic substrates using a felt-tip marker directly on the photograph. The resulting paper map, with the respective benthic types was scanned, and the image files were loaded into the GIS for geo-rectification. After georeferencing, each of the boundaries was traced using on-screen digitizing techniques that created polygons (shape files) of each of the benthic substrates (Figure 15.4) (Aswani and Lauer 2006a).

Then, a student researcher and local divers measured on a pre-printed PVC slate only the dominant benthic cover in accordance with

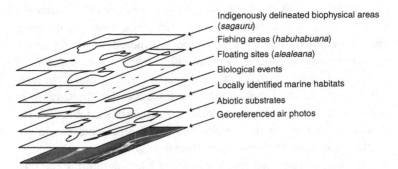

Indigenously delineated biophysical areas (*sagauru*)
Fishing areas (*habuhabuana*)
Floating sites (*alealeana*)
Biological events
Locally identified marine habitats
Abiotic substrates
Georeferenced air photos

Figure 15.3   Indigenous hierarchical cognition of the seascape as represented by layers (or themes) in the GIS (Aswani and Lauer 2006a).

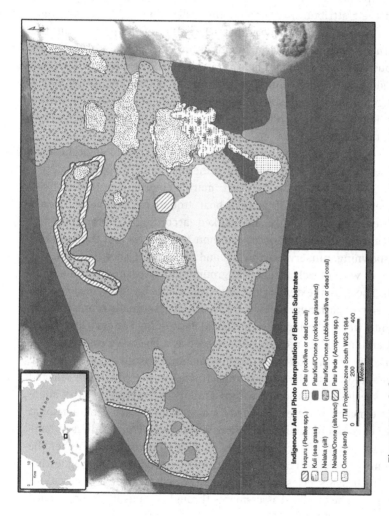

Figure 15.4 Informants' demarcation of predominant abiotic and biotic substrates on the aerial photographs of the Baraulu MPA, Roviana Lagoon (Aswani and Lauer 2006a).

367

a modified version (to suit local conditions) of the Australian Institute of Marine Science (AIMS) manual for underwater research (English, Wilkinson, and Baker 1997) to ground-truth this information. For the analysis, we compared the two datasets by using GIS to spatially display the substrate data collected in the marine science survey as one layer (points and their attributes), together with the layer (polygons and their attributes) created by the indigenous photo interpreters. Then we ran a spatial query that selected all of the points from the marine science survey layer found within each polygon of the indigenously defined dominant benthic attribute(s). The queries allowed us to add an attribute column to the benthic dataset indicating which indigenously defined benthic types were associated with each survey site. Finally, we ran a point-to-point comparison for an accuracy assessment of IEK.

Next, we mapped resident taxa and associated biological events of significance by interviewing fishermen and mapping the seascape as they conceptualized their marine environment (Figure 15.3). Fishermen guided us in a small boat around the perimeter of each named area, and named and ranked (according to abundance) the presence and distribution of common fish species and the locations of spawning, nursery, burrowing, and aggregating sites for particular species within each recognized ground and associated benthic habitats. The spatial extent of the area (represented as polygons) and the location of particular biological characteristics (usually represented as points) were collected with the Global Positioning System (GPS) receivers and imported into our GIS database as a layer. We conducted visual counts to ground-truth this information through a static 7-minute fish survey from the surface at each site, during which the selected fish species were observed within a radius of 5 meters. Relative abundance measures were calculated for all species in each general habitat type to compare their distributions across the MPA regardless of habitat size (rough cover percentage). Finally, to determine whether the Baraulu participants were significantly better than chance-guessing at which fish species were present in which areas, fish observations were matched to local assessments through various methods detailed in Aswani and Lauer (2006a).

Results for both analyses showed that equivalence between indigenous aerial photo interpretations of dominant benthic substrates and in situ quadrant field dive surveys ranged between 75 percent and 85 percent for a moderately detailed classification scheme of the benthos, which included nine locally defined abiotic and biotic benthic classes for the MPA seabed (Figure 15.4). The visual fish census showed a strong correspondence between the qualitative deductions of the indigenous informants and our quantitative analysis of non-cryptic species' general habitat distribution and relative abundance (Aswani and Lauer 2006b). This research showed the accuracy of local indigenous knowledge of dominant benthic substrates and specific resident taxa, and it also revealed that participatory engagements with local peoples can aid in successful implementation of MPAs.

Indigenous ecological knowledge and marine science

Coupling local or IEK with current marine science knowledge can help us to identify species and associated habitats that most urgently need management. In our studies, we sought to evaluate the commensurability of IEK with marine science for identifying ecological processes that support biodiversity, including the presence of species with significant ecological functions, vulnerable life stages, and inter-connectivity among populations of certain species. For instance, three main aspects of Roviana IEK were identified as being most relevant for the management and conservation of bumphead parrotfish (*Bolbometopon muricatum*) and as requiring study through a combination of marine science and anthropological methods. We studied (1) local claims that fishing pressure has had a significant impact on bumphead parrotfish populations in the Roviana Lagoon; (2) the claim that only small bumphead parrotfish are ever seen or captured in the inner lagoon and that very small ones are restricted to specific, shallow, inner-lagoon nursery regions; and (3) the assertions made by local divers that bumphead parrotfish predominantly aggregate at night around the new moon period and that catches are highest at that time.

First, we conducted and compared creel surveys of artisanal nighttime spearfishing in a heavily exploited area (Kalikoqu) and in the lightly fished site (Tetepare Island) in order to investigate the local claims that catch rates and mean size of the parrotfish captured in outer-reef and passage habitats have markedly decreased in the heavily exploited region over the last 20 years. Second, to test the hypothesis that the size distribution of bumphead parrotfish is structured by different lagoon habitats, we examined the size-frequency distribution of fish captured and recorded in inner-lagoon, passage, and outer-lagoon habitats. In addition, we conducted an underwater visual census (UVC) survey to independently assess the effect of lagoon habitat on structuring the size distribution of the bumphead parrotfish populations in six sites located in representative habitats. Finally, to test the proposition that bumphead parrotfish catches are higher during the new moon period, we compared the hourly catch rates of bumphead parrotfish taken on spearfishing trips conducted across each lunar stage.

Research results supported claims one and two, but did not support proposition number three. Overall, the results showed that in areas around Roviana Lagoon, where ecological changes have occurred within the lifespan of local fishers, knowledge regarding ecological transformation can be detailed and useful. More specifically, it allowed us to (1) verify that the bumphead parrotfish is a species in urgent need of protection, (2) aid in understanding how different habitats structure the size distribution of bumphead parrotfish; (3) help in identifying sensitive locations and habitats that need protection, including shallow inner-lagoon sites that serve as nursery areas, and (4) become informed about how lunar periodicity affects bumphead parrotfish behavior and catch rates. This information, in turn, allowed us to design MPAs that integrated local knowledge (see Aswani and Hamilton 2004 for further discussion).

DISCUSSION

Are social scientists (i.e., with natural science training) in a good position to achieve conservation projects that are socially and ecologically successful? There are a number of overriding social processes that drive the success or failure of environmental programs that are often missed by natural scientists, which can be identified more systematically by social practitioners. For instance, social scientists can study human–environmental interactions more fully and discern the social contexts in which MPAs are implemented, including existing conflicts among various stakeholders; differential forms of local resource governance (e.g., sea tenure); the role of conservation programs in enhancing or diminishing people's economic prospects, peoples' social values and aesthetic perceptions regarding the environment; and how conservation programs can empower or alienate coastal communities (e.g., Berkes, Colding, and Folke 2000; Christie 2004; Cinner, Marnane, and McClanahan 2005). For this reason, social scientists are in a good position to work with local and/or indigenous peoples to design conservation areas that represent locally cognized and delineated natural and social landscapes or seascapes. More generally, as this volume illustrates, social scientists have multiple qualitative and quantitative methods that can provide a fuller understanding of human–environmental relations.

For all this potential, however, conservation areas, such as MPAs, are generally designed by natural scientists who consider concrete biological data (which they often lack anyway) essential for designing marine conservation programs (e.g., an MPA optimal design may depend on studying patterns of larval recruitment and dynamics) (Bergen and Carr 2003). Marine scientists insist that selected sites should enhance spawning stock biomass, allow for larval dispersal and the export of adults to adjacent non-protected areas, maintain species diversity, preserve habitat, and sustain ecosystem function (Roberts *et al.* 2001; Russ and Alcala 1999). Yet, due to research bias and training, they ignore most of the socioeconomic processes that affect a targeted conservation site – processes that *really* determine the success or failure of a conservation project. This asymmetry has led to debates on how much attention should be paid to science- versus stakeholder-driven considerations when designing MPAs (e.g., Agardy 1997; Charles and Wilson 2009).

In the Solomon Islands example, we have attempted to combine targeted marine and social science research, local capacity building, and effective communication with local resource owners to conserve natural resources. The major objectives have been to integrate the socioecological research results into reserve design and existing reserve-management structures, and to provide local communities with long-term information regarding the benefits of community-based marine resource management in the region (Figure 15.5). For instance, by examining concrete actions and concomitant management strategies within each local customary management institution closely, we have found that even within small geographical areas these are shaped by, and are embedded in, particular cultural and historical contexts. Local customary management practices coalesce with foreign influences and localized socioeconomic transformations to generate varying forms of governance and management, including situations in which people are or are not able to solve collective-action problems. Then, there are villages where empowering customary management regimes through the establishment of community-based organizations (CBOs), coupled with the government's judicial protection of customary sea tenure, will be of critical importance for successful hybrid management. In contrast, there are sites in which this may not be as realistic, and alternative strategies that combine approaches

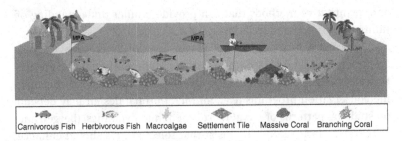

| Carnivorous Fish | Herbivorous Fish | Macroalgae | Settlement Tile | Massive Coral | Branching Coral |

Figure 15.5   Educational materials to show differences in fish, reef, and algal communities inside and outside of a marine protected area (MPA) in Nusa Hope Village, Roviana Lagoon. Tiles in the picture illustrate "healthy" (MPA) and "harmful" (outside MPA) algal communities (illustration by S. Albert).

like gear-based fishery management (McClanahan and Cinner 2008) with other managerial approaches, such as government-sanctioned spatiotemporal closures, may be more suitable to protect crucial biological resources and people's livelihoods.

Thus, what can social scientists do to design socially (and consequently ecologically) sustainable conservation programs? In the context of conservation areas in Oceania, for instance, we can do a number of things. First, managers will not achieve social and ecological sustainability and the protection of marine biodiversity unless they seriously consider local forms of governance and their adaptability to introduced management regimes. Second, it is unlikely that community-based conservation projects will succeed with only short-term expert guidance and financial support. People in developing nations have developmental aspirations that cannot be ignored. Hence, if local communities are to forfeit the exploitation of their resources, some form of alternative livelihood has to be furnished. Third, outside project leaders and funding agencies have to be prepared to accept the fact that local interest in conservation may wax and wane over time, particularly in places like Melanesia. Fourth, people's witnessing of actual conservation results (whether real or perceived) is the most effective means of environmental education – i.e., "seeing is believing." Therefore, even a poorly selected MPA (in ecological terms) can have tremendous educational and social benefits if people perceive positive environmental changes (e.g., more *Caulerpa racemosa*, which is eaten in many areas of the Pacific, yet not necessarily considered beneficial for coral reefs by marine scientists if too abundant). Once people believe in "MPAs," sites that are of more ecological significance can be selected with community compliance. Fifth, the participation of the local church leaders is of paramount importance. Local church support often furnishes the moral authority that politicians and local authorities sometimes lack. Finally, conservation programs should consider not only key biological and ecological parameters but also, as noted by Christie (2004), the characteristics and behaviors of all the stakeholders involved, the desires of different stakeholders, and the stakeholders' knowledge.

In other words, we should strive to develop *hybrid management* – that is, institutions that take advantage of both customary and modern governance (e.g., individual transferable quotas and sea tenure) and conceptual (e.g., marine science and IEK) systems to implement and manage natural resources. This includes (1) understanding and reflecting the patterns and scale at which resources are used and governed, (2) understanding and reinforcing local information exchange mechanisms, power structures, existing rules, and reasons for the rules, (3) providing a legal capacity to enact decentralized management (either through recognized sea-tenure institutions or village bylaws), (4) fostering cross-scale coordination with local institutions (i.e., government permitting such activities as the live reef fish trade for food or aquariums, or other commercial enterprises, which must be coordinated with and not undermine local regulations), and (5) embracing the utilitarian nature and goals of customary management institutions (Cinner and Aswani 2007: 212). That is, although preserving biodiversity and maintaining ecological resilience are often essential objectives of conservation, these must not overrule utilitarian community goals, such as allowing the occasional harvest of resources for feasts or rituals.

Social scientists using manifold methods and theoretical approaches are in a good position to envision multiple and comprehensive approaches to preserving environmentally critical and fragile ecosystems in Oceania and beyond. However, first they need to move beyond just promoting intellectual relativism and self-victimization (e.g., Peterson *et al.* 2009; West and Brockington 2006) and develop a set of empirical research tools (see Pollnac, Crawford, and Gorospe 2001 for an example of methods for evaluating MPA success) and policy guidelines that can be used by natural and social scientists alike for the integrated design and analysis of MPAs and terrestrial and marine conservation areas more generally. Simply, we need to demonstrate how socioecologically driven conservation programs are likely to be more successful socially and ecologically than purely biologically driven ones through our collaboration with natural scientists or, better yet, actual leadership of conservation projects.

CONCLUSION

In concert with those presented in this volume, this chapter offers social and ecological practitioners an opportunity to access multiple methods that transcend the artificial divide between natural and social sciences, and between quantitative and qualitative methods. Here I have outlined various research approaches that integrate social and ecological analysis for studying human–environmental relations, and for using these socioecological methods for designing natural resource management programs. From a local perspective, the systematic articulation of local ecological knowledge and cultural values through marine science and anthropology can better promote local participation in the design and development of community-based marine protected areas and produce a more inclusive approach to conservation. Community members can better understand the biological value and the use restrictions of a conservation program when it builds upon local cultural practices with which the community members are familiar – a situation that facilitates rule enforcement and monitoring. More generally, coupled studies of marine and social processes can foster management regimes that are more adaptive and effective and that move toward holistic ecosystem-based marine conservation.

ACKNOWLEDGMENTS

I wish to thank the people of the Western Solomon Islands for their continued support. The David and Lucile Packard Foundation (Grants 2001-17407 and 2005-447628-58080), Conservation International-GCF (Grant 447628-59102), the Pew Charitable Trust (through a Pew Fellowship in Marine Conservation, 2005), the John D. and Catherine T. MacArthur Foundation (Grant 60243), and the National Science Foundation (Grant NSF-CAREER-BCS-0238539; NSF-HSD-BCS-0826947) have generously provided funds for this research.

REFERENCES

Acheson, J. M. and J. A. Wilson, 1996. Order out of chaos: the case for parametric fisheries management. *American Anthropologist* **98**: 579–594.
Agardy, T. 1997. *Marine Protected Areas and Ocean Conservation*. Austin, TX: Landes Co.

Aswani, S. 1999. Common property models of sea tenure: a case study from Roviana and Vonavona Lagoons, New Georgia, Solomon Islands. *Human Ecology* **27**: 417–53.

Aswani, S. 2005. Customary sea tenure in Oceania as a case of rights-based fishery management: does it work? *Reviews in Fish Biology and Fisheries* **15**: 285–307.

Aswani, S. and R. Hamilton 2004. Integrating indigenous ecological knowledge and customary sea tenure with marine and social science for conservation of bumphead parrotfish (*Bolbometopon muricatum*) in the Roviana Lagoon, Solomon Islands. *Environmental Conservation* **31**: 69–83.

Aswani, S. and M. Lauer 2006a. Incorporating fishermen's local knowledge and behavior into Geographical Information Systems (GIS) for designing marine protected areas in Oceania. *Human Organization* **65**: 80–102.

Aswani, S. and M. Lauer 2006b. Benthic mapping using local aerial photo interpretation and resident taxa inventories for designing marine protected areas. *Environmental Conservation* **33**: 263–273.

Aswani, S. and A. Sabetian 2010. Urbanization and implications for artisanal parrotfish fisheries in the Western Solomon Islands. *Conservation Biology* **24**(2): 520–530.

Aswani, S., S. Albert, A. Sabetian, and T. Furusawa 2007. Customary management as precautionary and adaptive principles for protecting coral reefs in Oceania. *Coral Reefs* **26**: 1009–1021.

Bergen, L. K. and M. H. Carr 2003. Establishing marine reserves: how can science best inform policy? *Environment* **45**: 8–19.

Berkes, F., J. Colding, and C. Folke 2000. Rediscovery of traditional ecological knowledge as adaptive management. *Ecological Applications* **10**: 1251–1262.

Bernard, H. R. 2000. *Handbook of Methods in Cultural Anthropology*. Walnut Creek, CA: Altamira Press.

Charles, A. and L. Wilson 2009. Human dimensions of marine protected areas. *ICES Journal of Marine Science* **66**: 6–15.

Christie, P. 2004. MPAs as biological successes and social failures in Southeast Asia. In J. B. Shipley, ed., *Aquatic Protected Areas as Fisheries Management Tools: Design, Use, and Evaluation of These Fully Protected Areas*. Bethesda, MD: American Fisheries Society, pp. 155–64.

Chun, M. and K. Means 1997. Taking population into account in promoting conservation in Marovo Lagoon, Solomon Islands. SICDCD-WWF Report.

Cinner, J. E. and S. Aswani 2007. Integrating customary management into marine conservation. *Biological Conservation* **140**: 201–216.

Cinner, J. E., M. J. Marnane, and T. R. McClanahan 2005. Conservation and community benefits from traditional coral reef management at Ahus Island, Papua New Guinea. *Conservation Biology* **19**: 1714–1723.

D'Andrade, R. 1995. *The Development of Cognitive Anthropology*. Cambridge, UK: Cambridge University Press.

Diaz, R. J., M. Solan, and R. Valente 2004. A review of approaches for classifying benthic habitats and evaluating habitat quality. *Journal of Environmental Management* **73**: 165–181.

English, S., C. Wilkinson, and V. Baker 1997. *Survey Manual for Tropical Marine Resources*, 2nd edn. Townsville, Australia: Australian Institute of Marine Science.

Habyarimana, J., M. Humphreys, D. N. Posner, and J. M. Weinstein 2007. Why does ethnic diversity undermine public goods provision? *American Political Science Review* **101**: 709–725.

Hauert, C. 2006. Cooperation, collectives formation and specialization. *Advances in Complex Systems* **9**: 315–335.

Henige, D. P. 1974. *The Chronology of Oral Tradition: Quest for a Chimera.* Oxford, UK: Clarendon Press.

Henrich, J., R. Boyd, S. Bowles, *et al.* 2005. "Economic Man" in cross-cultural perspective: economic experiments in 15 small scale societies. *Behavioral and Brain Sciences* **28**: 795–855.

Hughes, T. P., D. R. Bellwood, and S. R. Connolly 2002. Biodiversity hotsposts, centres of endemicity, and the conservation of coral reefs. *Ecological Letters* **5**: 775–784.

Jentof, S., T. C. van Son, M. Bjørkan 2007. Marine protected areas: a governance system analysis. *Human Ecology* **35**: 611–622.

Johnson, A. W. 1975. Time allocation in a Machiguenga community. *Ethnology* **14**: 301–310.

McClanahan, T. R. and J. E. Cinner 2008. A framework for adaptive gear and eco-system-based management in the artisanal coral reef fishery of Papua New Guinea. *Aquatic Conservation of Marine and Freshwater Ecosystems* **18**: 493–507.

Neumann, K. 1992. *Not the Way it Really Was: Constructing the Tolai Past.* Honolulu: University of Hawai`i Press.

Pelto, P. J., and G. Pelto 1978. *Anthropological Research: The Structure of Inquiry*, 2nd edn. Cambridge, UK: Cambridge University Press.

Peterson, R. B., D. Russell, P. West, and J. P. Brosius 2009. Seeing (and doing) conservation through cultural lenses. *Environmental Management* **45**(1): 5–18.

Pollnac R., B. Crawford, and M. Gorospe 2001. Discovering factors that influence the success of community-based marine protected areas in the Visayas, Philippines. *Ocean and Coastal Management* **44**: 683–710.

Roberts, C. M., J. A. Bohnsack, F. Gell, J. P. Hawkins, and R. Goodridge 2001. Effects of marine reserves on adjacent fisheries. *Science* **294**: 1920–1923.

Rogers, B. L., and N. P. Schlossman, eds. 1990. *Intra-Household Resource Allocation.* Tokyo: United Nations University Press.

Russ, G. R. and A. C. Alcala 1999. Management histories of Sumilon and Apo marine reserves, Philippines, and their influence on national marine resource policy. *Coral Reefs* **18**: 307–319.

Santos, F. C., M. D. Santos, and J. M. Pacheco 2008. Social diversity promotes the emergence of cooperation in public goods games. *Nature* **454**: 213–216.

Smith, E. A. 1991. *Inujjuamiut Foraging Strategies: Evolutionary Ecology of an Arctic Hunting Economy.* New York: Aldine de Gruyter.

Solomon Islands Government 1999. Report on the census of population 1999. Honiara, Solomon Islands: Statistics Office.

Stephens, D. W. and J. R. Krebs 1986. *Foraging Theory.* Princeton, NJ: Princeton University Press.

West, P. and D. Brockington 2006. An anthropological perspective on some unexpected consequences of protected areas. *Conservation Biology* **20**: 609–616.

Index

Printed in the United States
by Baker & Taylor Publisher Services